W9-BIZ-031

— PIGS —

A Handbook to the Breeds of the World

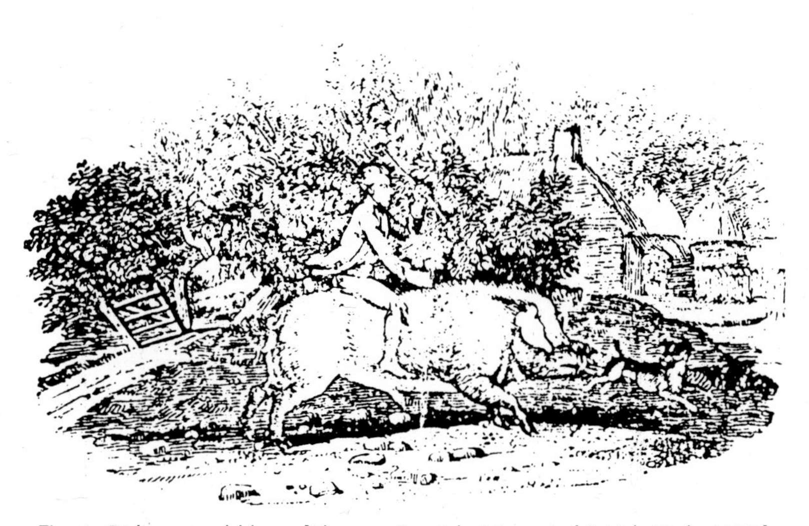

Fig. 1. Riding an old boar [Thomas Bewick, *History of British Birds*, 1797]

Other books by Valerie Porter include:

Cattle: A Handbook to the Breeds of the World (Helm 1992)
Practical Rare Breeds (Pelham 1987)
The Southdown Sheep (Southdown Sheep Society 1991)

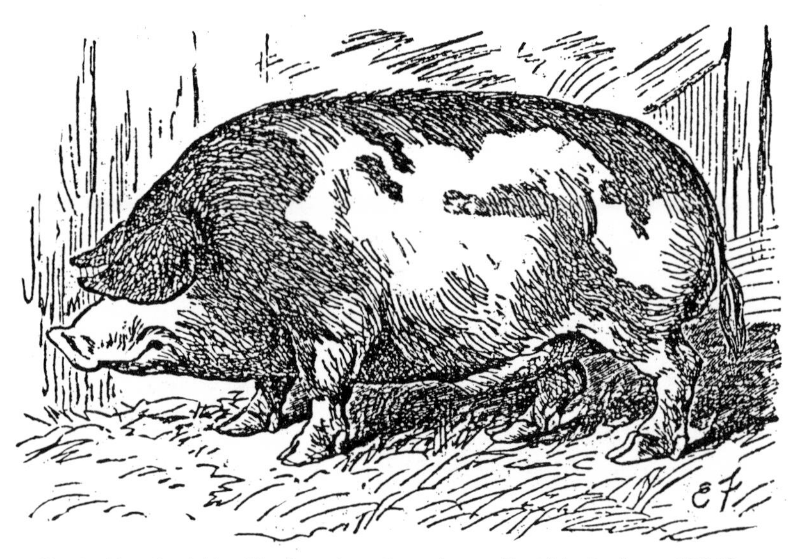

Fig. 2. Herefordshire Pig [Loudon, *Encyclopaedia of Agriculture*, 1825]

— PIGS —

A Handbook to the Breeds of the World

Valerie Porter

Illustrated by
Jake Tebbit

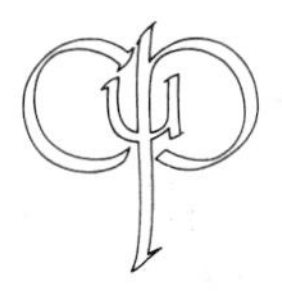

COMSTOCK PUBLISHING ASSOCIATES
A Division of CORNELL UNIVERSITY PRESS
Ithaca, New York

International Standard Book Number 0-8014-2920-X
Library of Congress Catalog Card Number: 92-56193

CONTENTS

ACKNOWLEDGEMENTS

A book of such scope would not have been possible without the worldwide network of pig breed experts who have so generously provided guidance and detailed information. It is impossible to name all of them here but I should particularly like to thank the following.

Above all, my deepest debt is to Mr Ian L. Mason, author of the long-running, immaculately researched and constantly up-dated *World Dictionary of Livestock Breeds*, and editor of *Evolution of Domesticated Animals*. With the utmost kindness and courtesy, he has lent me the keys to so many doors and has unstintingly shared new information to ensure that this book is right up to date at the time of writing - though of course the pig industry evolves so quickly that there are new developments almost daily.

Secondly my thanks are due, as always, to the Rare Breeds Survival Trust at Stoneleigh, especially Lawrence Alderson and Pat Cassidy, and the many members of RBST who contribute their views and the outcome of their own research to that invaluable monthly journal, *The Ark*.

Thirdly, I have received much support and advice from the major pig breeding companies in the United Kingdom and their various agents in other countries. In particular I would like to thank Maurice Bichard (PIC); David Curtis, Roger Widdowson and Dr Jon Mercer (NPD), Dr Rex Walters (Masterbreeders), Dr John Webb and Martin Looker (Cotswold), Eric Oakes (Peninsular), Philip Robins (Premier) and Ian Brisby (Newsham).

Breed societies, government departments and universities all over the world have readily supplied information about the pigs of their own countries. Space does not allow for them all to be listed in these acknowledgements but, again, the book would not have been possible without them. Finally, there are certain individuals who have contributed more than most to the contents of the book and I should like to extend a special note of thanks to them, including:

Professor V.G. Arganesa (Philippines)
Robert Ball
Dr H.J. Bauer
Donald E. Bixby (AMBC)
Dr Imri Bodó
Dr W. Derek Booth (British Wild Boar Association)
Tim Brigstocke (BOCM-Silcock)
Professor I. Lehr Brisbin Jr.
Walter S. Craven
Danish Bacon and Meat Council
Dr C. Devendra (Singapore)
Olafur R. Dýrmundsson (Búndarfélkag Íslands)
Fédération National des Éleveurs de Porcs de Belgique
Dr Stefano Feroci
Luis Dos Santos Ferreira (DSEMA, Lisbon)
Dr Gustavo Gandini (Milan)
P.A. Mario Grazi (Associazione Senese Allevatori)
Dr Christopher S. Haley (IAPGR, Edinburgh)
K.S. Harris (British Pig Association)
Tim Harris (Harris Associates, Redhill)
Elizabeth Henson
Eric Hindson (Barcelona)
Marie Iles
David L. Kennett (Calabria)
Jan Košlacz (Warsaw)
Gustavo J.M.M. de Lima (EMBRAPA, Brazil)
Nils Lundehelm (Swedish University of Agricultural Science)
Dr George Malynicz
R. Mani (SSZV, Sempach)
Donald McLean
Dr Ir J.W.M. Merks (Nederlands Varnkensstamboek)
Anne Merriman (Oxford Sandy-and-Black Pig Society)

Dr Klaus Meyn
Museum of English Rural Life
Dr Ifor L. Owen (Papua New Guinea)
Dr J.T.R. Robinson (Vleisraad/Meat Board, Arcadia)
J.P. Runavot (Institut Technique du Porc)
Philip Ryder Davies
David E. Steane (FAO)
Muriel Smith
Alexander Temple (Monterchi)
Bjarne J. Trodahl (Norsvin)
Sam Walton (Pig World)
Eleanor Ford West (Ossabaw Foundation)
Dr John V. Wilkins (Bolivia)

LIST OF ACRONYMS

ABRO: Animal Breeding Research Organisation
AMBC: American Minor Breeds Conservancy
BLUP: Best Linear Unbiased Prediction
F_1: first generation (of a cross)
FAO: Food and Agricultural Organisation (United Nations)
FCE: feed conversion efficiency
FCR: feed conversion ratio (ie. weight of food consumed for each unit of weight gain)
INRA: Institut national de la recherche agronomique
ITP: Institut technique du porc
MLC: Meat and Livestock Commission
PIDA: Pig Industry Development Authority
PiGMaP: Pig Gene Mapping Programme
PSE: pale soft exudate
RBST: Rare Breeds Survival Trust
USDA: United States Department of Agriculture

LIST OF MAPS

LIST OF PLATES

As far as possible, the breeds are all to scale to highlight size differences worldwide.

PLATE 5: UNITED KINGDOM, Breeding Companies

PIC: Camborough and Camborough 12
Masterbreeders: Westrain, Sovereign and 555
NPD: Hamline boar and Manor Ranger
Newsham: HC , Duroc and N32
Cotswold: 90 and Gold
Peninsular: Hampen
Premier

PLATE 6: ORIGINAL LANDRACES

Danish Landrace
Jutland
Dan-Hybrid
German land pig
Improved German Landrace
German Landrace "B"
Finnish Landrace

PLATE 7: LANDRACES

Norwegian Landrace
Swedish Landrace
British Landrace
Dutch Landrace
Belgian Landrace
Swiss Landrace

PLATE 8: FRANCE AND BELGIUM

Piétrain
West French White
Normand
Gascony
Limousin
Basque Black Pied
Corsican

PLATE 9: PORTUGAL, SPAIN AND ITALY

Alentejana
Extremadura Red
Black Iberian
Andalusian Spotted
Siena Belted
Siena Grey
Romagnola
Calabrian
Casertana
Neapolitan

PLATE 21: NORTH AMERICA, Major Breeds

Canadian Yorkshire
Canadian Landrace
American Yorkshire
American Landrace
Chester White
Spotted
Poland China
Hampshire
Duroc

PLATE 22: NORTH AMERICA, Minor Breeds

Lacombe
American Berkshire
Gloucester Old Spots
Large Black
Mulefoot
Tamworth
Guinea hog
American feral
Ossabaw Island
Froxfield Pygmy
Texas Razor-back
Hereford
Beltsville No. 1
Montana No. 1
Minnesota No. 1
Minnesota No. 2

PLATE 23: BRAZIL

Pirapetinga
Macau
Canastrinho
Caruncho
Canastrão
Nilo
Piau
Canastra
Pereira
Moura

PLATE 24: LATIN AMERICA

Haiti Creole
Sino-Gascony x Guadeloupe Creole
Pelón
Bolivian
Yucatan
Guadeloupe Creole
Costa Rican
Brazilian village

PEOPLE

Certain names feature frequently in the text, especially the following authors, whose works are given in the Bibliography:

Baxter: Sussex publisher of agricultural encyclopaedia, 1830s
Coburn: F. D. Coburn, *Swine in America*, 1909
Gaál and Gunst: L. Gaál and P. Gunst, *Animal Husbandry in Hungary*, 1977
Harris: Joseph Harris, *Harris on the Pig*, 1870 (USA)
Long: James Long, agricultural professor and author in 19th and early 20th century - *The Book of the Pig*, 1906 (2nd ed.); also produced special reports for governments in Canada, USA and New Zealand; Professor of Dairy Farming in the Royal Agricultural College.
Low: David Low, Professor of Agriculture at University of Edinburgh; compiled 2-volume work *The Breeds of the Domestic Animals of the British Islands*, 1842; commissioned William Shiels to paint all the notable breeds in oils (half life-size for pigs), many of which were engraved by Nicholson for Low's books.
Loudon: John C. Loudon, *An Encyclopaedia of Agriculture*, 1831
Mayer and Brisbin: John J. Mayer and I. Lehr Brisbin, Jr., *Wild Pigs of the United States*, 1991
Sidney: Samuel Sidney, *The Pig*, 1871.
Towne and Wentworth: Charles Wayland Towne and Edward Norris Wentworth, *Pigs from Cave to Corn Belt*, 1950.
Youatt: W. Youatt, *The Pig*, 1847 - and also *The Complete Grazier*, frequently reprinted and updated.
Young: Arthur Young (1741-1820), writer on agriculture, Secretary to the Board of Agriculture in England; also his contemporary, the Reverend Arthur Young, who reported to the same Board on the agriculture in several counties.

FIGURES

INTRODUCTION

> "It is frequently said there is no 'best breed', but that
> is not quite true. There is a best breed for every man, but,
> inasmuch as there are many types and classes of men, it is
> but natural that there are various breeds and types of
> swine. Each breed preserves some characteristics, marketable
> or ornamental, to recommend it, but one man's taste may be
> another's dislike."
>
> [F.D. Coburn, *Swine in America*, 1909]

This is an unashamedly ambitious book which seeks to draw attention to the immense diversity in the pigs of the world. Essentially it is a guide to breeds and types of domesticated pig but it also looks at their wild ancestors and relatives in considerable detail. For at least 40,000 years, pigs have been a major source of animal protein in the human diet, and they have also played an essential role in some societies far beyond that of providing meat and manure or turning the soil for the planting of crops.

Far from being merely a breed catalogue, therefore, this book paints the setting in which pigs of all kinds exist - whether wild, domesticated or feral - and the factors that have shaped them. These include the natural environments to which they have adapted themselves; the historical movements of pig-keeping cultures and hence the spread of pig domestication; the arrival of domesticated pigs in unlikely places in the company of the old navigators and explorers; the importance of pigs in certain cultures as well as in agriculture; historical and current national pig industries, and the often complicated and intriguing detective stories about the history of different breeds.

Above all, the book takes a *global* look at pigs—a context which gives a much broader perspective to their development and also emphasises the internationality of the pig.

Notes

Breed names throughout are in accordance with Ian L. Mason's *World Dictionary of Livestock Breeds*; names used in the native language, where they differ markedly, are given in the breed entries, and synonyms are listed alphabetically in the Appendix for ease of reference. It should be borne in mind that, in the past, breeds have often changed their names, and that the names of particularly influential breeds or types have often been borrowed for pigs which have no right to that name and might have no blood connection with the original breed.

Performance figures, where given, must be regarded with due circumspection. Conditions vary so greatly in different regions, whether in climate, disease status or general management systems, that it is misleading to compare performance unless environmental factors are taken into account. In addition, the pig is such a malleable species that its performance can be improved rapidly and statistics quickly become out of date. Equal caution should be applied to population figures, which can fluctuate wildly from year to year and which also depend on sometimes unreliable sources of information.

Metrication units have been used except in the case of historical data for the United Kingdom and current data in the United States of America. As a rough guide, a weight of 100 pounds equals 454kg (or 100kg = 220 pounds), one inch equals 2.54cm (1cm = 0.39 inches), and one acre equals 0.4 hectares (1ha = 2.47 acres).

THE WILD PIGS

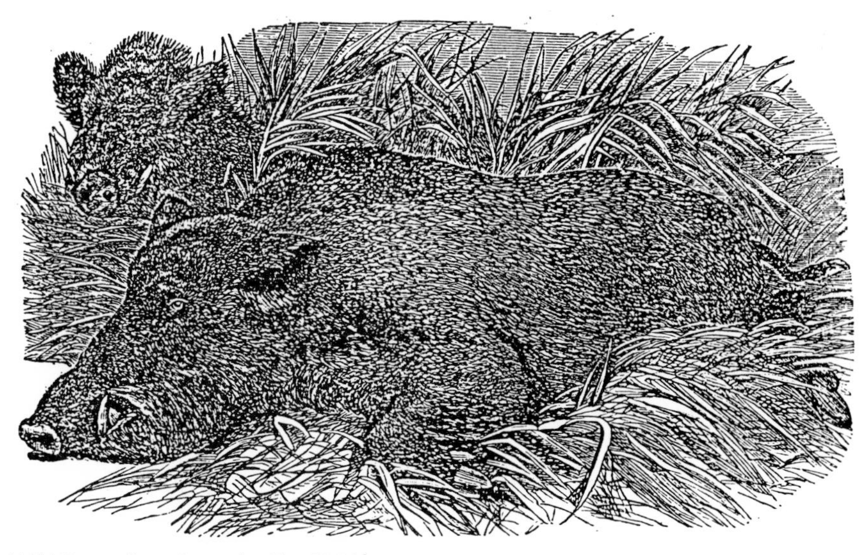

Fig. 3. Wild Boars [*Harris on the Pig,* 1881]

MAP 1. Wild Species of South East Asia

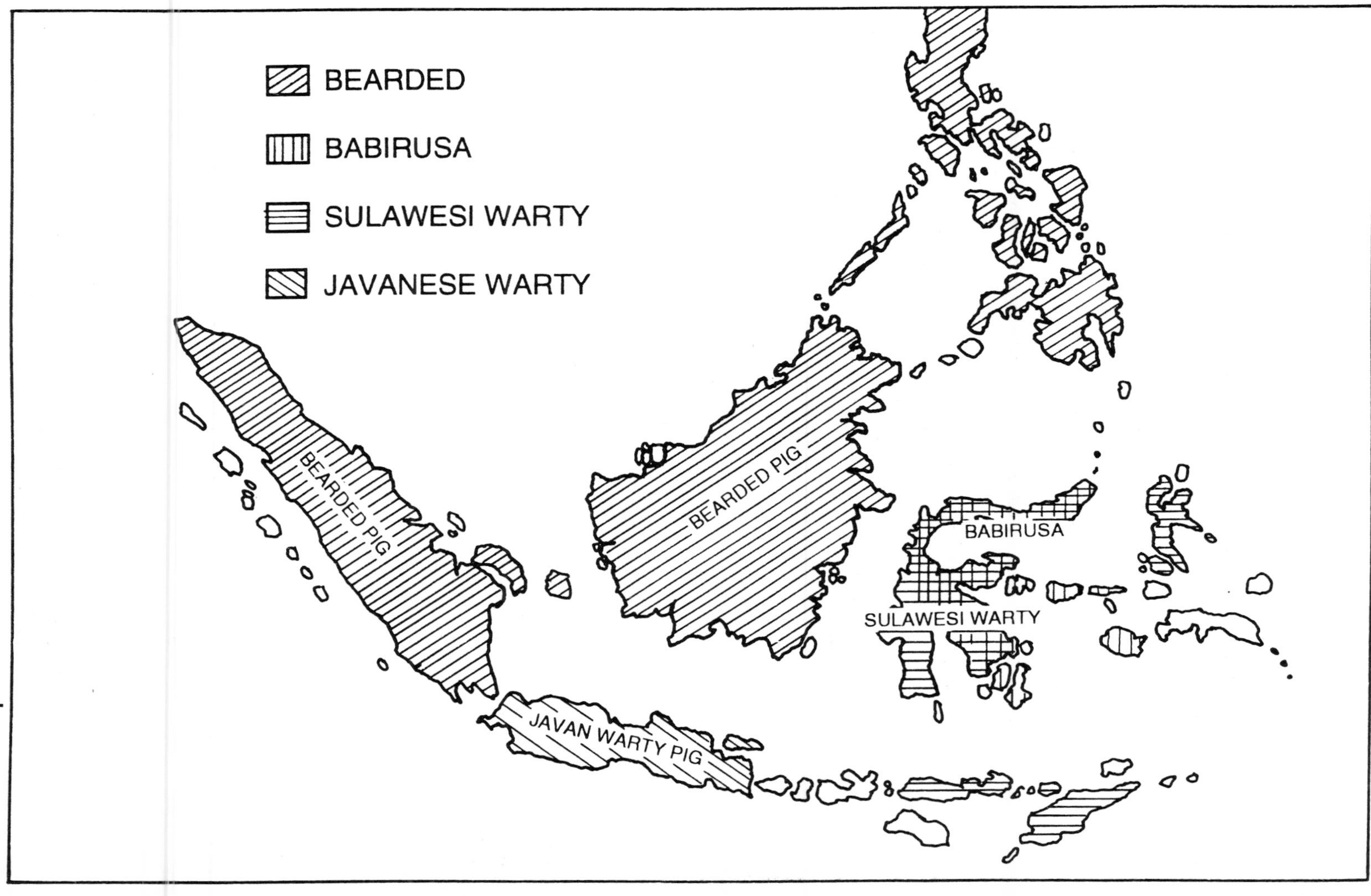

THE WILD PIGS

Domesticated pigs are marvellously diverse in shape, size, features and colours. The sway-backed, pot-bellied, wrinkle-skinned lard pigs of south east Asia are in sharp contrast to the long, lean white breeds of western Europe; the thick, curly coat of eastern Europe's Mangalitsa defies its relationship with the hairless miniature *cuino* of Central America. Comparing the squashed face of an English Middle White with the long, tapering snout of an Iberian in Spain or Italy is like comparing the profile of a Pekingese dog with that of a wolf. Yet nearly all the widely different pigs of Asia and of Europe share the same wild ancestor, a single species within a diverse family of wild pigs.

THE PIG FAMILY

Pigs, whether wild or domesticated, are even-toed ungulates: they belong to the order Artiodactyla, which also embraces ruminants such as deer, sheep, goats and cattle. However, pigs are not ruminants and they form a separate sub-order, Suina, which is divided into three families: the hippopotamuses of tropical Africa, the little American peccaries and, between the two, all kinds of swine (Suidae). The latter family is formed of nine species within five genera, as shown in Table 1 and illustrated in Plate 1.

TABLE 1: THE WILD PIG FAMILY

Order: Artiodactyla (even-toed ungulates)

Suborder: Suina (hippopotamuses, pigs, peccaries)

Family: Suidae (pigs)

1. Genus: *Sus*
   - *S. barbatus* Bearded pig [Malaya, Sumatra, Borneo]
   - *S. celebensis* Sulawesi Warty pig [Sulawesi]
   - *S. salvanius* Pygmy hog [S.E. Nepal, Assam]
   - *S. scrofa* Wild Boar [Europe and Asia]
   - *S. verrucosus* Javanese Warty hog [Java, Sulawesi, Philippines]
2. Genus: *Babyrousa*
   - *B. babyrussa* Babirusa [E. Indonesia]
3. Genus: *Hylochoerus*
   - *H. meinertzhageni* Giant Forest hog [Central Africa]
4. Genus: *Phacochoerus*
   - *P. aethiopicus* Warthog [subSaharan Africa]
5. Genus: *Potomochoerus*
   - *P. porcus* Bushpig or Red River hog [subSaharan Africa, Madagascar]

The species have much in common. They are omnivorous; though largely vegetarian, they are opportunists and most will eat a wide range of food of animal origin as well, including carrion. Their digestive systems are similar to those of that other opportunistic omnivore, the human. And therein lie the seeds of potential conflict between the two.

Most of the species fashion nests for their litters and most have multiple litters. A noticeable behaviour pattern in almost all the wild pigs is the formation of "sounders" - groups based on one or more matriarchal sows and their daughters. Males live either in bachelor groups or as solitary mature boars: they may be sexually mature by, say, 18 months of age, but do not reach full physical maturity until perhaps four years old, by which time they might be strong enough to claim their own sows. Meanwhile the sounders, often including several generations, tend to share territory and resources with related sounders and it is common for sows within a group to share piglet-rearing duties as well.

The sows have an appropriate number of teats for their litter sizes. Newborn piglets characteristically make a determined effort to locate and "claim" a particular teat for themselves and will always use that nipple thereafter - a hierarchy is established within minutes of birth. The young of the wild pig species are born with striped coats, and the range of adult colours among the Suidae includes shades of red-brown, yellow-brown, black, grey, brown, blackish brown and fawn. The adult coat is rarely patterned, except for gradual shading or, in the case of the Bushpig and Bearded pig, definite white markings on the face, and in the case of the Wild Boar a frosted effect (especially as a face "saddle") of coloured bristles tipped with white or pale colouring. All the nine species tend to have stiff, coarse bristles rather than the smooth, fine hair coat of a ruminant, but some also have scant, coarse hair-coats and some have a dense undercoat in certain environments. Males often have a more vigorous growth of bristles forming a ridge or crest along the back and neck.

The preferred environments of the wild pigs are forest, woodland or bushland, and savanna, in both tropical and temperate climates, according to species. The family's omnivorous inclinations, however, help most of them to be adaptable and they have had to be so: several species are now under threat of extinction because of pressures created by humans who not only compete directly for food (and hence frequently hunt wild pigs to protect food supplies) but who also clear-fell the natural habitats, pushing the pigs up into the hills and deeper into the remaining forests. The tiny Indian Pygmy hog is now one of the most endangered mammal species in the world.

Table 1 reveals certain geographical constraints in that all the wild pigs are species of the Old World. Three of the genera are African and most of the species in the other two genera are east Asian (within a very limited area). The range of the Wild Boar, *Sus scrofa,* however, still stretches right across Eurasia from the Pacific Ocean in the east to the Atlantic coast of Portugal in the west, and from the Mediterranean shores of North Africa in the south to the fringes of the great conifer belts of northern Europe and Siberia. Although it probably never ventured further north than about 57 degrees N, in recent centuries the Wild Boar has disappeared from the extremes of its range - notably the United Kingdom and Ireland, southern Scandinavia, the coastal lowlands of North Africa and the whole of the Nile valley. Elsewhere, in spite of many, many centuries of European hunting and general loss of habitat, the Wild Boar has been remarkably persistent and has long outlived the wild aurochs (the ancestor of domesticated cattle) which once shared all its range.

The wild pigs can have an effect upon local domesticants in that in many places they will interbreed with them. Several of the wild species are of interest as potential domesticants themselves.

THE WILD PIGS OF AFRICA

Giant Forest Hog (*Hylochoerus meinertzhageni*) <Plate 1>

Central Africa, Congo basin, parts of west and east Africa - tropical rainforests, and intermediate zone between forest and grassland.

This is the largest of the wild pigs: it can be more than 2m in length and weighs up to 275kg, but is smaller in lowlands. It has a coat of brown and black bristles, and facial warts; sows have three pairs of teats and a gestation period of 149-154 days. It is a grazer, seldom digging with its snout, and is one of the least well known pig species. Despite its size, it seems to be rather shy.

Warthog (*Phacochoerus aethiopicus* and *P. africanus*) <Plate 1>

Subsaharan Africa - savanna woodland and grassland.

Named for the very obvious facial warts covering its huge head, this species lives almost entirely on grass and makes use of all parts of grass plants - the leaves and the stems, the seeds and the rhizomes. It does not use its large tusks to dig out food but scoops grass roots out of baked soils in the dry season with the tough upper edge of its nose. Like the Giant Forest hog, it is active in the daytime. It is up to 135cm long and weighs up to 110kg, and lives for 12-15 years. It has grey-brown skin with black or white bristles, small erect ears and an unforgettable face with a flat, wide look to it. The legs are long and it is a fast mover, characteristically running with its tail erect. Sows have two pairs of teats and their gestation period lasts from 170-175 days; they do not build the typical pig nest but use a den already dug out by another animal, especially the aardvaark. The *africanus* is the common Warthog, while the *aethiopicus*, confusingly, is or was the Cape Warthog, which no longer exists in South Africa but might be represented in northern Kenya and Somalia.

Bushpig (*Potamochoerus porcus* and *P. larvatus*) <Plate 1>

Subsaharan Africa and Madagascar - forests, moist savanna woodlands and grasslands.

An interesting wild pig looking much more like the domesticated pig than the other African species. The latin name means "river pig" and there seem to be two types: the Red River hog in west and central Africa (*P. porcus*) and the Bushpig (*P. larvatus*) of the east and south east.The Red River hog is quite common on the grasslands and in the rainforests of its region, where it is regularly killed for its meat: it has a coat of bright orange hair with a white stripe along the back, and a black and white mask on the whiskery face (the male has warts); the young are born striped. Its ears are erect with long tufts of hair hanging down from the tips The profile of the face is straight and long, with a mobile snout. The pigs weigh up to 120kg and are up to 150cm long. Sows have three pairs of teats and the gestation period is 127 days. The animals can live 10-15 years. The Bushpig of the eastern grasslands and savanna woodlands is similar but more bristly, of a muddy colour with greyish bristles, and slightly bigger. The diet of both types is similar to that of the Eurasian Wild Boar and includes a wide range of plant species and parts, and also insect larvae, earthworms and small vertebrates. They are adept rootlers.

THE WILD PIGS OF ASIA

Babirusa (*Babyroussa babyrussa*) <Plate 1>

East Indonesian islands: Sulawesi, Taliabu, Buru, Mangole - tropical rainforests.

This extraordinary pig takes its name from the Malay words *babi* (hog) and *rusa* (deer);its French name *cochon-cerf* (pig-stag) refers to the male's self-destructive tusks. There are two pairs of them: a set of elongated lower canines curving upwards, and a dramatic upper pair which grow up right through the flesh of the snout and then arch so strongly that they can literally gore the animal's forehead in due course. It is not one of the larger species - it weighs up to 90-100kg and is up to 110cm long and 80cm tall (male); the conformation is lighter than that of a domestic pig of similar size. It has no facial warts. The skin is grey or brownish-grey with sparse, short white or grey bristles; there is a hairier subspecies with a light coat of creamy to sandy or black hair. Sows have only one pair of teats and produce only one or two piglets a year (rarely three), after a gestation period of about 158 days, but can be sexually mature at 5-10 months old. One captive animal lived to the age of 24 years and the species is easily tamed - there is a long tradition of capturing the young and raising them for their tasty meat and their tusk ivory, and they will breed in captivity - if they can be caught in the first place (they are fast runners and good swimmers).

They are sociable animals, moving in groups, and they like to be near water, usually living in the marshes and swamps and in dense jungle. The preferred diet is fruits and grass, and the stomach has an extra sac which possibly helps them to digest cellulose - they often browse foliage, and will also eat roots and grubs but are not as ardent rootlers as domestic pigs.

Pygmy Hog (*Sus salvanius*) <Plate 1>

Northern India: Himalayan foothills, Assam and south east Nepal - tall savanna grassland.

This tiny pig weighs only 6-10kg and is perhaps 58-66cm long with a little 3cm tail, and standing perhaps 25cm high at the shoulder. Its skin is greyish-brown, with a good coat which is brown on the sides, darkening along the back. The face has a band of short, dark hair under each eye and there are no facial warts. Given the chance, it can live for 10-12 years; but it is one of the world's rarest mammals and its environment is under constant threat through the deliberate burning-off of long grass in the interests of agriculture. Two very small populations are in protected reserves in Assam and the species probably numbers less than a hundred in total; it is further endangered by the activity of armed rebels controlling one of the reserves. The Pygmy is omnivorous, living on all sorts of plant material, insects and earthworms, and also taking eggs and carrion. Sows have three pairs of teats and a gestation period of about 100 days, after which they give birth to 2-6 young, usually at the onset of the rainy season in April and May. It is a shy and nervous species which has probably never been domesticated but can be tamed.

Javanese Warty Pig (*Sus verrucosus*) <Plate 1>

Java, Sulawesi, the Philippines - forests, lowland grasslands, swamps.

There are several "warty" pigs in this region, under various names - the Bearded pig (below) is also well endowed with warts, for example. The Javanese Warty is usually up to 135cm long and 90cm tall, and mature males weigh 80-120kg, with females only half as heavy. The large warts on its long face are obvious. It has a coat of black-tipped red or yellow hairs. Its reproductive traits and longevity are much like those of the Wild Boar, with which it seems to interbreed where the ranges of the two overlap (the Java pig's diploid chromosome number is 2n=38). It had been thought extinct in the pure form in the wild until a herd was discovered in 1981. Sow litters range from 2 to 8 and are born at any time of year. The animals tend to remain below altitudes of 800m, preferably with very few humans around and plenty of open grassland, and are omnivorous.

The **Philippine Warty pig** is sometimes given its own species name, *Sus philippensis*, or it is sometimes regarded as a type of the **Sulawesi Warty pig** (described below). There is also a ***Visayan Warty pig*** in the central Philippines, recently dubbed *Sus cebifrons*, though originally considered to be a subspecies of the **Bearded pig** (see below). It is now very rare.

Sulawesi Warty Pig or Celebes Wild Pig (*Sus celebensis*)

Indonesia: Sulawesi, and introduced to other islands, also domesticated - lowland and upland tropical rainforest.

This is one of possibly only two wild pig species to have been domesticated and it is a village or household pig on some of the islands of south east Asia. It was also bred long ago with *Sus scrofa* domesticants to form the common pig of New Guinea and parts of the Moluccas. Native to Sulawesi and neighbouring islands, it has been deliberately introduced elsewhere and is widespread and common in eastern Indonesia, except where its numbers have been controlled by hunting or loss of habitat. Wild, domesticated or feral, it is an adaptable pig: its natural environments include grassland, rainforest, mountain forests and agricultural areas, and although mainly vegetarian (preferring fruit, young shoots and leaves) it also eats earthworms and aquatic invertebrates, and will take birds, rodents and carrion.

It is quite small, about 60cm tall and weighs up to 70kg (boars larger than sows). Boars have three pairs of prominent facial warts, but the sows are often clean faced. Both sexes have tusks but those of the boar are longer (about 10cm). After a four-month gestation, sows give birth to 2-8 striped young, usually in April or May, and the adult colour is reddish-brown, with a clearly marked underside of white and yellow. The coarse hair is scanty, and there is a ridge of stiff bristles along the back which are erected in alarm. Older animals have a 3cm round white spot on each cheek.

Bearded Pig (*Sus barbatus*) <Plate 1>

Malaya, Sumatra, Borneo - tropical forest, mangrove swamps.

Yet another warty pig: adult males have facial warts, but they are less obvious because of the general hairiness of the face, including the bushy white cheek tufts that give the species its name but are more like an overgrown moustache and sideburns than a beard. The snout is very long and flexible.

Sows are smaller than the boars, which can be up to 160cm long and 1m high and might weigh 150kg or more. the colour ranges from pale reddish-brown or yellow-brown to black, including dark brown-grey. Reproduction traits are similar to those of the Wild Boar, with which the species interbreeds to produce fertile offspring of both sexes. It is a potential domesticant.

Like the Sulawesi Warty, the Bearded pig is an adaptable animal, eating seeds, fruit, banana stems, roots, herbs and earthworms, with a few turtle's eggs for variety. Its main habitat is evergreen forest but it will live where it can, whether in the upland rainforests or even down on the beaches. It lives in groups, usually remaining in one area, but sometimes gathers in large herds in search of seasonal food (probably a certain type of acorn), for which the herds will swim across rivers in their thousands - ready prey for hunters.

THE EURASIAN WILD BOAR (*Sus scrofa*) <Plate 1>

The Wild Boar is the animal known in heraldic English and in French as *sanglier.*

With such an extensive original range throughout Europe and Asia, many regional subspecies of *Sus scrofa* evolved. There have been endless arguments about the classification of the subspecies but most now recognise at least two dozen, the majority of which are in eastern Asia. Full descriptions of all the world's subspecies, along with their many synonyms, are given by John J. Mayer and I. Lehr Brisbin Jr. in their recent book, *Wild Pigs of the United States: Their History, Morphology, and Current Status.* Another very useful reference is the paper *Introduced and Feral Pigs,* presented at the 1982 Workshop on Feral Mammals (Helsinki) by William L.R. Oliver of the IUCN/SSC Pigs & Peccaries specialist group.

The main differences beween the subspecies seem to be in size, in skull shapes and, to a lesser extent, in the colour of the pelage. In the context of domesticated pigs, the most interesting are also the most divergent of the subspecies: the European Wild Boar (*Sus scrofa scrofa*) and south east Asia's Banded pig of Malaysia and Indonesia (*S.s. vittatus*). Another which is often mentioned in the context of domestication is the Indian Wild Boar or Jungle pig (*S.s. cristatus*).

Taking the species *Sus scrofa* as a whole, the natural habitat of the Eurasian Wild Boar includes broadleaf woodland or forest and steppelands, in a wide range of climates - moist European maritime to arid Eurasian steppe, Siberian continental to tropical rainforest.

The bristles are generally described as fuscous (brownish-grey) and are often tipped with cream or white, giving a grizzled appearance, while in several subspecies pale-tipped bristles create patterns on the face, especially in the form of a "saddle" or as a "mouth streak". Looking more closely at the subspecies, there is quite a variety of coat colours. The basic colours described in Mayer and Brisbin for the animals' backs and sides include fuscous, dark greyish-brown, black, burnt umber, drab, blackish-brown, snuff brown, dusky brown, olive black, olive grey, blackish-grey, and yellowish; while the bristle tips may be white, cream, buff, fawn, cinnamon, russet, golden, burnt umber, antique brown, yellowish-brown, yellow or grey. Sometimes the undersides are cream or white but in most subspecies the colouring extends over the whole body, shading to darker areas but generally without any obvious coat pattern. Occasionally, there is a dark stripe along the back. The "points" such as ears and limbs are often either darker or lighter than the main coat but there are no spotted, patched or belted patterns in the wild species, nor are any of an overall cream or white.

The length and density of the bristles vary. Animals in colder climates may have a dense underfur beneath the bristles, its colour including dark brown, drab, fawn, smoke-grey, cinnamon, burnt umber and cream.

Unlike several other *Sus* species, the Wild Boar has no facial warts. Facial profiles vary from flat/concave to convex, the latter seen in Asian subspecies, which has led some taxonomists to suggest that they belong to a separate species, generally termed *S. cristatus.* Current opinion places all Wild Boar within *S. scrofa.*

The skulls of many Asian subspecies tend to be generally shorter, with a higher appearance than the long ones of the Europeans. The main element is the "lacrimal index", a term which comes up frequently in the arguments and which refers to the proportional length to breadth of the lacrimal bone (just in front of the eye socket, along the snout), which is much shorter and thus proportionately wider in the south east Asian subspecies, and is also different between the Wild Boar (much longer than broad, with an index of more than 2) and the domesticated pig (index of less than 1). However, there seems to be almost as much variety between different subspecies as between each continental group, and there is a traceable reduction of the index in direct proportion to the increasing degree of domestication.

The same applies to body size differences, which have also been cited as evidence of a separate Asian species of Wild Boar. Body length ranges from about 90cm in the Taiwanese to twice that size in northern Europe, and average mature weights from about 50kg to more than 200kg. The general trend is for the boars to be larger than sows in the same subspecies, and for the largest subspecies to be in Europe, gradually decreasing in size over the geographical range eastwards. The European Wild Boar (*S.s. scrofa*) can be up to 180cm long and can weigh twice as much as the Indian (*S.s. cristatus*), which is perhaps 115-150cm in length, with the Indonesian *vittatus* perhaps 100-150cm long. The trend also runs from north to south: the European, found in north European countries from France to Czechoslovakia, is larger than the southern Iberian peninsula subspecies (which might be 120-140cm in length), or the Turkish (*S.s. lybicus*) and the Middle East Wild Boar (*S.s.*

attila), which are both about 130cm long. The North Chinese (*S.s. moupinensis*) can be even bigger than the European. In general, the size difference is a gradual geographical shading, and it does not seem a valid reason for splitting the European and Asian into two different species. It is only when, say, the Indonesian *vittatus* is compared in isolation against the geographically distant European *scrofa* that the former seems so markedly smaller and lighter, with a shorter cranium and finer tusks. The difference would not be so noticeable if intervening geographical types were brought into the reckoning.

This is not merely an academic argument. It has been used as the basis of a theory that European and Asian domesticated pigs are not of the same species, which is important in relation to hybrid vigour when the two are crossed. There is another factor to consider: the (diploid) chromosome number#(2n), which is often used to differentiate between species and to predict their ability to interbreed and produce fertile offspring - a very important factor in the context of livestock breeding. Insofar as information is available it seems that, for the great majority of *Sus scrofa* subspecies, 2n=38. This figure is the same as that for domesticated pigs and also for some of the other *Sus* species such as the Javanese Warty pig and the little Pygmy hog. However, the European Wild Boar appears to be polymorphic and has been reported variously as 2n=36 or 38. The French, for example, claim that the only pure form of their Wild Boar has a (diploid) chromosome number of 2n=36, and that this is found in the majority of Spain's wild population as well.

Yet most, if not all, of the subspecies appear to interbreed successfully with each other and with the domesticated pig, and can also breed with one or two other species; for example, the first-generation (F_1) offspring of a cross between Wild Boar and the Bearded pig (*S. barbatus*) are fertile in both sexes. In theory it would be possible to cross Wild Boar with the Pygmy hog of India but in practice the latter species is much too rare for such experiments and, more important, there is a substantial size difference between the two.

Farming Wild Boar

The Wild Boar remains widespread and is still hunted for its meat, and for sport, as it has been for some 40,000 years. In several countries it is now being "farmed", either by selective hunting in a controlled environment or by confinement and eventual slaughter as if it was a domesticant in a livestock system.

In France, Wild Boar are often regarded as agricultural pests but their meat became in such high demand as a gourmet dish that the French were importing as many again as they could produce from hunting and culling. Hence in the 1980's there developed a considerable interest in the idea of exploiting the "pest" by farming it. More than 800 Wild Boar farms were established and the French learned a great deal about the species. They noted that it is a seasonal (photoperiodic) breeder in temperate regions; the rut, taking place as daylength shortens in the autumn, coincides with the pannage season. Sows tend to be anoestrous from July to September, partly because they are lactating or, rarely, are pregnant with a second litter. Most of the young *marcassins* are born between February and May and the typical litter is of six striped piglets. After three days the young leave their nests and the litters mingle, often suckling other sows. Weaning might be completed by the time they are 3-4 months old.

In the United Kingdom, Wild Boar meat is regarded as healthily low in cholesterol. Initially, farmers crossbred the wild with domesticted pigs but the meat was too much like pork and lacked the distinctive texture and flavour of pure Wild Boar meat. However, one enterprise successfully produced a "Wild Blue", which was a first cross from Wild Boar x outdoor blue domesticated sow.

Fig. 4. A Wild Boar [*Harris on the Pig*, 1881]

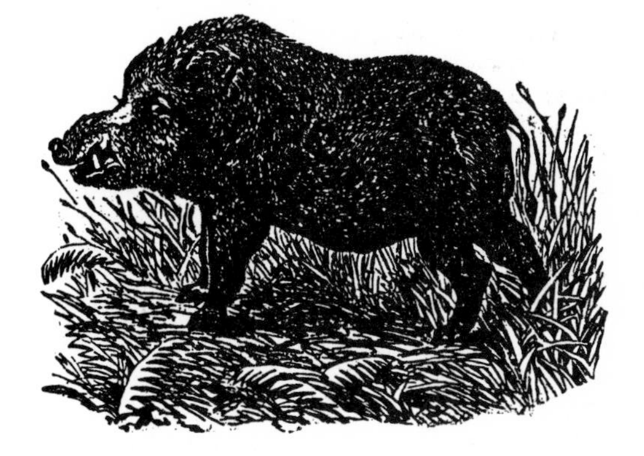

TAMING THE WILD

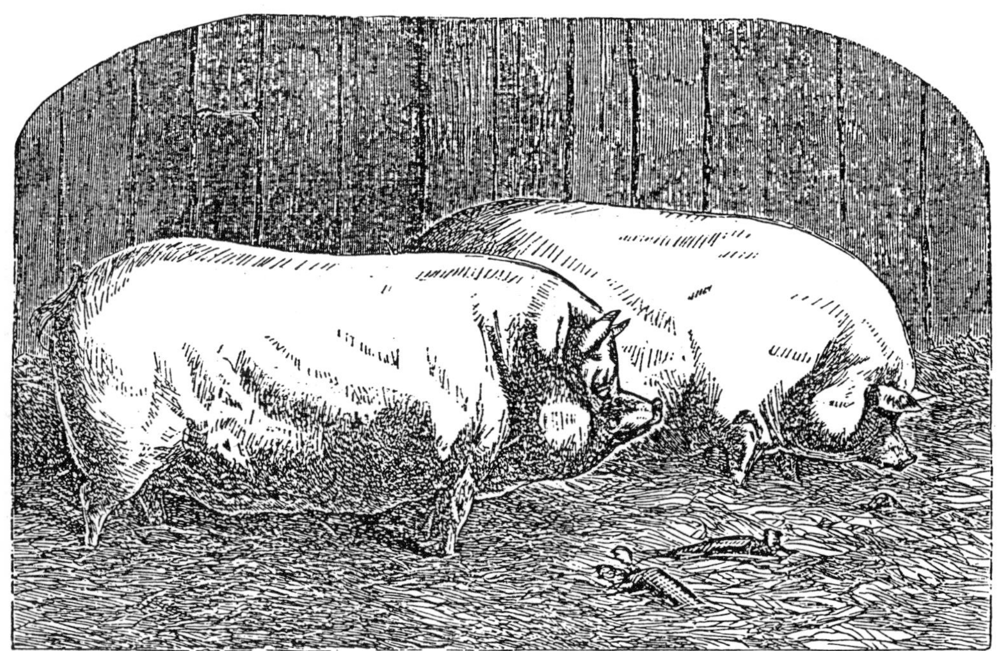

Fig. 5. Small White Leicester [*Harris on the Pig,* 1881]

TAMING THE WILD

When humans began to domesticate useful species for their own purposes, it would seem that they had plenty of choice among the Old World's widely distributed wild pig species. But there were practical limitations. The Pygmy was perhaps too small and too nervous. The easily tamed and long-lived Babirusa bore only one or two young each year. Litter sizes were also restricted in the Warthog, which has only four teats, and in the African Bushpig and Giant Forest hog, with only six teats each. The Javanese and Sulawesi Warty pigs and the Bearded pig of Indonesia were very local.

The Eurasian Wild Boar, however, offered everything. It was widespread and abundant. It had twelve teats (females produce three or four in the first litter, but subsequently can give birth to up to 15 fast-developing young). It could live for up to 20 years if it managed to avoid the hunters, and the very act of hunting produced, often intentionally, orphaned young which could then be reared in captivity, to which they seemed to adapt quite readily - a first step in domestication. And the meat was plenteous and good.

It was the Wild Boar, *Sus scrofa*, that became the source of almost all the domesticated pigs of Europe and Asia, apart from very local domestications of the Sulawesi Warty hog. And it was the innate variety in the many geographical subspecies of the Wild Boar that was and continues to be the source of invaluable variety in the domesticated pig.

Domestication of an animal species tends to occur independently in different parts of the world, contemporaneously or otherwise. It is not usually possible to state that a particular species was first domesticated by a certain group or race of people in a particular region at a particular time and this is probably as true of pigs as of cattle or dogs. However, as is so often the case with livestock, it is likely that the earliest domestication was within the "fertile crescent" of south west Asia. The Near East was the birthplace of the world's settled farming practices from about 10,000 BC and the archaeological evidence suggests that the earliest domestication of the pig was already underway there some 9,000 years ago. Evidence in Anatolia, Mesopotamia and northern Iraq, for example, includes figurines dating back to the sixth and seventh millennia BC as well as bones. Pigs became popular subjects for statuettes in ancient Persia, especially during the fourth and third millennia BC, a period during which there is contemporaneous evidence from the bones of domesticated pigs in China as well.

It seems that the domesticated pig soon radiated from its south west Asian cradle. It spread southwards, into ancient Syria, into the Jordan valley's Jericho and into Palestine. Pork was still on the menu for Jewish religious rites during the Bronze Age. By the end of the fifth millenium there were domesticated pigs in Egypt, and there were large herds being bred in the Nile Valley around 1500 BC. From ancient Egypt the domesticated pig went into Sudan, where it was still common in 1173 AD.

From its original cradle, the pig had also spread westwards, into Greece and south east Europe, and accompanied migrating humans via the Carpathian basin and southern Ukraine into the rest of Europe during the Neolithic period. But there are two strange features of this spread. The pig, unlike other livestock, is the animal of the settled farmer rather than the nomad. It is easy to imagine nomadic pastoralists taking their ruminants with them on their travels but the herding of pigs for such journeys was a more awkward manoeuvre altogether. Surprisingly, it appears that people did move the pigs, rather than simply spreading the technique of domestication so that locals could domesticate their native Wild Boar - a practice which came later. So, looking at the various subspecies, it seems likely that Turkey's *S.s. libycus* was the wild source of many of the old pigs of Europe, western Asia and northern Africa. The range of the Turkish Wild Boar includes central and western Turkey, Syria, Lebanon, Jordan, Israel and possibly Yugoslavia and the Nile delta: the animal's colouring is fuscous, with cream to buff hair tips on the back and sides, and touches of cinnamon, burnt umber and buff on the extremities, and dense drab-coloured underfur. Specimens from Turkey have been measured at about 130cm long, 75-95cm tall, weighing 125-185kg (see Mayer and Brisbin).

At that stage much of Europe was still well

forested with deciduous trees - the ideal environment for a pig - and apparently the precious domesticated imports thrived wherever they were taken.

Meanwhile, pigs were also being domesticated in eastern Asia. In China, they were already numerous in the third millenium BC. In recent years Chinese archaeologists have claimed that pigs have been domesticated there for 7,000 years, from the evidence of carbon-14 dating of pig bones at sites spread widely over the country. There is a special claim for domesticated pigs at Zengpiyan in South China some 10,000 years ago - which is a thousand years before the Anatolian evidence. Presumably, therefore, those domesticants were based on an east Asian subspecies of the Wild Boar, most of which have convex profiles with short lacrimal bones.

In 3486 BC emperor Fo-Hi of China decreed that swine should be bred and raised - and he also advised his subjects to import domesticated pigs from the west. His compliment was repaid in full some five thousand years later when pigs from China and Indo-China had a considerable influence in the improvement of local European types.

Some say that, a thousand years before *Sus scrofa* was domesticated by anybody, anywhere, in the west or in the east, the small Sulawesi Warty pig (*Sus celebensis*) had already been tamed locally. It found its way to other islands and a few thousand years later it was still there, both domestic and feral or wild, ready to greet and breed with European domestic pigs dropped off by exploring navigators. The pigs of New Guinea, in particular, are descended from these hybrids and the people of that large island have a "pig culture" as strong as any African cattle culture. This unusual relationship between pig and human is looked at more closely in the section on south east Asia.

The Domesticated Pig

The process of domestication brings about morphological and behavioural changes in all species and it is possible to deduce from archaeological evidence whether bones are from a wild animal or from its domesticant.

In the early stages of deliberate breeding, the head tends to become smaller, the legs shorter, but the body proportionately longer. The next stage seems to be that the skull itself is changed in shape: a pig's becomes shorter and broader than the long skull of the Wild Boar. This is especially noticeable in the shortening of the face and mandibles, and the lacrimal bone becomes shorter and shorter. Meanwhile the profile of the face changes froM straight to "broken", as seen in a domesticated dog like the spaniel, with an angle between muzzle and forehead.

Another feature of pig domestication is a change in the coat. The Wild Boar has very coarse bristles, and a marked crest along the back. Domestication refines the bristles and reduces their density (to almost naked in some cases). Pigs also begin to show non-wild colours which can be "fixed" by deliberately selective breeding.

It is not only by their bones that prehistoric domesticants can be recognised. Artistic representations also give clues. It was only after domestication that pigs gained curly tails or lop ears. The Wild Boar has a straight tail and prick ears. When a figurine shows what otherwise seems to be a tusky, bristle-crested wild animal, the creature's curled tail immediately denotes its domesticity. However, even modern breeds in China and south east Asia sometimes have straight tails.

European Pigs

During the Neolithic period, the domesticated pigs of central and eastern Europe were not unlike the wild type. They had the typical long head and were generally primitive, but small. It has been suggested that local differences were due to a combination of importation from south west Asia (by way of south east Europe) and interbreeding with local wild pigs. It was a period in which the gene pool of the domesticant was being constantly replenished and invigorated with wild blood.

The domesticated pig spread northwards. As early as 3000 BC immigrant pigs had reached Sweden, where they were much smaller than the local Wild Boar and showed no signs of having been bred from or with it. There is evidence of pigs in Denmark some 3,500 years ago - not necessarily fully domesticated, but certainly living in close association with human settlements.

In the Roman era, husbandry and breeding techniques improved dramatically for all livestock. Pigs began to grow larger and pig rearing became more deliberate. The principles of fattening were understood; methods of curing ham and bacon were known, and sausages were sold in Roman cities. Local people, however, continued with their old ways and their pigs remained small, even while an "advanced" neighbour's pigs grew large. Those small European pigs are the ones that are often described as turbary pigs, like those found at Neolithic lakeside village sites in Switzerland. With the fading of the Roman empire, the husbandry and breeding techniques were lost until medieval times.

Whatever its shortcomings, the pig was an important animal in medieval Europe. The poorer inhabitants of rural areas rarely saw any meat other than from the pig. Even up to the Second World War, rural workers used to keep a couple of backyard pigs for family consumption. It was perhaps because of the pig's close association with the peasantry that the livestock improvers of the 18th century virtually ignored the species. Yet in 1643 the Hungarian archbishop, György Szelepcsény, had said of his pigs: "In every farm of mine I keep animals of a different colour, in one the blond ones, in another the piebald, the black and white or spotted ones, and again in another the black ones." Selection for colour is one of the major, if superficial, steps in creating and consolidating a breed.

The Development of Breeds

The domesticated pig, just like the ancestral Wild Boar, adapted to its local environment and diversified accordingly, so that, in due course, a wide range of regional types developed, affected to some extent by factors such as climate and natural resources, but more by local husbandry methods and the degree of interbreeding with wild subspecies. Considering the geographical variation in the latter, it is not surprising that the domesticants could show morphological differences. Very gradually, pigs were selected on the basis of physical features such as colour and particular characteristics such as hardiness, docility, fertility, good mothering, and the ability to produce lard or whatever was deemed important locally. But it was a long, long process and inevitably hit-and-miss until the curtain that masked the understanding of genetics was drawn aside by Mendel and the breeding of livestock could become more methodical.

The regional types that preceded the deliberate improvement and standardisation of recognised breeds owed as much to natural selection on a Darwinian basis as to human control. From a combination of archaeological findings and early art, and later documentary evidence, some of the main types to emerge were these:

Ancient Egypt (c1500-1000BC): Long head with straight profile and pointed snout; short erect ears; twisted tail; strong ridge of bristles along the back and neck; a black pig.

Neolithic in central and eastern Europe: Local differences from degree of domestication, extent of breeding with local wild subspecies, and earlier domesticants imported from south west Asia. **Turbary type:** Small, slender and leggy; small head with flat forehead, shortened jaws, crowded teeth, and shorter lacrimal bone than wild type; relatively refined. **Larger Neolithic European:** Larger, coarse-boned pig with long legs, long head, flat ribs, high back, late maturity; more evidence of domestication from local wild subspecies, plenty of interbreeding between large domesticant and local wild.

Roman Empire: Larger than the turbary (better conditions and conscious breeding); diminishing dentition but larger limb bones. Contemporary small local pigs widespread around villa settlements in colonies. There has been speculation that Roman pigs were based on imports from China (low-legged and fleshy) but the proof is lacking.

Very broadly, it seems that the European pigs eventually fell into two main categories: a smaller pig with erect ears, and a larger with hanging ears. The latter feature proved to have advantages in husbandry, in that the ears acted as blinkers and the sows were usually more docile, though sometimes the boars were more dangerous. In many European countries these lop-eared pigs were seen as the indigenous type and came to be called land pigs, developing into the long, lean, lop-eared Landrace breeds. In Britain, however, many were "improved" with the help of Chinese, IndoChinese and Neapolitan (Iberian/Chinese) blood and often became prick-eared, dish-faced and earlier maturing as a result of that infusion.

The Unclean Pig

Finally, there is a huge gap in the pig world which partly accounts for the divergence between the breeds of East and West. Of the world's major religions, those who follow Islam, Judaism or Hinduism eat no pork or pig meat products of any kind. Sikhs eat little pork. The pig is considered unclean and unhealthy, and so is the swineherd.

Neanderthal man would eat any kind of meat he could catch. Over the ages, different cultures began to develop different prejudices about what animals they would and would not eat - the British and Americans, for example, do not eat either horses or dogs, nor do they eat insects, whereas all these are welcomed as food somewhere in the world (though it is relatively unusual for humans to eat other carnivores). There is a theory, expressed by Dr Robert Sallares at the 1992 annual meeting of the Classical Association at Oxford, that any species of animal that could not be integrated into an ancient economy became suspect and ultimately regarded as "unclean" meat. Pigs were awkward to herd and therefore in due course became regarded as unclean by nomadic societies. There is a second theory that pig meat not only harbours unpleasant parasites if inadequately cooked but also turns bad quickly in hot climates - though this theory makes no allowances for the pig's huge popularity in the tropics and subtropics of South East Asia.

Whatever the reasons (and no doubt they also had much to do with the fact that pigs are excellent scavengers whose omnivorous tastes include human bodily wastes), the pig has been regarded as a taboo animal in a large part of Asia for many centuries, and is also ignored in many parts of Africa except as a wild animal to be hunted. In some places the taboo has proved to be the pig's redemption, in a strange way. For example, in India, where pigs are largely taboo as food, there are countless ferals in the villages that perform the role of street cleaners and are given special protection for their services.

What is a Breed?

A breed is not the same as a general type or even as a local type. Juliet Clutton-Brock has carefully defined a breed as: "A group of animals that has been *selected by man* to possess a *uniform appearance* that is *inheritable* and *distinguishes it* from other groups of animals within the same species." (My italics.)

Apart from the first criterion, the description could define a species, or more precisely a subspecies, but the latter evolve in the wild by natural rather than human selection. A species, as described by Clutton-Brock, is a group of actually or potentially interbreeding natural populations that are reproductively isolated from other such groups - though within the species there are individual variances, and also geographical ones (subspecies are geographically and morphologically separated but can interbreed with other subspecies should they meet).

Clutton-Brock points out a contrast: a species develops a set of characteristics that improve its chances of survival, whereas the characteristics of a breed are developed by humans for their own ends (aesthetic, ritual, social status, economic etc.) and do not necessarily improve the type's ability to survive - in fact they sometimes decrease that ability dramatically by so altering the physiology that, for example, breeding or breathing become awkward, or the animal becomes too dependent on man and would not thrive without special management. However, except in extreme cases in which the actual anatomical structure has been altered, most of the characteristics of a breed are fairly superficial and relatively evanescent. They leave no trace in the archaeological record, and indeed - especially in pigs, with their multiple litters and quick generation - can be deliberately altered in a very short time, which is one reason why pigs have become the favourite subject of commercial breeding companies today.

It should also be noted that a breed can be artificially selected to resemble a much more ancient type but that the resemblance is entirely superficial: there need be no direct ancestral link between the two, or at least no closer relationship than with any other breed. Thus it is possible on the one hand for similar-looking breeds to evolve in widely separated regions or areas, with a genetic relationship no closer to each other than to any other breed - and it is also possible for a breed to be deliberately produced to resemble another, perhaps an extinct breed, but again only superficially: it might look very much the same but it does not have the continuous link with the original that proves its pedigree, nor does it necessarily have all or even any of the original's special qualities.

Appearances can be deceptive: *never* judge a pig breed by its coat! For example, the once famous Berkshire pig of England was during its peak (and remains today) a black pig with white points, prick ears and a dished face. Yet in the early 19th century it was a larger and more colourful animal with a red-and-black spotted coat and big lop ears. The only reliable way to trace a breed is through its pedigree - and that, in most cases, is virtually impossible further back than the establishment of pig breed societies and herdbooks in the late 19th century.

However, essentially a breed relies on being visually recognisable from a combination of features such as colour, ear carriage, face shape and general conformation which, to the experienced eye, immediately identify it as a member of that breed or as having a trace of some specific breed in its past.

Worldwide, the domesticated pig diverged into two major extremes: the European "Wild Boar" type, which was coarse in bone and shape, the back tending to arch, with a coarse coat—an agile, alert and muscular animal whose fat was mixed with the muscle in streaks and marbling; and the Asian type, whose fat was put down in thick, blubber-like layers under the skin, whose nature was much more docile, and whose bones were light and fine, and back low. There came a time when there was considerable potential for hybrid vigour when the two extremes could be crossed.

The geographical sections look more closely at regional types and how different countries developed their own breeds.

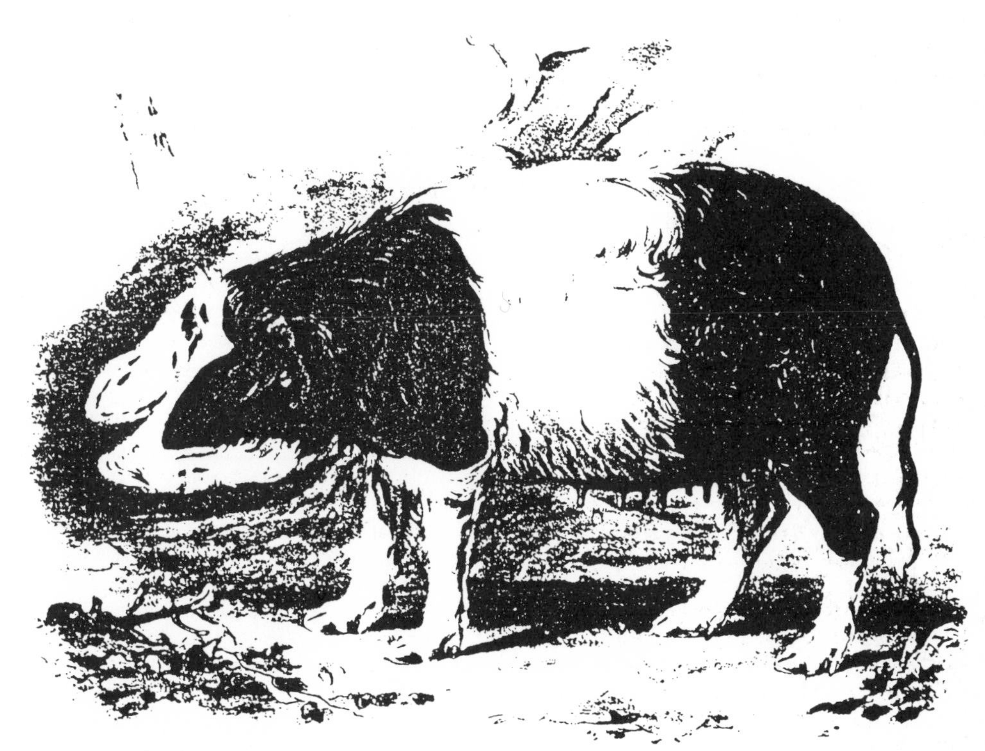

Fig. 6. Old English [Low, 1842]

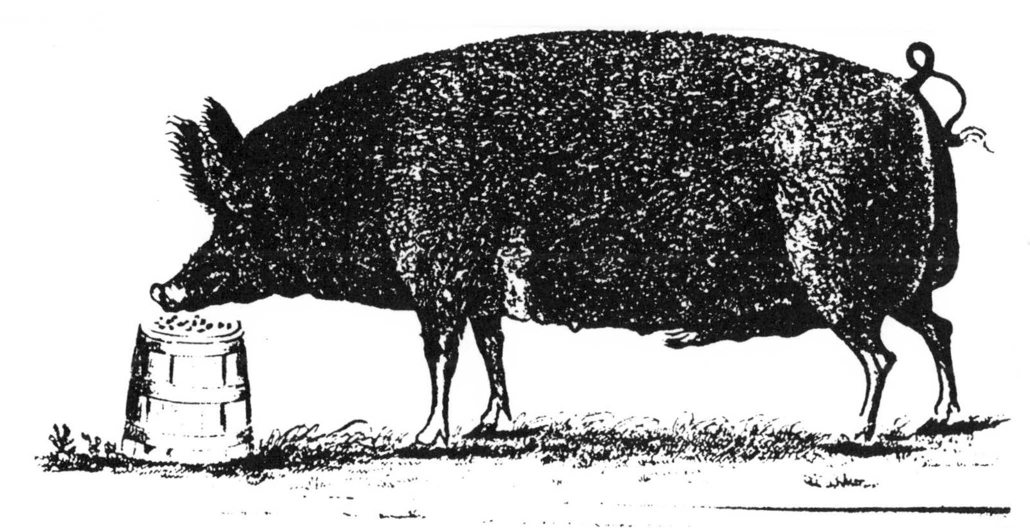

Fig. 7. Essex Half-black, Mr. Western's boar [Young, *General View of the Agriculture of Essex*, 1807]

PIG BREEDING

PIG BREEDING

The essence of controlled breeding is to fix and enhance desirable charecteristics while, if possible, eliminating or reducing the undesirable. It is a delicate balance and it is only very recently that enough has been understood about the structure of DNA to be able - in theory - not to lose something of secondary value, or potential value, in the pursuit of the primary goal.

The main factors which breeders have sought to manipulate fall broadly into categories such as appearance, productive performance, hardiness and behaviour. The first proved to be the easiest for the early breeders to control, and hence came the development of definitive breeds with standards which were based almost entirely on what the animal looked like - its colour and its shape. Colour (and pattern) are for the most part governed by quite simple genetic relationships, likewise features such as the carriage of an ear, but less visible traits such as behaviour and performance are often controlled by a more complex combination of genes, and are sometimes of very low heritability, which is to say that the chance of a trait being passed to the offspring is relatively low. Geneticists use all their skill and knowledge to harness some of the desired commercial traits and combine them in such a way that they do not conflict with each other or with the aims of the breeder and the producer. And they are gradually winning that particular battle, mapping the gene structure in the pig and preparing for a transgenic future in which pieces of DNA will be virtually like goods in a supermarket, packaged and identifiable so that they can simply be picked off the shelf and transferred to a shopping-basket bundle of genetic material that becomes the perfect pig for whatever purpose the breeder has in mind.

In the meantime, however, breeders must also admit that there is a lot more to it than genetics, and that greater understanding of the pig in all its aspects - including its normal behaviour patterns as well as its physiology - are the essential tools of better management and, as a result, better performance. At the same time a new element has recently crept into the equation - probably for the first time in the history of commercial pig management - and that is public opinion about such management. For years the main criteria for breeders have been to meet the demands of producers, who in turn have been guided largely by market returns and the pursuit of efficiency. Now, however, the consumer is beginning to indicate that the quality, quantity and price of the product are not the only factors to be considered. There is also the quality of life for the individual animal.

SIMPLE GENETICS

Gregor Johann Mendel, son of a Silesian peasant, was born in 1822 and was ordained a priest in 1847 after entering an Augustinian monastery. He studied science in Vienna during the early 1850's and became a biologist as well as a monk. In 1868 he became abbot at Brünn, where he continued his remarkable research into plant breeding - in particular, hybridisation. The principles of inheritance which his painstaking studies revealed became the basis of modern genetics.

The essence of those principles is the existence of pairs of genes which control the inheritance of specific traits, in animals as well as plants. When reproductive cells are formed, the paired elements separate and each egg or sperm cell contains only one gene of each of the chromosomal string of pairs that together make up the genotype of an individual. Thus a parent transmits to its offspring a sample half of its own inheritance, and when the samples from two parents are combined at fertilisation, the embryonic cell begins life with a proper complement of two genes in each pair, one from each parent. It seems to be pure chance which of a pair of genes in any one parent becomes the single gene in the reproductive cell, and the potential combinations are considerable.

At its simplest, a gene is expressed in two forms, or *alleles*: one is termed dominant and the other recessive. If both genes in a pair for a characteristic are dominant, then that dominant characteristic is expressed in that individual. If one of the genes is dominant and the other recessive, the dominant characteristic is expressed and the individual appears to be the same as if both those genes were of the dominant allele, but the individual retains the ability to pass on the masked recessive characteristic which remains in its genotype. If both genes are of the recessive allele, then the recessive characteristic is expressed in the individual. Thus it is easy to fix a recessive characteristic in a breed by always breeding from those showing the recessive trait and culling animals showing the dominant one, but not so easy to eradicate completely the recessive in favour of the dominant.

The usual shorthand gives a capital letter to the dominant allele and a lower-case letter to the recessive - for example "*B*" and "*b*". Thus a pair of homozygous (similar) dominant alleles would be designated "*BB*", a pair of homozygous recessive alleles as "*bb*", and a pair of heterozygous alleles as "*Bb*".

If an individual whose genotype includes a dominant pair of genes *BB* for a certain trait is mated with another who also has the dominant pair *BB*, then all the offspring will be of the *BB* genotype. Likewise if both parents are *bb*, so too will all the offspring be *bb*. But if one parent is *BB* and the other is *bb*, the first generation offspring will be of the heterozygous type *Bb*,expressing the *B* characteristic but able to pass on the *b* type to offspring. If those *Bb* offspring are interbred, the likely genotypes will be in the proportions (more or less) of one *BB*, two *Bb* and one *bb*. Their phenotypes (the expression of the genotype) will therefore be three with the dominant trait to one showing the recessive. It can be seen that it is only in the mating of two *bb* types that you can be (almost) certain that all the offspring, and all *their* offspring if they are bred with each other, will also be of the *bb* type. But if a recessive allele remains masked by a dominant one, it will one day re-emerge in a future generation.

That is the simplest scenario. However, there are many complications. For a start, dominance is not necessary complete. Secondly, very few traits are controlled by just a single pair of genes, and the more genes involved the more combinations are possible. Thirdly, various bits of DNA cross over and generally confuse the issue by throwing up completely unpredictable genotypes. If they did not, nothing much would ever change in the long run.

Bearing those complications in mind, here are some of the usually simple patterns of dominance and recessiveness in the pig:

Ears

Generally, lop is dominant and prick recessive. Wild pig species all have erect ears, of various sizes but none of them large. If a homozygous lop-eared pig is mated with a prick-eared pig, all the offspring have lop ears but are heterozygous - they still carry the prick-eared gene, so that if they in turn are interbred there will be roughly three lops to one prick-eared in the second generation but two of the three lops still carry the prick-eared gene.

Colour

The main types of coat colour in pigs are wild or agouti, uniform black, uniform red, black spotting, black with white points, belted, shiny white, and dirty white.

WHITE is due to a single dominant gene. The Large White and the Landrace are generally homozygous for that gene, which inhibits the production of black and yellow pigments. Coloured breeds such as the Berkshire, the Large Black and the Poland China are homozygous for the recessive gene. However, if a Landrace is crossed with a Hampshire, there is a possibility of a third allele which sometimes produces roans. (Roan = mixture of coloured and white individual hairs.)

BLACK, BLACK SPOTTING and RED are three alleles at the same locus, at which uniform black is dominant and uniform red is recessive. The order of dominance is black, black spotted, red. Large Black and Hampshire are homozygous for the dominant black allele; the Duroc is homozygous for the recessive red allele; the Piétrain is homozygous for the intermediate black spotted allele. The black breeds with white points (e.g. Berkshire and Poland China) are examples of an extended form of black spotting.

WHITE BELTS are probably due to the action of another dominant gene.

In summary: white is dominant over colour; black is dominant over spotted; spotted is dominant over red, and belting is dominant over non-belting. In the case of skin colour, in general white is dominant and black recessive but the relationship is not simple.

The wild colouring is described as AGOUTI. Its relationship with other colour genes is not well understood - all sorts of interesting things happen in crosses between wild pigs and red or black breeds. But it can be reasonably assumed that most domestic pigs carry the recessive non-agouti allele. Mayer and Brisbin describe the wide range of colours and patterns in America's free-breeding feral pigs.

People have had fun over the years cross-breeding different colours to see what comes out, and sometimes being greatly surprised (it is a good method of discovering past crossing in a supposedly pure breed). The first generation of Large White x Berkshire are all white; that of Landrace x Berkshire tend to have some spotting; that of Berkshire and Tamworth crosses produce sand-and-black spotted (with prick ears); that of Saddleback x Tamworth produce saddleback with no obvious trace of Tamworth. Hampshire x Middle White produced blue-and-white patches (like a Wessex/Large White cross) in one litter but piglets identical to the Hampshire in another; later they developed into what were described as "Berkshire Saddlebacks" with a perfect white saddle like the father and the white points and dark eyes of the Berkshire, with the latter's stocky conformation. The Large White x Tamworth usually produces pure white in the first generation, but very occasionally blue-and-white spotted; the "blue" being white hair over dark pigmented skin. A Poland China (black with white points) crossed with an Oxford Sandy-and-Black (orange to tan with random black markings) produced 56% identical in colouring to the dam, 44% to the sire; the same OSB sows were crossed with Berkshire and the colours of the offspring were in roughly equal proportion to those of the two parents; the same sows were then crossed with the OSB-marked boars from the Poland China/OSB original cross and produced two OSB to every one Poland China in colour.

Quite apart from personal aesthetic preferences and the desire to use colour and pattern as the most obvious badge of a breed, there have been various colour prejudices over the ages. For example, in the UK during the 19th century it was still possible to divide the country geographically by the colour of its pigs: those of the southern counties of England tended to be black, those of the midlands, especially the west, were coloured, and those of the north and east were usually white. Sometimes there was a certain amount of logic in the preferences: it was said that white pigs suffered from sun scald in the warmer climate of south west England, for example, and it is still a fact that those who dress carcasses dislike coloured pigs in which the pigmented hair roots leave their mark. Consumers often object to coloured skin in a product for which the rind is retained (for example, bacon), though in the past in many regions they prefered the coloured rind as an indication of better meat. Colour has also been associated with fattiness, in that outdoor breeds are usually coloured and they need an extra lining of fat as protection against the climate.

But there is a lot more to a pig than its colour.

COMMERCIAL BREEDING

Commercial pig producers have certain demands to make of the pig. They are interested in particular in efficiency - which includes ease of management and a good return on investment. Thus they tend to concentrate on qualities such as predictability of performance; faster growth in the lean parts; a quicker time to slaughter weight; lower maintenance and feed costs; resistance to disease to avoid veterinary expenses, and an acceptable carcass at the abattoir. Breeders attempt to meet these needs by looking for the best possible growth rates (daily weight gains); feed conversion efficiency; sow prolificacy and mothering qualities; and a higher lean proportion in the carcass, preferably weighted towards the more expensive cuts. The meat trade demands easily dressed and uniform carcasses and, increasingly, a better "eating quality" in the meat - a vague term. The consumer is concerned about meat quality, too, including taste and flavour, texture and tenderness, succulence and perhaps colour. The consumer is now also concerned about too much fat, the possibility of additives in the meat and the price in the shops. More recently, consumers have expressed increasingly strong views on environmental pollution by slurry, and on animal welfare.

The perfect breeder takes all these demands into consideration but can fairly point out that it is not *all* down to good breeding. For example, the number of pigs reared per sow per annum might initially depend upon genetic factors such as the number of eggs a sow releases, and on partly environmental factors such as the abilty of the boar to fertilise them, and the ability of the sow to maintain the viability of the embryos and give birth to a high number of live piglets. After that much depends upon her ability to rear the piglets to weaning - a function of her own mothering instincts and milk supply, encouraged by good stockmanship, good nutrition and a happy environment free from disease and stress.

Feed conversion efficiency (i.e. the ability to turn feed into saleable meat, usually defined in terms of the ratio or FCR between the amount of feed consumed by the pig and its liveweight gain) depends partly on breeding and appetite; partly upon the type, amount and cost of feed and the length of time it takes the pig to convert the feed to slaughter weight. It can be improved by better breeding; but a clear understanding of a pig's needs, tastes and digestive system is as important. Pigs need to eat a lot in order to grow quickly, and they need the right type of feedstuffs and the right timing to convert them into lean meat without producing too much fat.

The eating quality of the meat is difficult to test and quantify, because tastes vary. For example, an increasing proportion of pig meat is processed before being eaten, rather than being consumed as fresh pork, and the chemical composition of the meat is an important factor for successful processing, especially the protein content and the ability to retain moisture. Breeders have successfully striven to reduce the thickness of backfat in pigs to barely a whisper, in comparison with the thick layers of lard demanded of the 19th century pig, and they are now turning again to coloured pigs like the Duroc for "marbled" meat. Fat, however, is a traditionally rich source of energy for those who consume it. The change in diet preference away from fat in some modern cultures highlights an important aspect in pig breeding: the demands for various pig products have varied in different cultures and ages. Pig types have needed to vary as well to meet those demands. Fortunately for producers, pigs are far more prolific than other mammalian livestock and they also reach sexual maturity quickly. Thus they are ideal material for those who wish to change the animal's phenotype to meet new markets in the shortest possible time and the greatest possible numbers.

Geneticist John Webb (of the Cotswold Pig Breeding Company) made the point recently that 90% of a tasting panel's preferences could be attributed to what happened to the pig *after* it left the farm. "Genetic differences", he explained, "played such a small part that it would not be cost effective to include them in selection programmes at present". Growth patterns, nutrition and age at slaughter were all contributory factors but more important was freedom from stress during transport and in the lairage at the abattoir. All the good work of the breeder and the producer could be wiped out by the inducement of fear in what is probably the most intelligent of all livestock species.

Breeders are also well aware that they are playing a delicate game in manipulating genetic material. It is all too easy to upset the balance, by concentrating on a particular trait and failing to appreciate its link with another characteristic. The classic example of the latter is the halothane gene, described below. A topical example is the European use of the Taihu group of breeds from China to improve prolificacy: they do indeed have high litter numbers but they also have fat carcasses, and the trick is to incorporate the one without the other into western hybrids.

There are countless equations which need to

be balanced by the geneticist in the search for a pig perfectly matched to the demands of the market, and there are still many unknowns in how characteristics are inherited.

One of the basic facts, which has been exploited almost as far as it can be, is that the depth of backfat is a highly heritable trait. Another is that breeds with low mature weights (i.e. early-maturing) are more developed, and therefore fatter, at a particular slaughter weight - fatness increases as development progresses. Another is that fat is an uneconomical product: an animal produces a unit weight of lean for a quarter of the energy from its feed intake as the same weight in fat.

During much of the 20th century, commercial pig farmers capitalised on the 19th century work of those who had improved local types and fixed them as breeds with recognisable and heritable qualities. Producers could choose from different lines within breeds or, if a breed did not meet their needs, they could switch to another that did or would grade up existing stock by using improved sires to cross with local sows so that, in no time at all,the proportion of the new blood in the herd became high.

Because of the pig's high reproductive rate, there is a great deal of material available quickly for assessment, comparison and selection in the interests of general improvement, either on a breed or a regional or national basis. Such co-operation is hard to achieve in regions where the majority of pig farmers have very small herds which are incidental to other enterprises. There are financial constraints on the farmers, and there is the problem of distributing quite complicated information about genetics to a large number of people, some of them with little interest. Where pigs are the sole or main enterprise, the farmer is eager to improve returns and therefore is alert to new ideas that might achieve that end. Where the pigs are farmed in large herds by a company or a co-operative venture with the resources and drive to maximise investment, the desire for breed improvement is obvious. The larger the number of pigs you work with, the larger the database and the more quickly it can be assessed and exploited.

Denmark was the leader in pig improvement on a national scale with its Landrace, and other nations have since followed its example. In recent years the trend in many countries has been towards a specialisation within the pig industry which has led to the development of major pig breeding companies that produce highly improved stock for the farmers. Most of the companies rely heavily on crossbreeding, exploiting what is known as heterosis.

Heterosis

Crossbreeding is the mating of two animals of substantial genetic difference, commonly using the boar of one breed with a sow of another breed, or at least of a different line within the breed. The aim might be to produce a better breeding sow, to produce a better slaughter generation, or perhaps to bring together useful traits from different breeds or lines. In the case of the first two, the aim is achieved as a result of *heterosis*, or hybrid vigour, in which the offspring of a cross show a greater degree of certain traits than the mean of the performance of the breeds used in the initial cross. The greater the genetic difference between the two, the greater the degree of hybrid vigour seen in the offspring.

In particular, hybrid breeding sows tend to mature earlier (and therefore can begin to breed younger), be more obvious in their heat, have a better conception rate and generally have a longer productive life and produce more piglets. Crossbred piglets (again comparing to the mean of their parents) are better able to survive whether as embryo, foetus or piglet, through the various stages from implantation to birth and from farrowing through weaning to finishing.

The art of commercial crossbreeding includes selecting the parents so that the desirable traits from each come together ("nick") and are enhanced in the offspring but their less desirable traits do not. However, in the meantime, the breeding stock should also be continually improved . A widely divergent gene pool must be maintained - a case for the conservation of as many breeds as possible, regardless of whether or not their qualities seem desirable at present. It is impossible to forecast when those traits might suddenly be required.

There is a danger in the trend to the universal use of favoured breeds, the spread of which has been greatly accelerated by the use of artificial insemination and the improvements in transport that allow easier exportation and importation of breeding livestock. For example, a few years ago many countries seized upon the unique "double-muscling" of the Belgian breeds, especially the Piétrain and the Belgian Landrace. Here is a cautionary tale.

The Halothane Gene

The Piétrain is an extreme breed in two respects which are now known to be closely linked. Its most obvious characteristic is the bulging double-muscling (*culard*) in its hams, a source of heavy weights of very lean meat. Its second well known characteristic is a tendency to drop dead, quite suddenly, under stress. Submit it to the anxiety of being mixed with unfamiliar animals, or of being boxed for transport, or incite it to violent exercise or the possibly less violent exertion of mating or farrowing, and its temperature begins to rise, irreversibly. There are other problems including reduced feed intake (which can reduce the growth rate and upset feed conversion efficiency), a shorter carcass, poorer reproductive performance and, more important, a high frequency of PSE (pale, soft, exudative muscle tissue), in which the muscles at slaughter are unappetisingly pale, or two-toned, and suffer from high drip-loss, causing problems during curing.

All these effects, in many cases, can be traced to a single recessive gene, and in general the more obviously compact and muscular the pig, the higher its extreme reaction to the porcine stress syndrome. The gene is known as the *halothane* gene because stress-susceptible pigs can usually be identified with accuracy at 10 weeks old by their reaction after inhaling halothane, an anaesthetic gas. Susceptible pigs lie with rigid, extended legs; others, the non-reactors, are completely relaxed in this anaesthetised state.

As the gene is recessive, heterozygous animals will carry it without showing symptoms. If they are then mated with similar carriers, the offspring can inherit the gene from both parents and will therefore be stress-susceptible. The breeds with the highest incidence of the gene are the Piétrain and some of the Landraces. At the other extreme, the British Large White and the Duroc show no incidence of the gene.

The gene can now be detected by a commercial DNA probe but it is not thought desirable to eradicate it completely. Rather, the breeders identify lines which carry the gene and limit it to the sire line to boost performance and carcass quality in the slaughter generation.

Chinese Prolificacy

The high prolificacy of the Chinese Taihu group relies on a combination of factors, including early puberty (average age and weight of gilt, 64 days and 15kg) and sexual maturity (3-5.5 months), high ovulation rates (15-16 for gilts, 21-29 for sows) and high oestradiol levels (50 % higher in, say, Jiaxing Black than in Large White).

To produce a large litter, a sow must first of all produce a large number of eggs and must then ensure a high rate of fertilisation and subsequent viability. In most domestic pigs, about 30% of embryos (i.e. fertilised eggs) die during the sow's pregnancy and it seems that the percentage which survive decreases as the number of eggs initially produced increases. Inspired by news of record litters such as one sow producing 31 piglets (30 born alive) in one litter, and another producing a litter of 42 (40 born alive) in her eighth parturition with an average of 22 live per litter and a total of 215 (200 born alive) up to her 9th parturition, it is hardly surprising that Europe has shown so much interest in the Taihu pigs.

The British concentrated their investigations on the **Meishan** as apparently the most prolific of the Chinese breeds. The Americans took an active interest in several Chinese breeds, importing **Meishan**, **Fengjing** and the North China **Min**. In 1990, the French led the field by publishing a book summarising their latest research into Chinese pigs.

The Meishan research in the United Kingdom is a joint venture, partially funded by a consortium of five pig breeding companies. In 1987, eleven male and twenty-one female Meishans were imported from China and established initially at the Institute of Animal Physiology and Genetics Research at the Edinburgh research station in Roslin. Staff who have handled the Edinburgh Meishans comment that they (and Chinese pigs in general) are much more docile and lazy than western pigs - in fact, so lazy that it can be quite difficult to move them around, though they can also be snappy when in the mood. It was noticed that the Meishan's oestrus lasted a day longer than that of European breeds and to such a strong degree that the sows could not be shifted.

In a report (to the 4th World Congress at Edinburgh) Agaro, Haley and Ellis gave details of performance testing on a total of 453 animals comparing Meishan, Large White and both reciprocal F_1 crosses. They observed relatively slow growth rates and high subcutaneous fat levels in the Meishan; the crossbred females showed significant heterosis for feed intake and growth rates but not for subcutaneous fat levels. Previous studies had shown that the Chinese breeds were superior in aspects of reproductive performance, and that through heterosis this trait in European x Meishan F_1 sows was similar to that of the purebred Meishan; but French studies showed that the Meishan achieved poorer growth rates and carcass performance.

In the Edinburgh study, growth rates of the crosses were up to 250g per day higher than those of purebred Meishan; the first cross with Large White grew as quickly as pure Large White, and backfat levels were between those of each breed. Growth rates were the same between Large White males and females, but in the Meishan the male growth rate was slower than that of the female.

It was prolificacy that was of greatest interest, of course. Many crossbreeding programmes have been tried in various countries to harness that good trait without the disadvantages of the Taihu's excessive fat, lower rate of weight gain and poorer feed conversion efficiency.

Looking at prolificacy in the Taihu, while they do produce large numbers of eggs and large numbers of piglets born alive, they do not have a high survival rate to weaning. Out of 940 litters in one study, the average born was 16.10 (14.2 born alive) but the weaning rate was only 12.10.

At Edinburgh, crossbred sows produced up to four more live piglets than British Large Whites. Pure Meishan females produced more eggs than the Large Whites, and also 20% more of their embryos survived - litter size seemed to be controlled by genes acting in the female rather than in the embryos.

The British pig breeding companies who formed part of the original consortium each explored their own ways of exploiting the Meishan's fertility and in the early summer of 1992 one of them took the industry a little by surprise when it launched its own Meishan synthetic, the **Manor Meishan** <Plate 15>. However, the French already have at least two Meishan synthetics: the **Sino-European** line, developed since 1985 by France Hybrides of Evry, Ile de France, from a basis of Meishan, Jiaxing, Landrace and Large White; and the **Tia Meslan** line in Brittany, developed during the 1980s by the Pen ar Lan breeding company of Maxent, using (Meishan x Jiaxing) boars on European sows.

Gene Mapping

The IAPG Meishans have become part of PiGMaP (Pig Gene Mapping Project) along with the genetically very distant European Large White and the Wild Boar (*Sus scrofa scrofa*). Polymorphic markers are being mapped in the F_2 crosses between the two domestic breeds, the aim being to identify, understand and exploit the action of individual genes which contribute to economically important traits in the domestic pig, and ultimately to study the evolutionary relationship between pigs and other mammals, including humans. Among farm species, the pig has several advantages in such a project: it has a well defined karotype, short generation interval and large full-sib families. Diverse genetic stocks (such as the Meishan and Large White) are available for study and, when those studies are complete, there is a professional breeding industry advanced enough to be able to exploit the results.

This massive and far-reaching project has the support of Britain's government and also collaborates with laboratories in the United Kingdom, France, Germany, the Netherlands, Belgium, Denmark, Norway and Sweden. It is funded by the European Community and co-ordinated from Edinburgh. The results are awaited with great interest.

PLATE 1. WILD PIGS

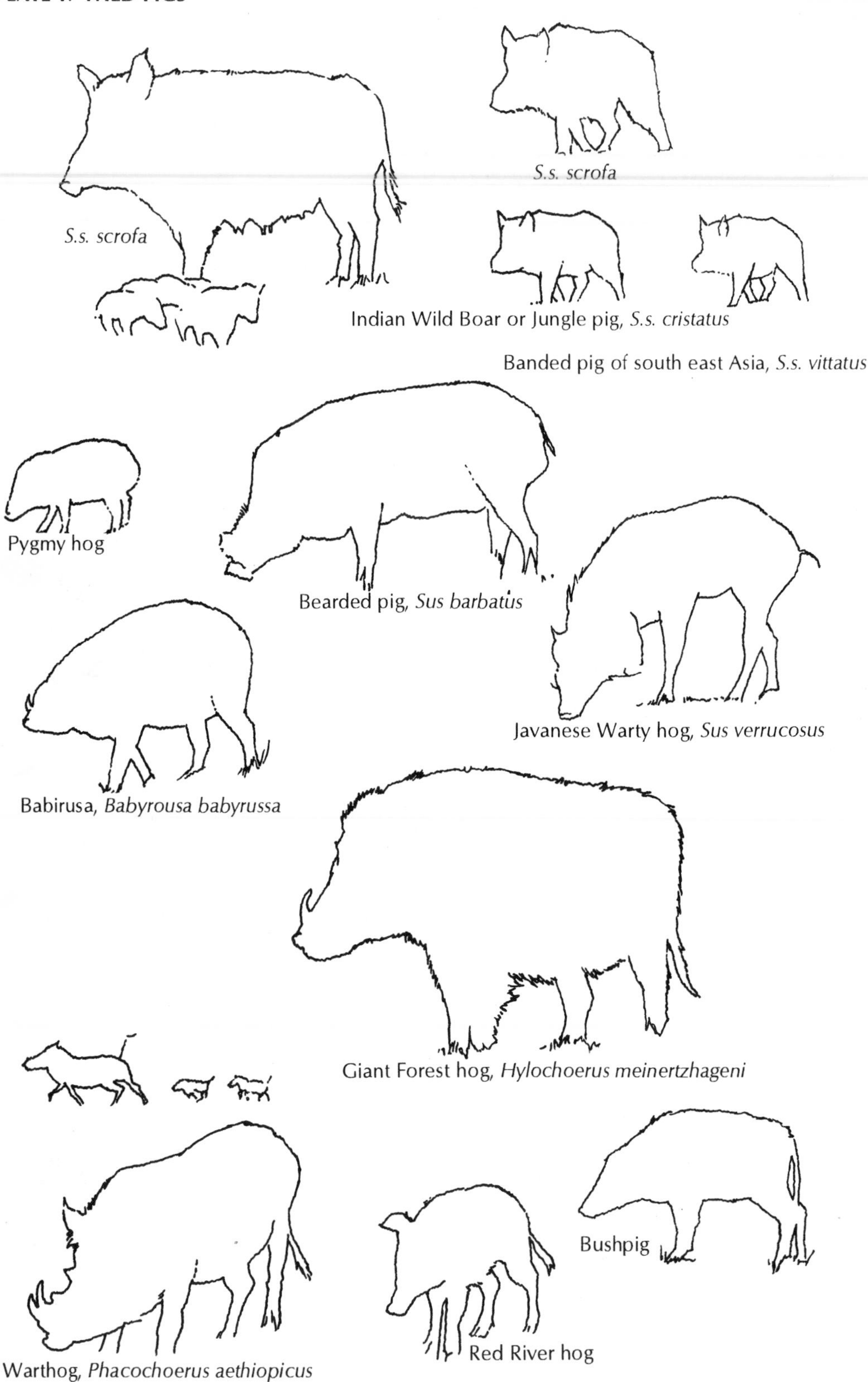

S.s. scrofa
S.s. scrofa
Indian Wild Boar or Jungle pig, *S.s. cristatus*
Banded pig of south east Asia, *S.s. vittatus*
Pygmy hog
Bearded pig, *Sus barbatus*
Javanese Warty hog, *Sus verrucosus*
Babirusa, *Babyrousa babyrussa*
Giant Forest hog, *Hylochoerus meinertzhageni*
Bushpig
Red River hog
Warthog, *Phacochoerus aethiopicus*

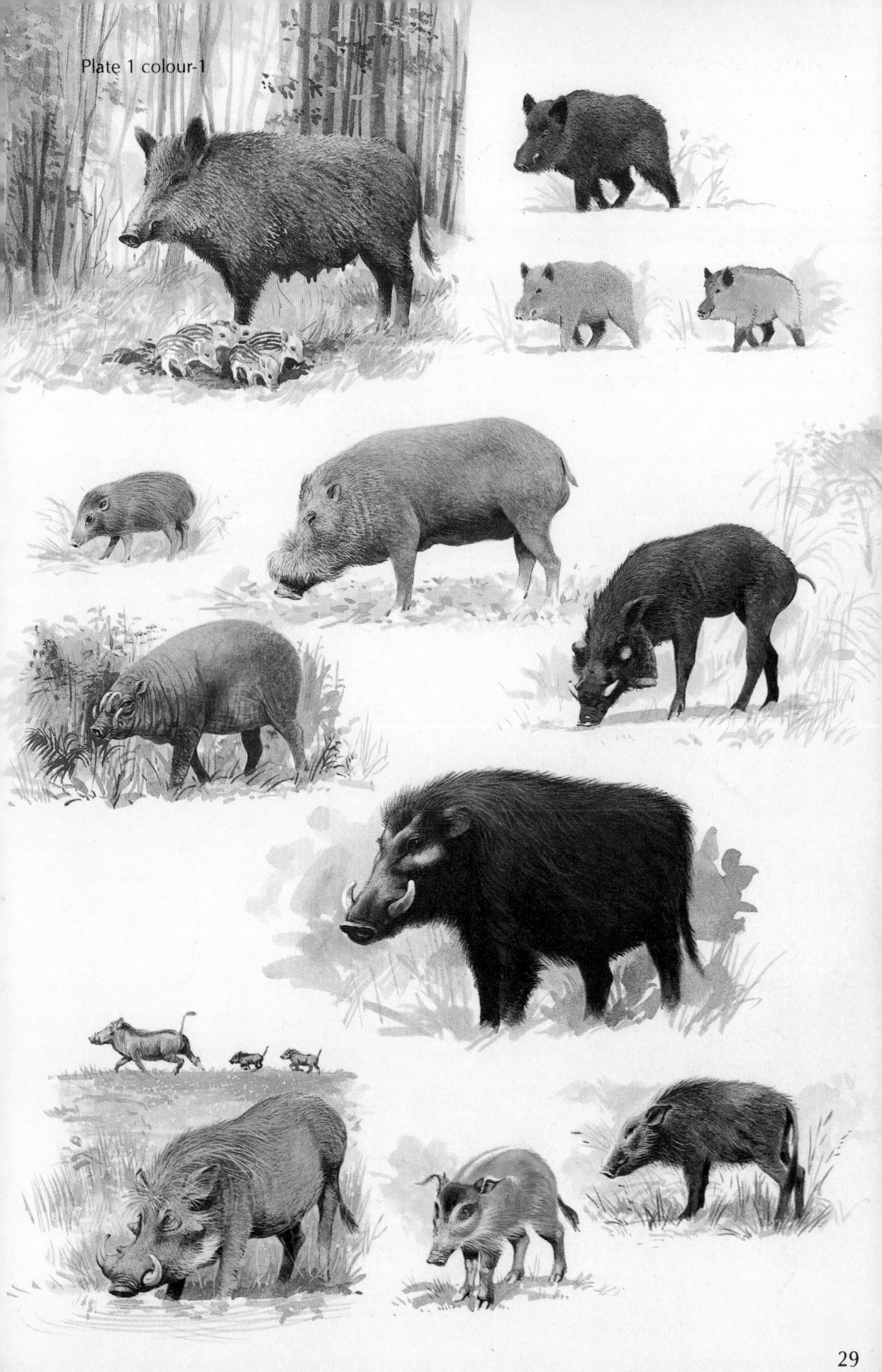
Plate 1 colour-1

PLATE 2: UNITED KINGDOM, Coloured Breeds

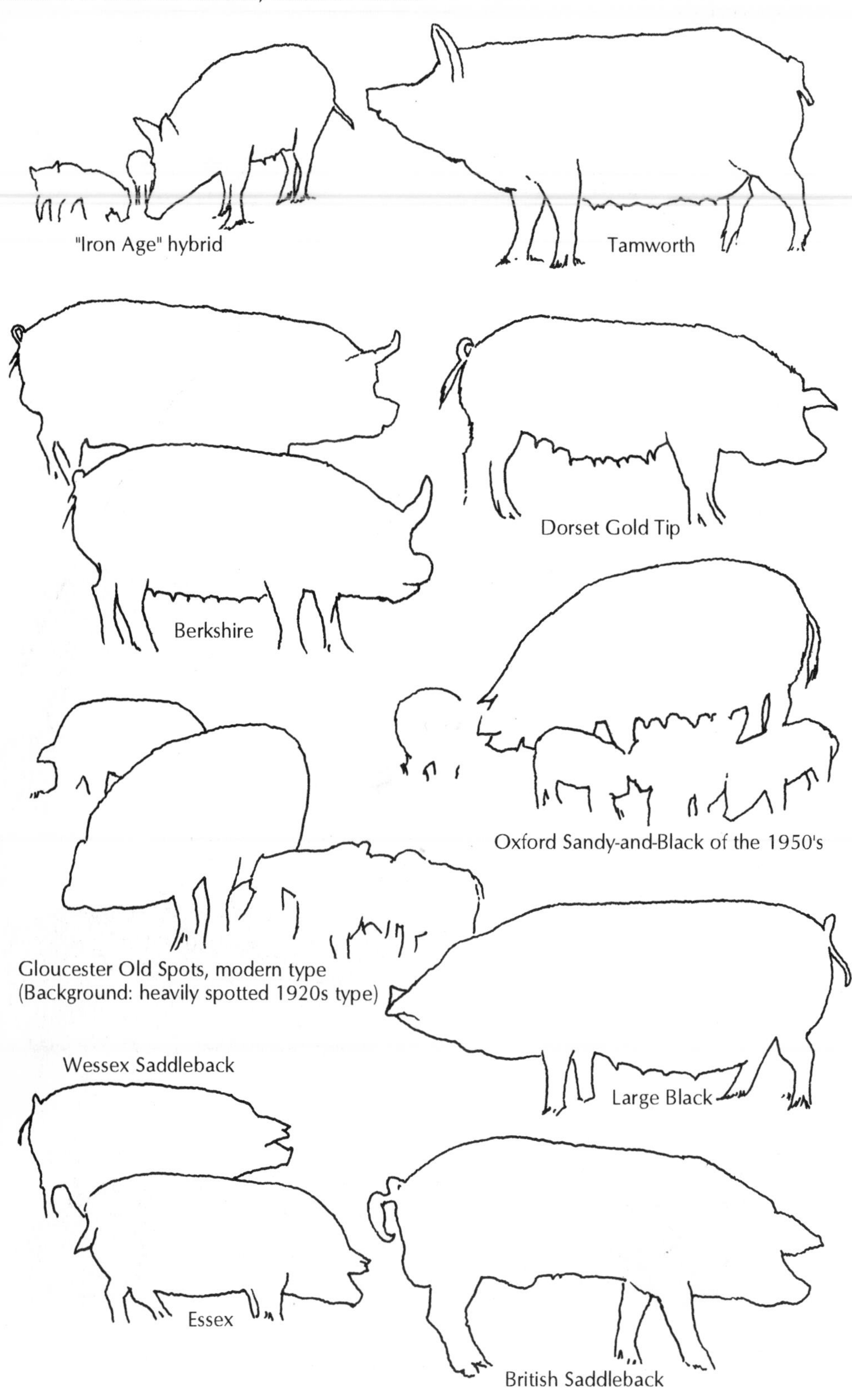

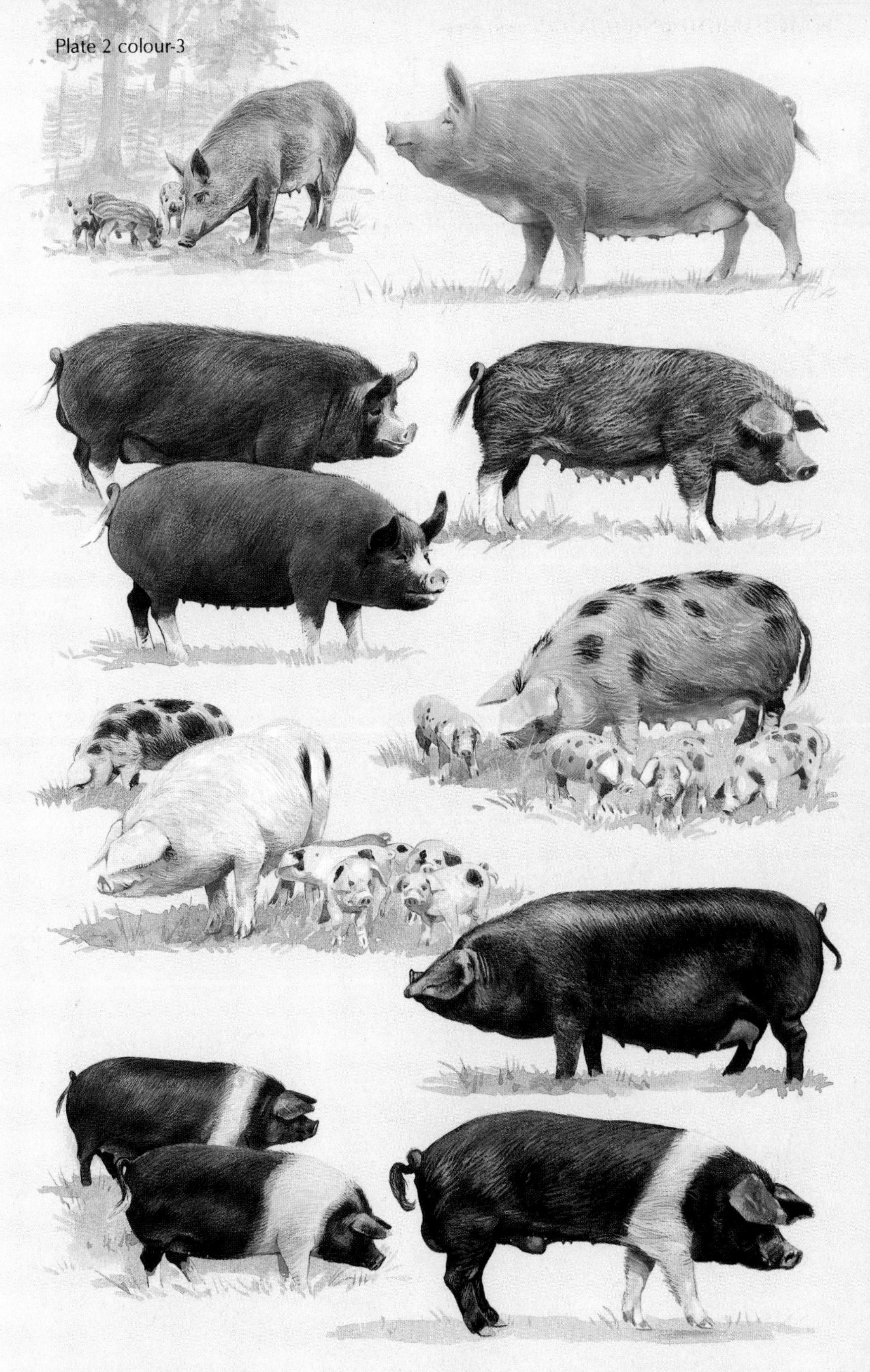

PLATE 3: UNITED KINGDOM, White Breeds

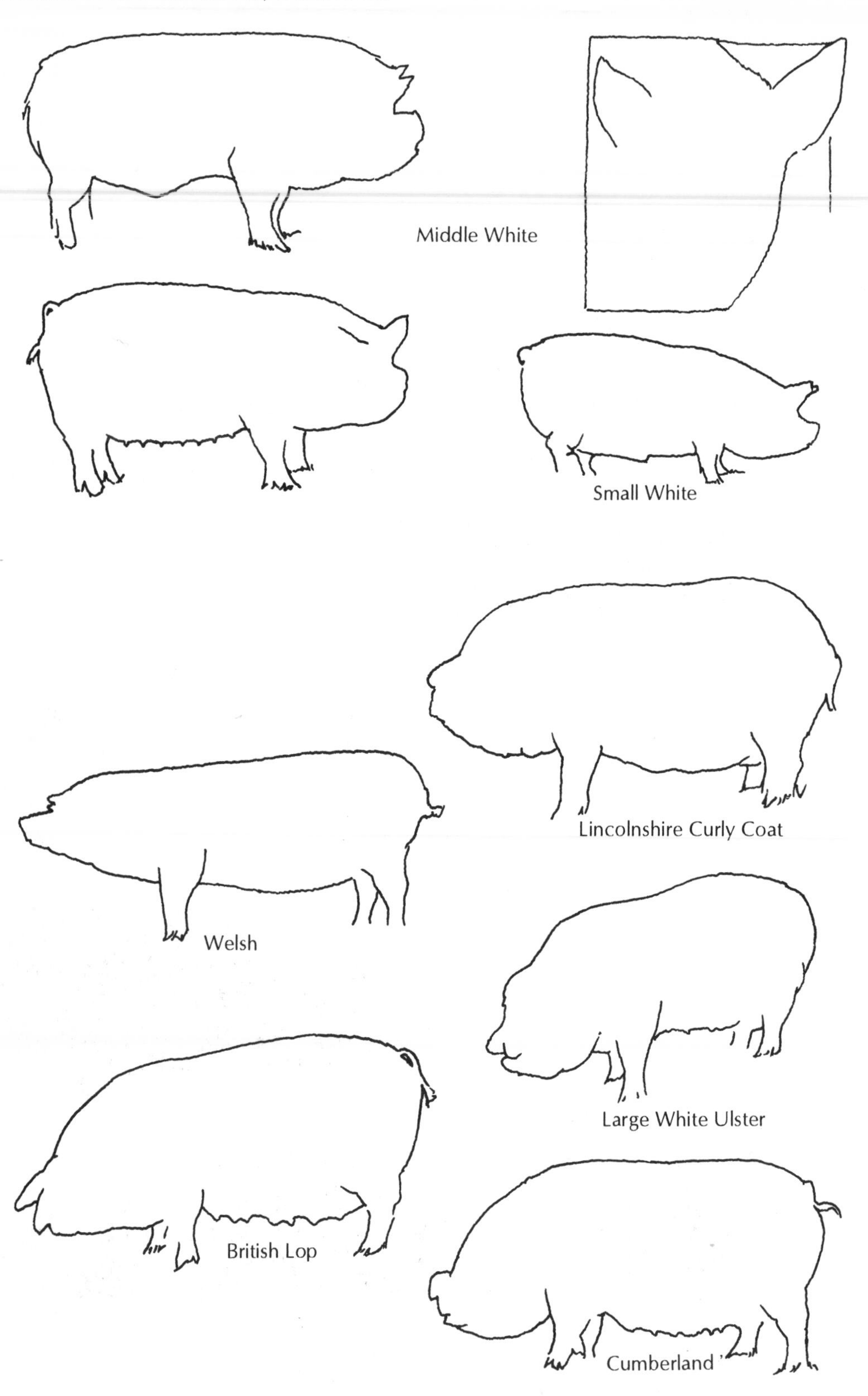

Plate 3 colour-5

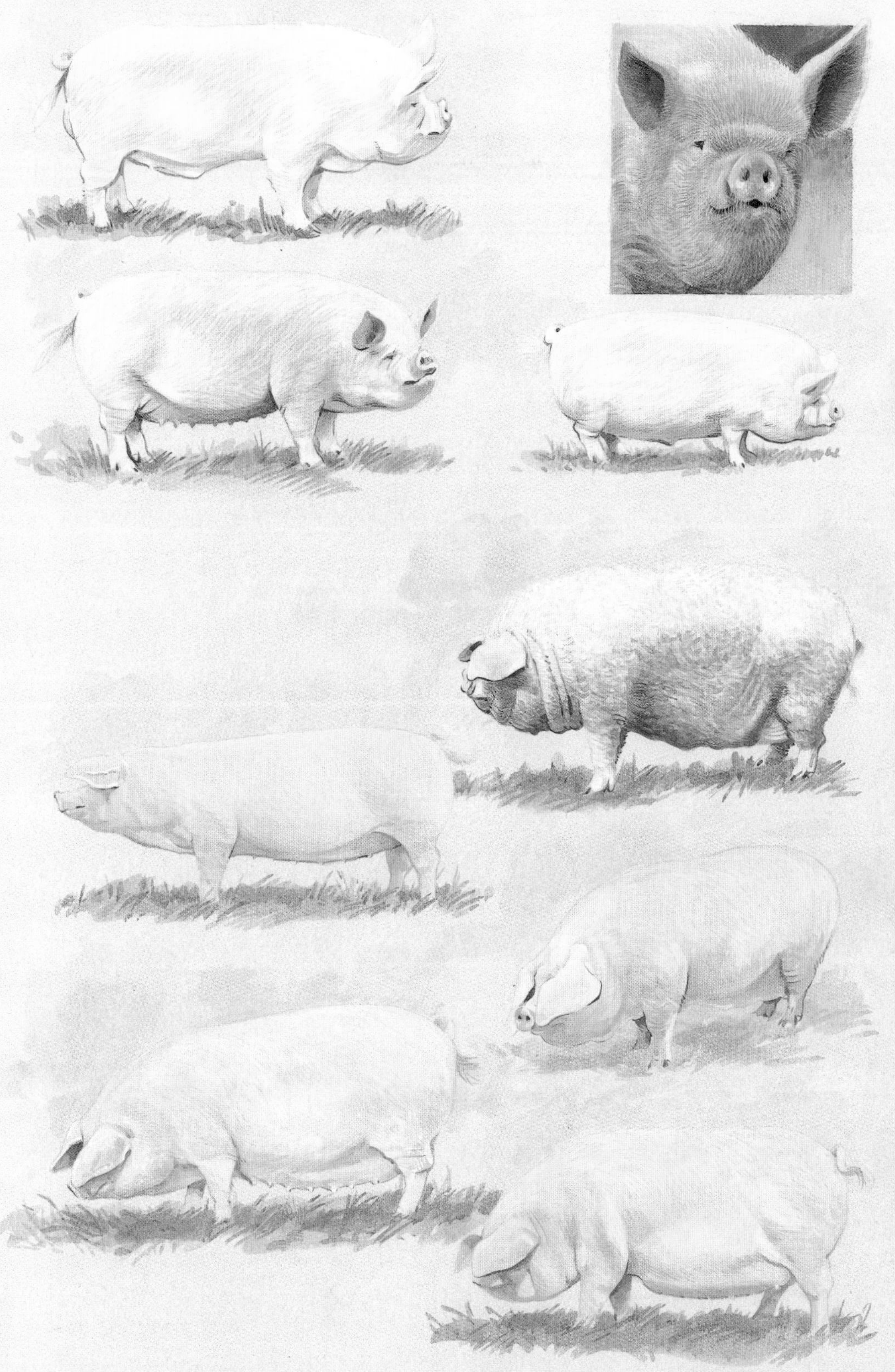

PLATE 4: EUROPEAN YORKSHIRES

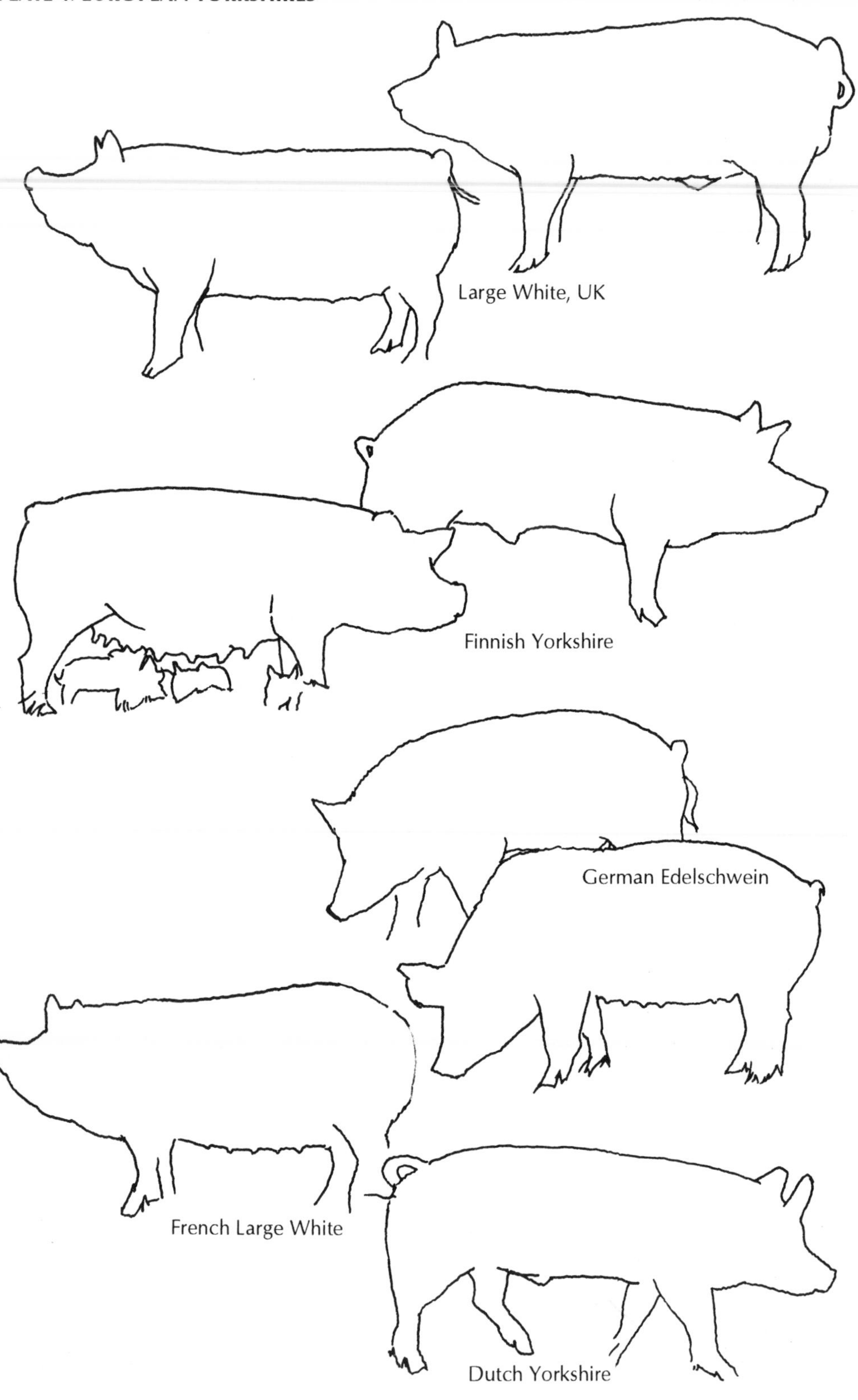

Plate 4 colour-7

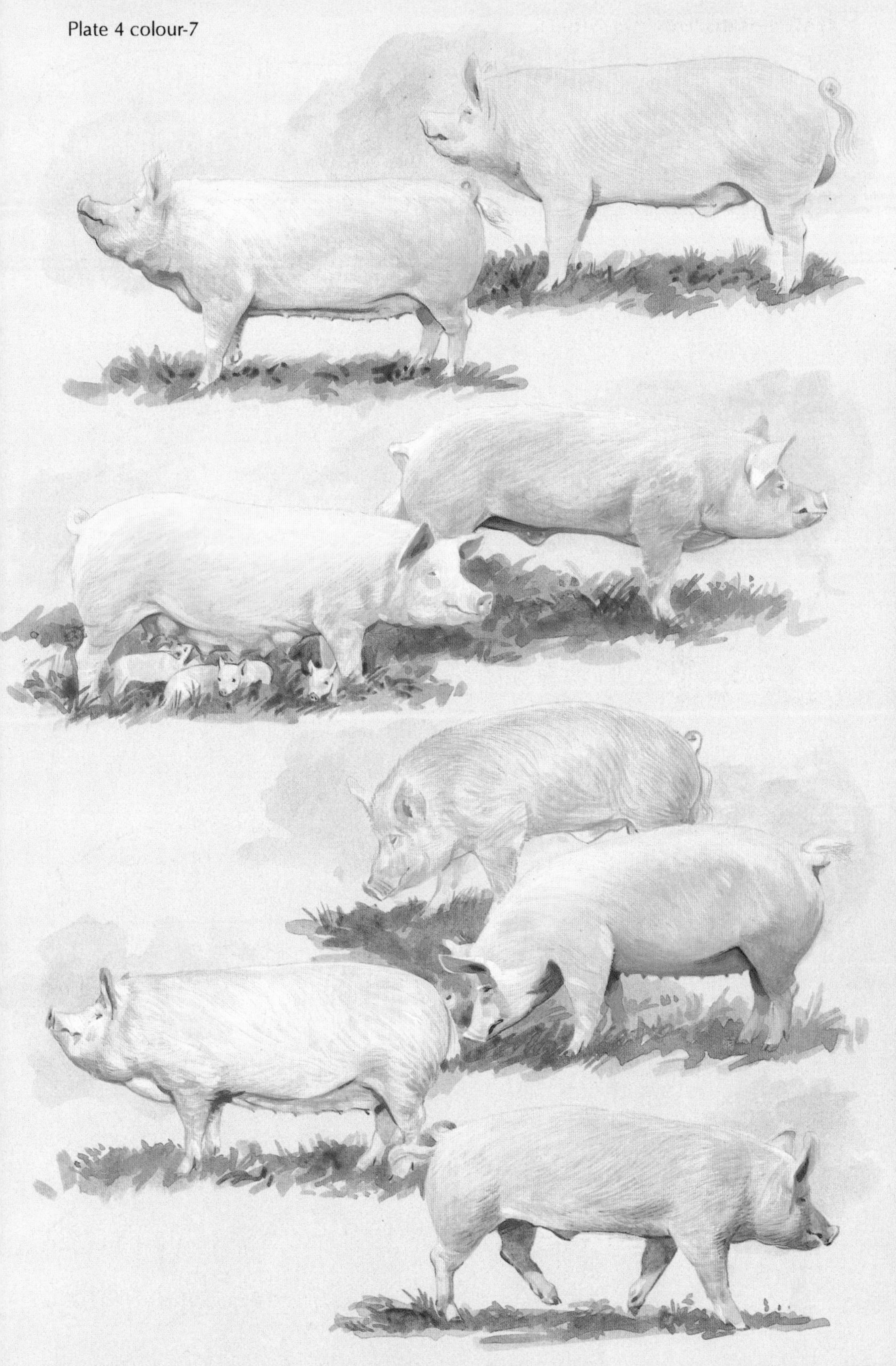

PLATE 5: UNITED KINGDOM, Breeding Companies

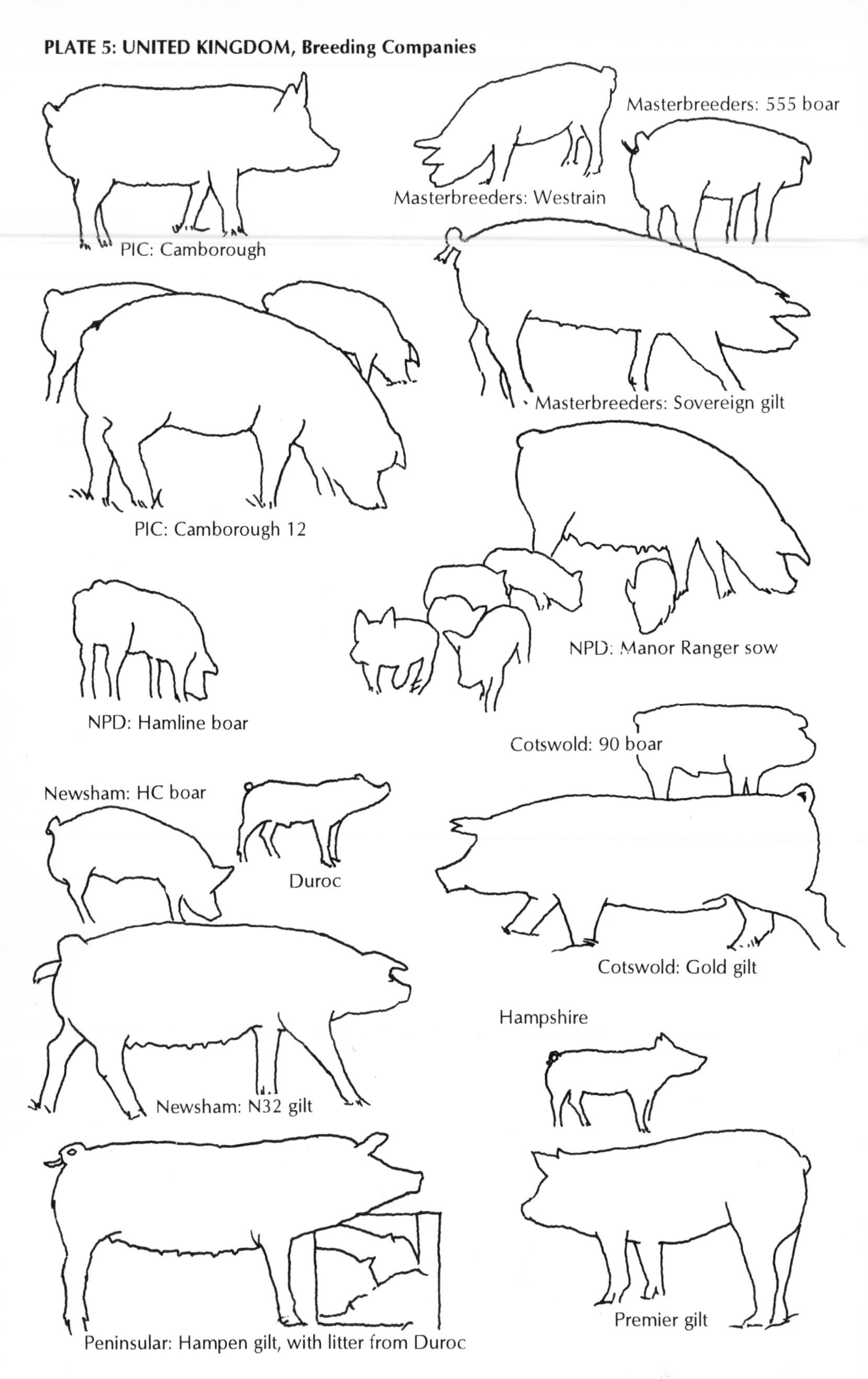

Plate 5 colour-9

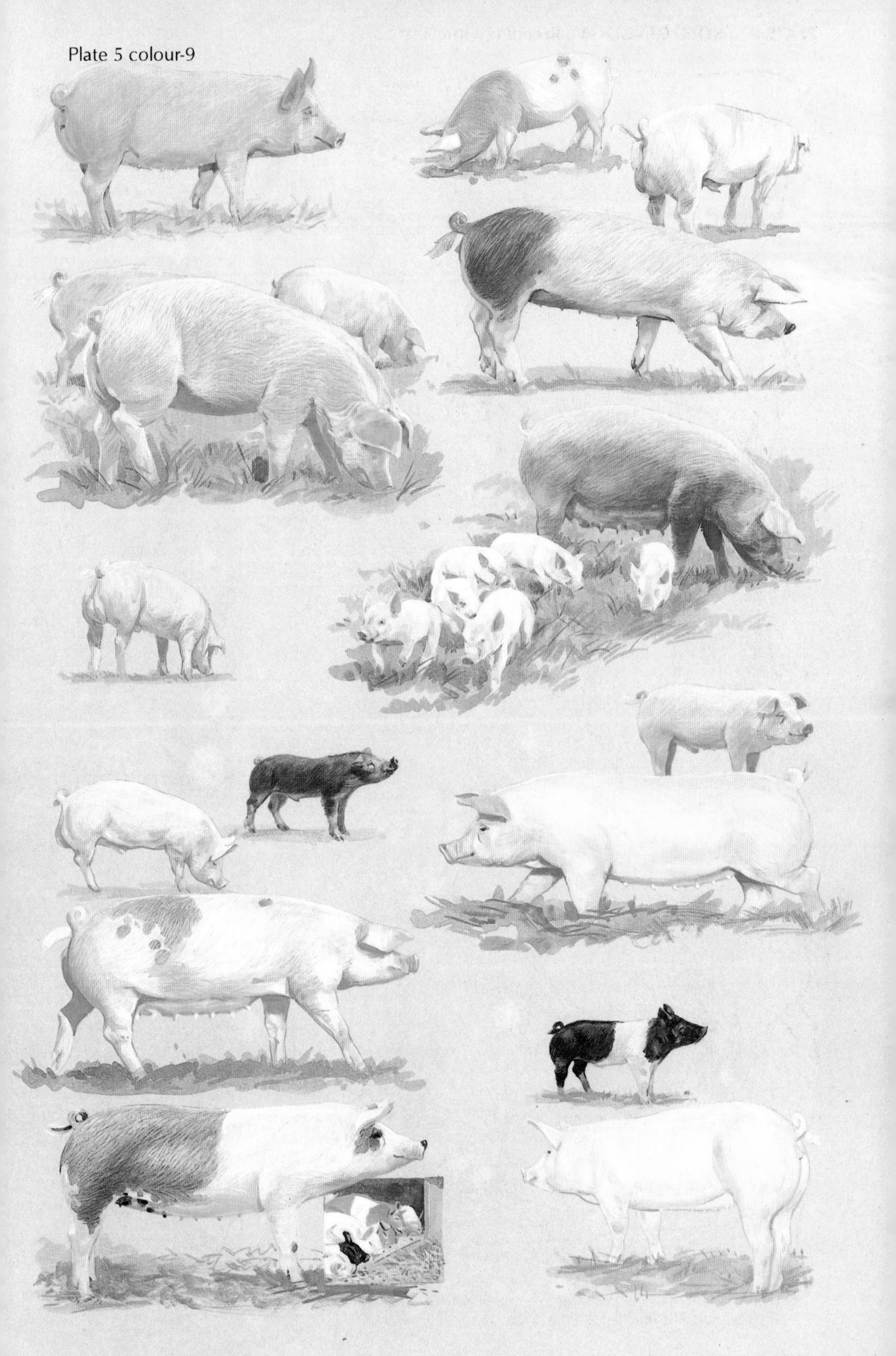

PLATE 6: ORIGINAL LANDRACES

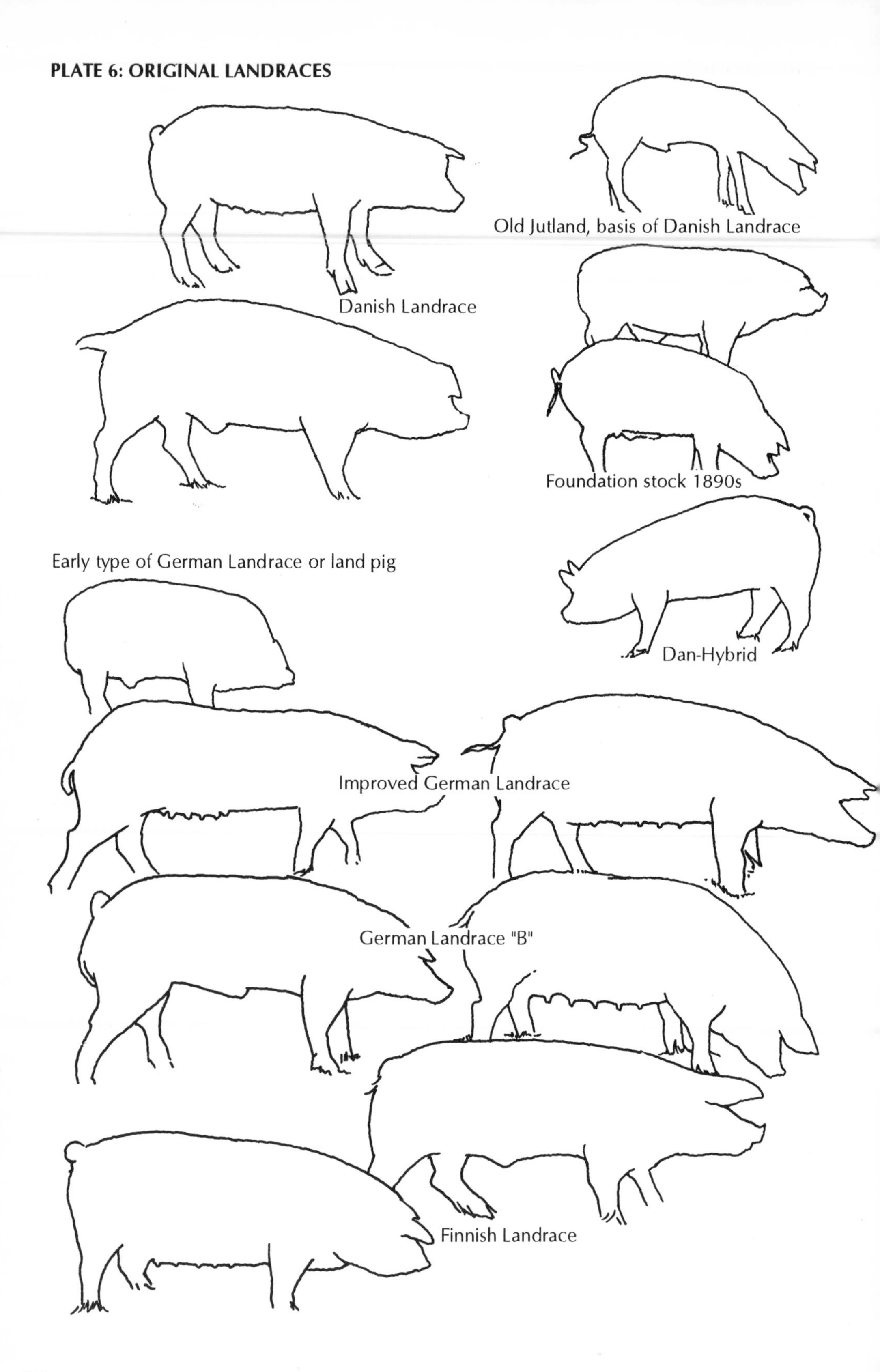

Plate 6 colour-11

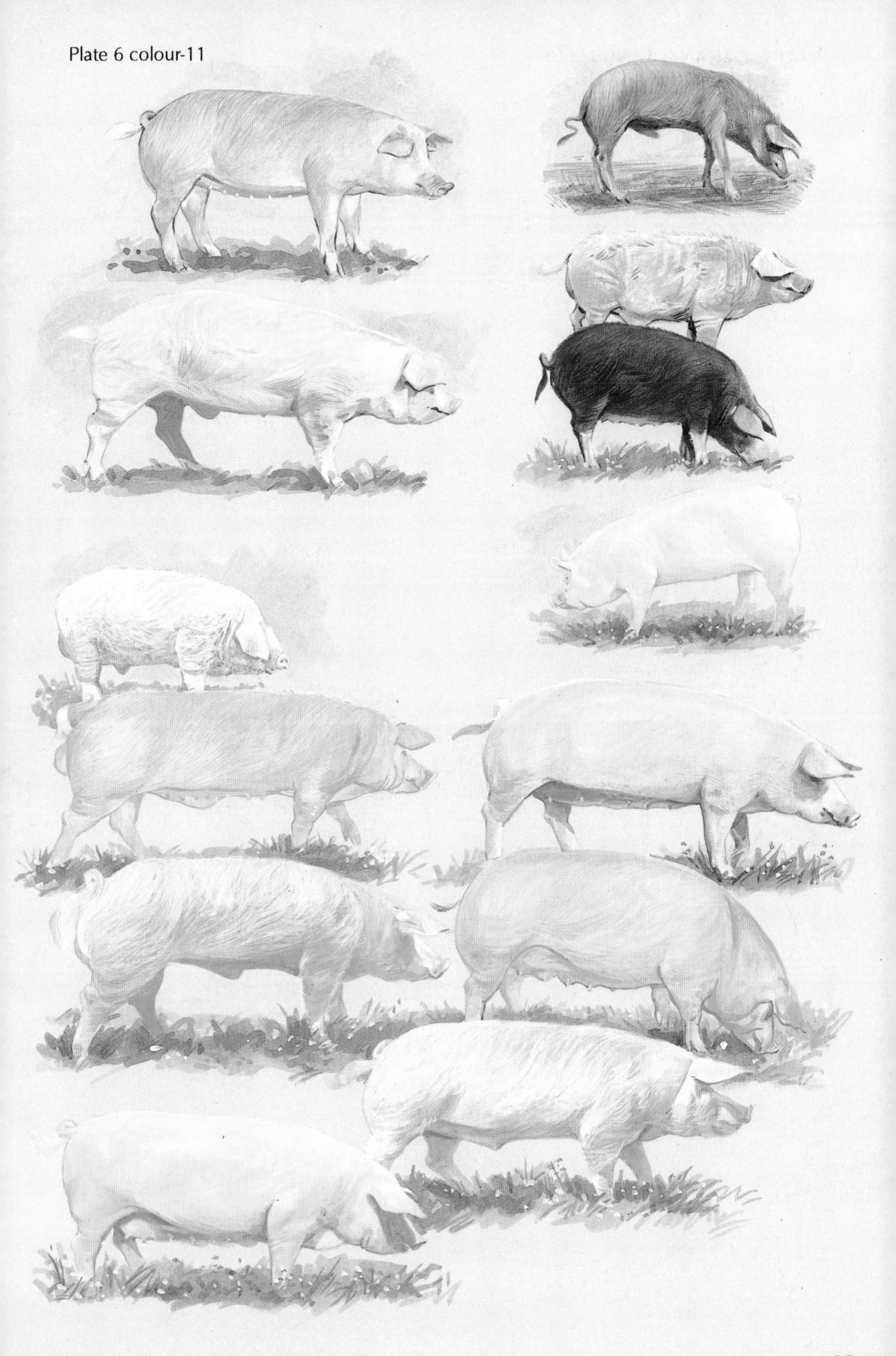

PLATE 7: LANDRACES

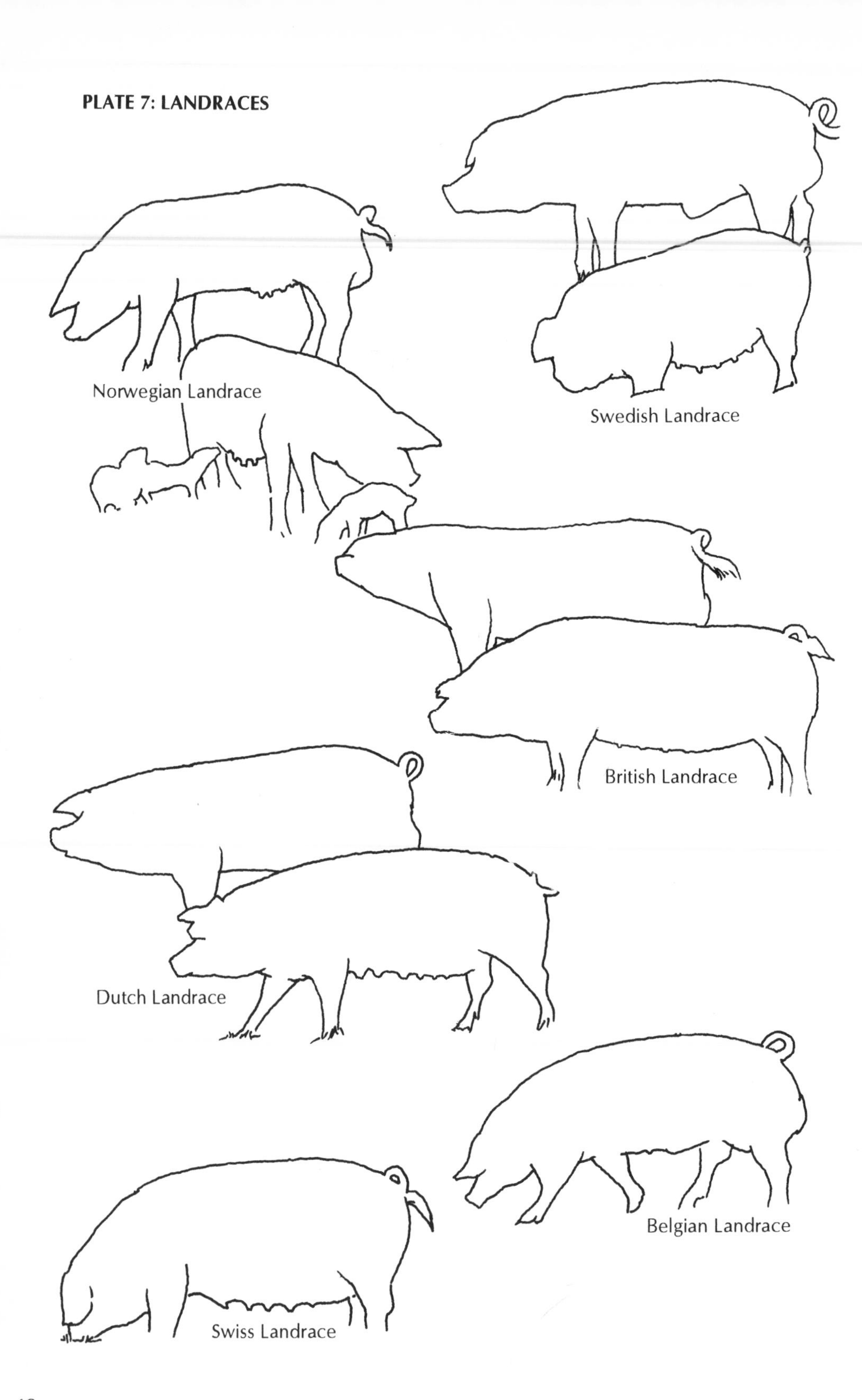

Plate 7 colour-13

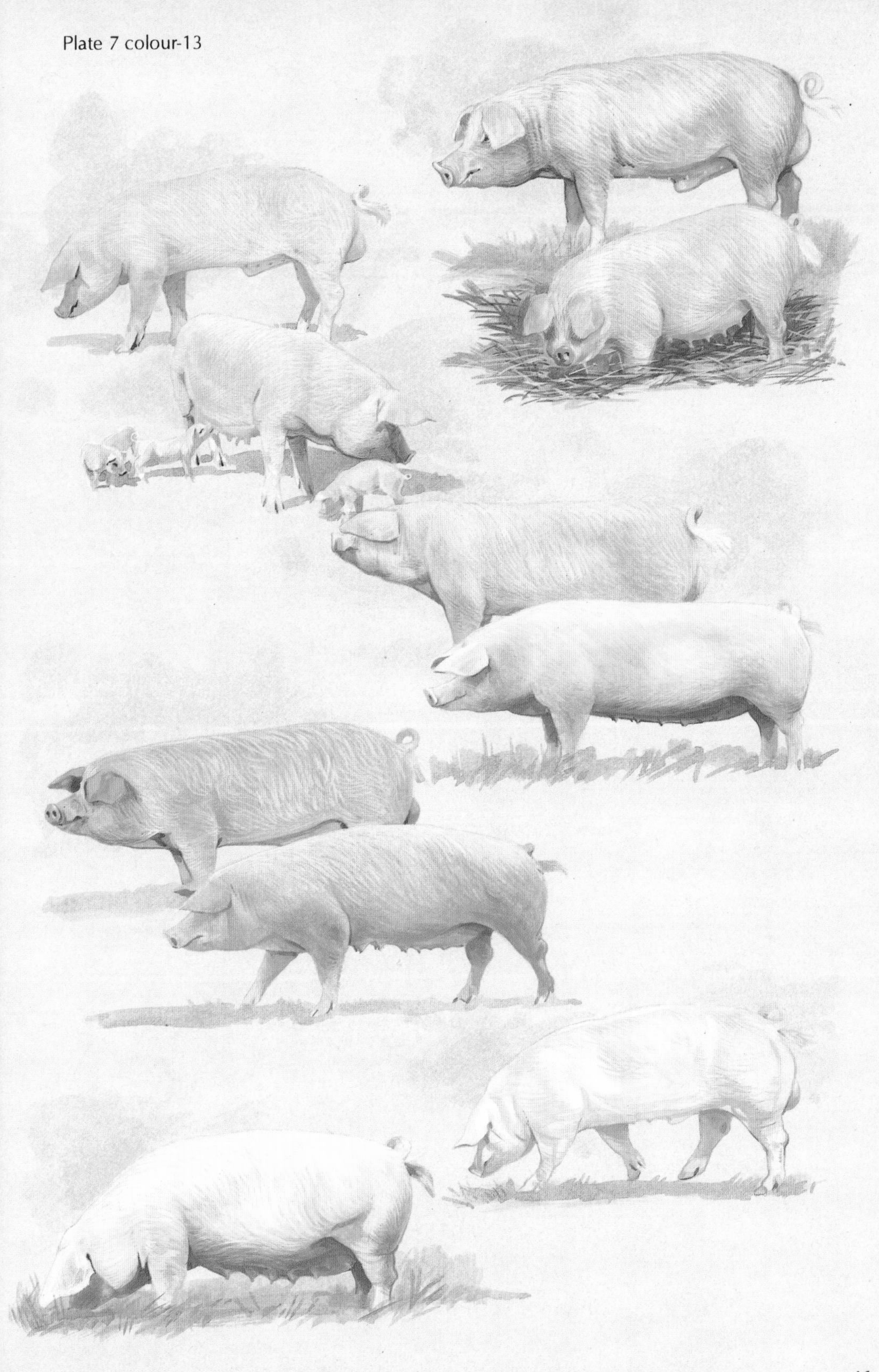

PLATE 8: FRANCE AND BELGIUM

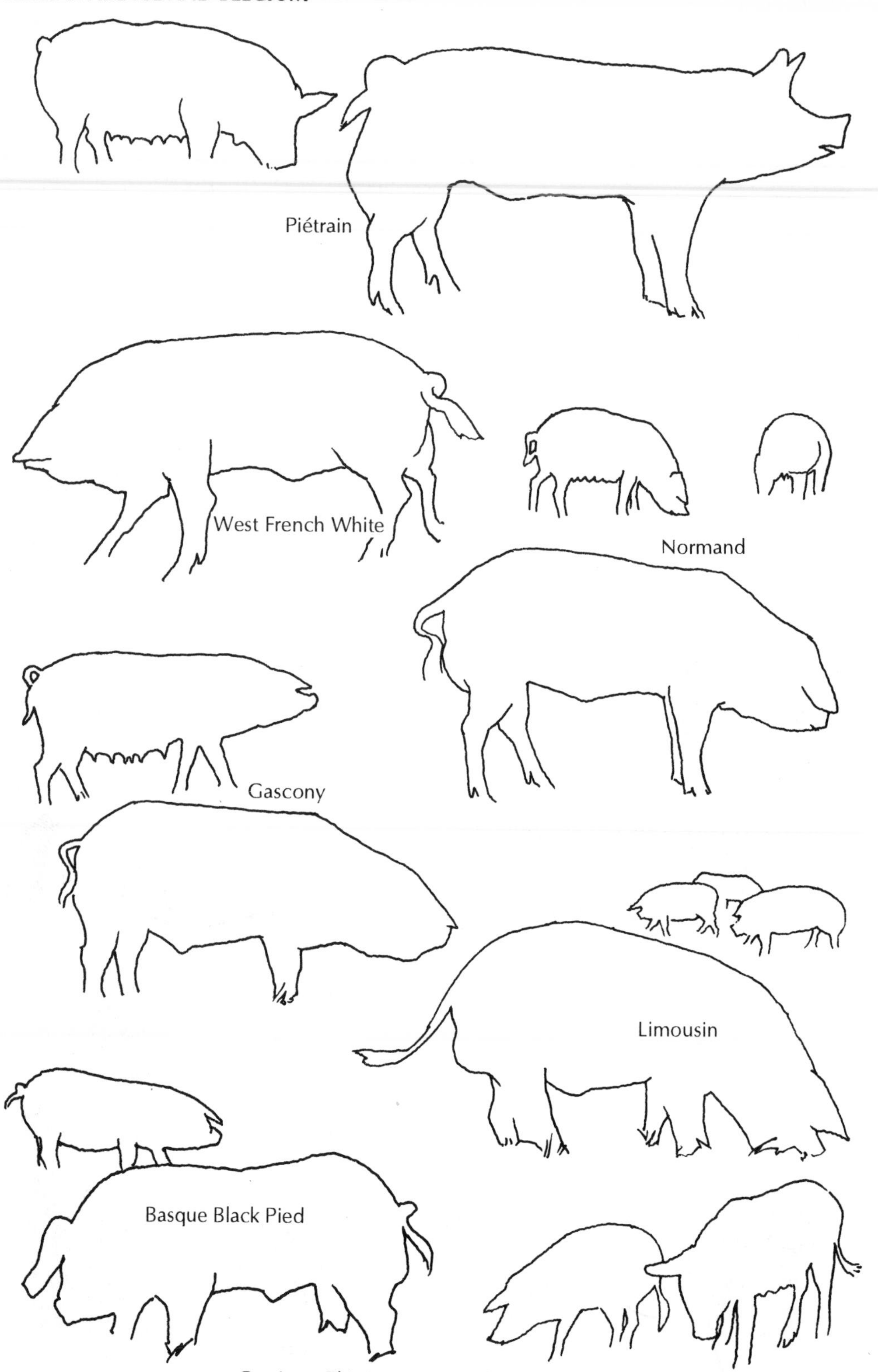

Corsican. This is one example of a wide range of colours in Corsican pigs.

Plate 8 colour-15

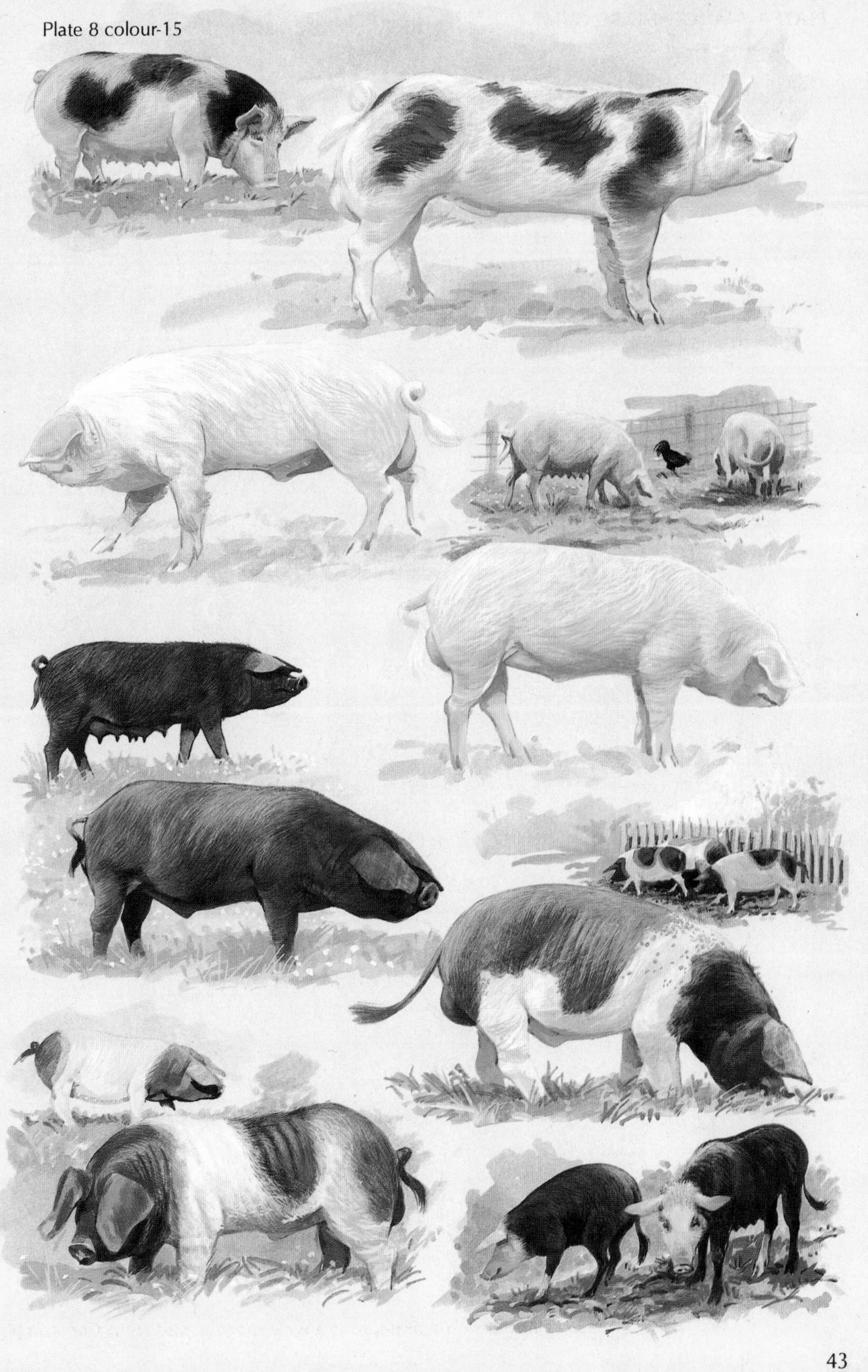

PLATE 9: PORTUGAL, SPAIN AND ITALY

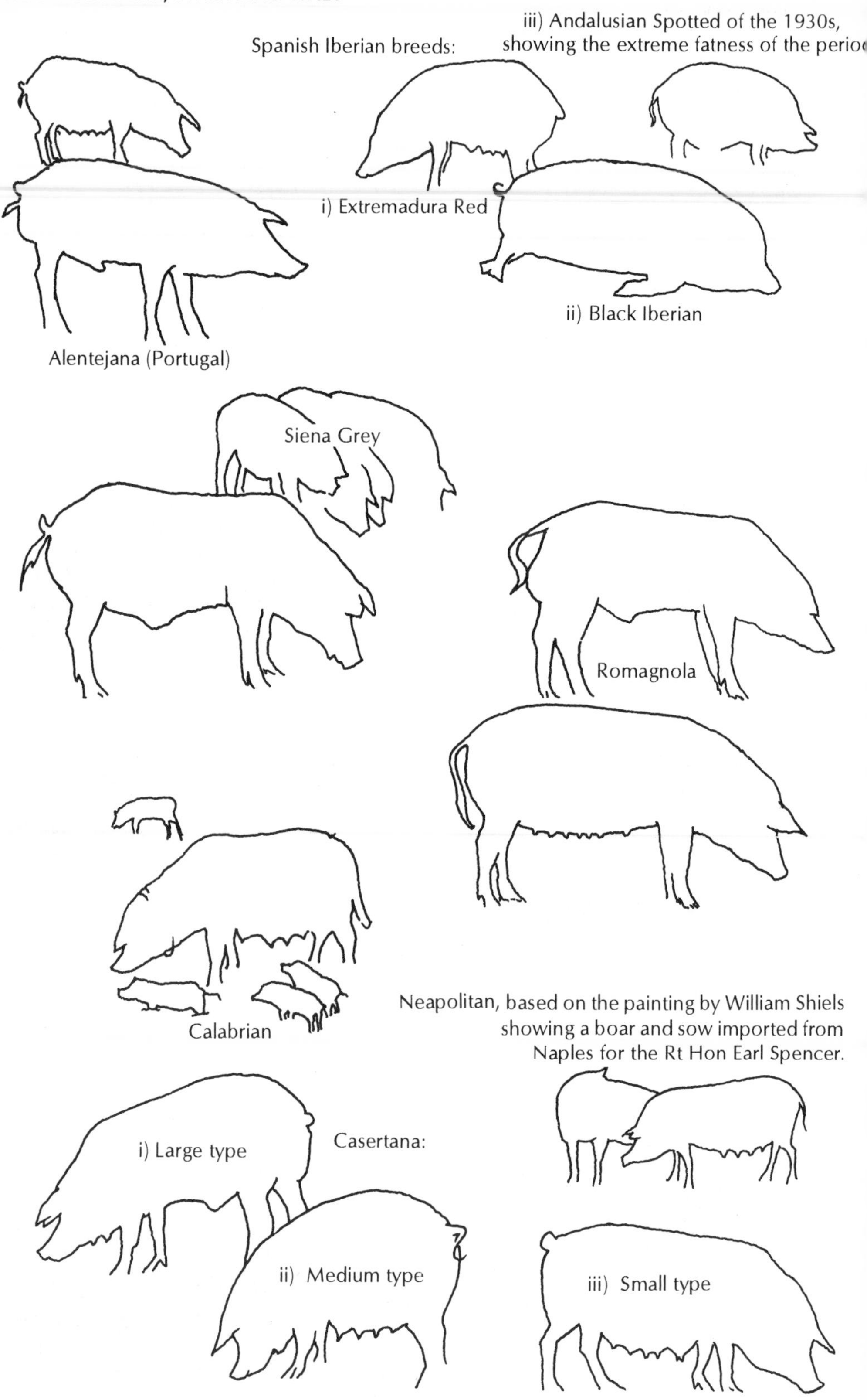
Spanish Iberian breeds:
iii) Andalusian Spotted of the 1930s, showing the extreme fatness of the perio
i) Extremadura Red
ii) Black Iberian
Alentejana (Portugal)
Siena Grey
Romagnola
Calabrian
Neapolitan, based on the painting by William Shiels showing a boar and sow imported from Naples for the Rt Hon Earl Spencer.
Casertana:
i) Large type
ii) Medium type
iii) Small type

Plate 9 colour-17

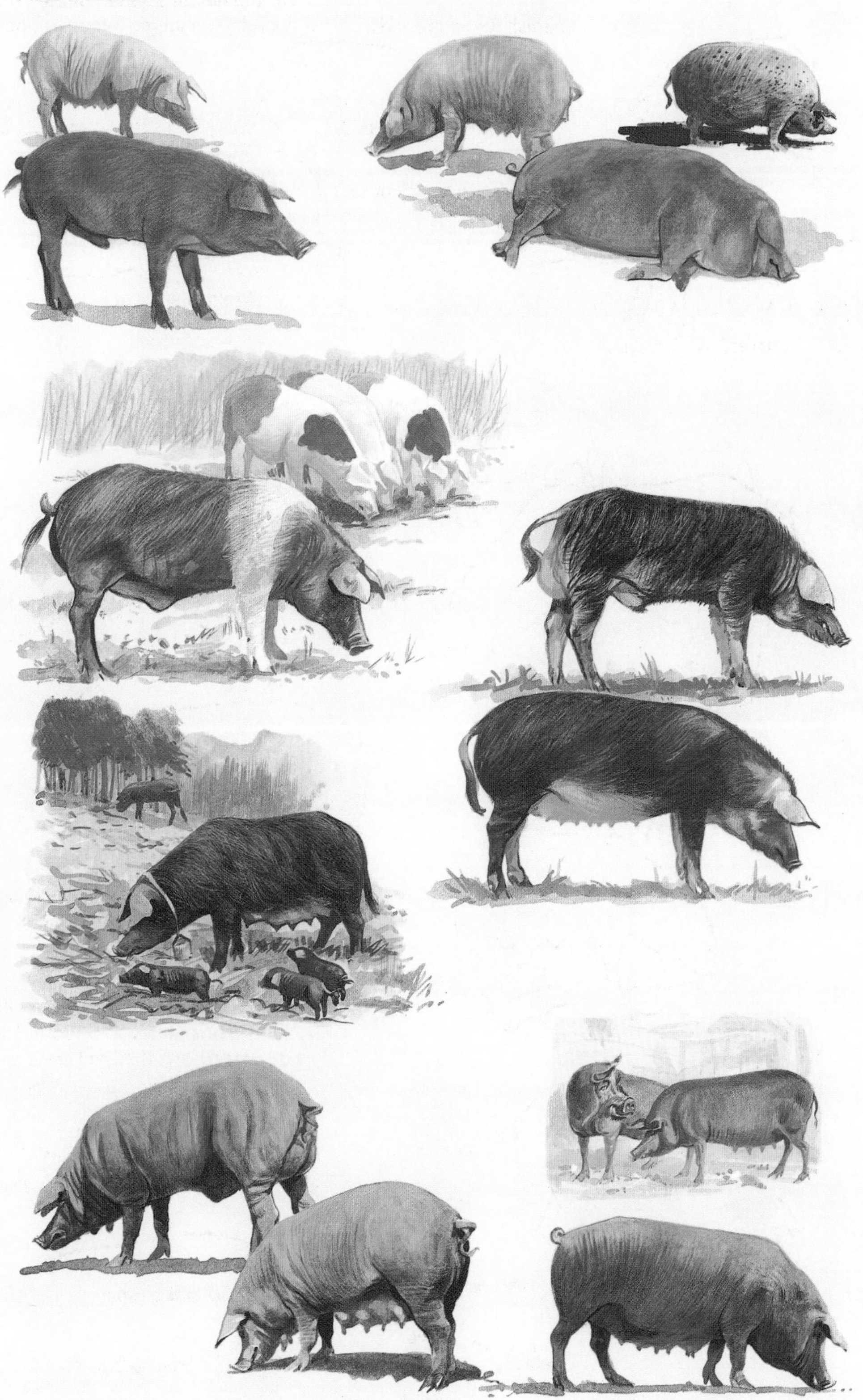

PLATE 10: GERMANY

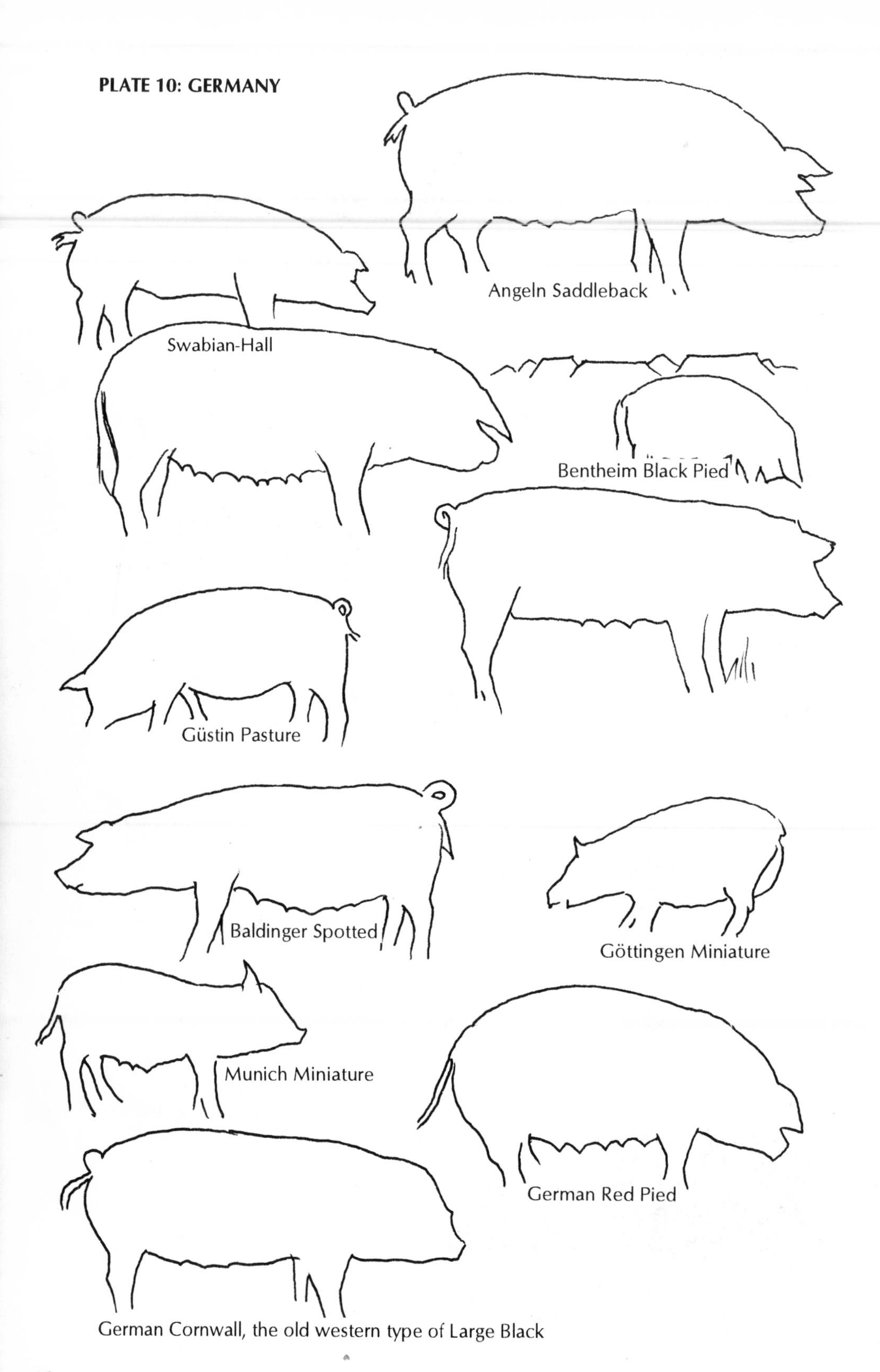

Angeln Saddleback
Swabian-Hall
Bentheim Black Pied
Güstin Pasture
Baldinger Spotted
Göttingen Miniature
Munich Miniature
German Red Pied
German Cornwall, the old western type of Large Black

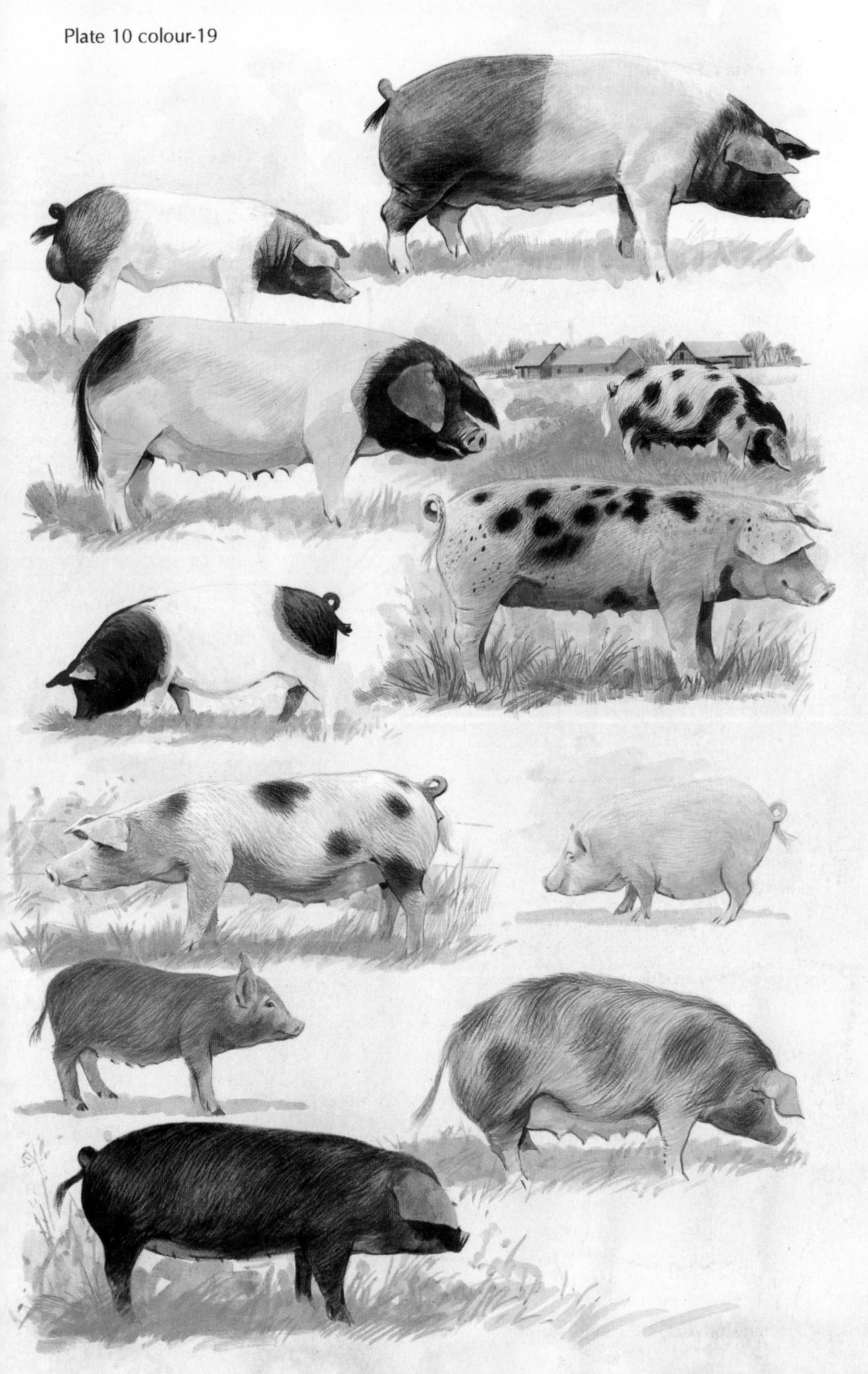

PLATE 11: EASTERN EUROPE, Coloured Breeds

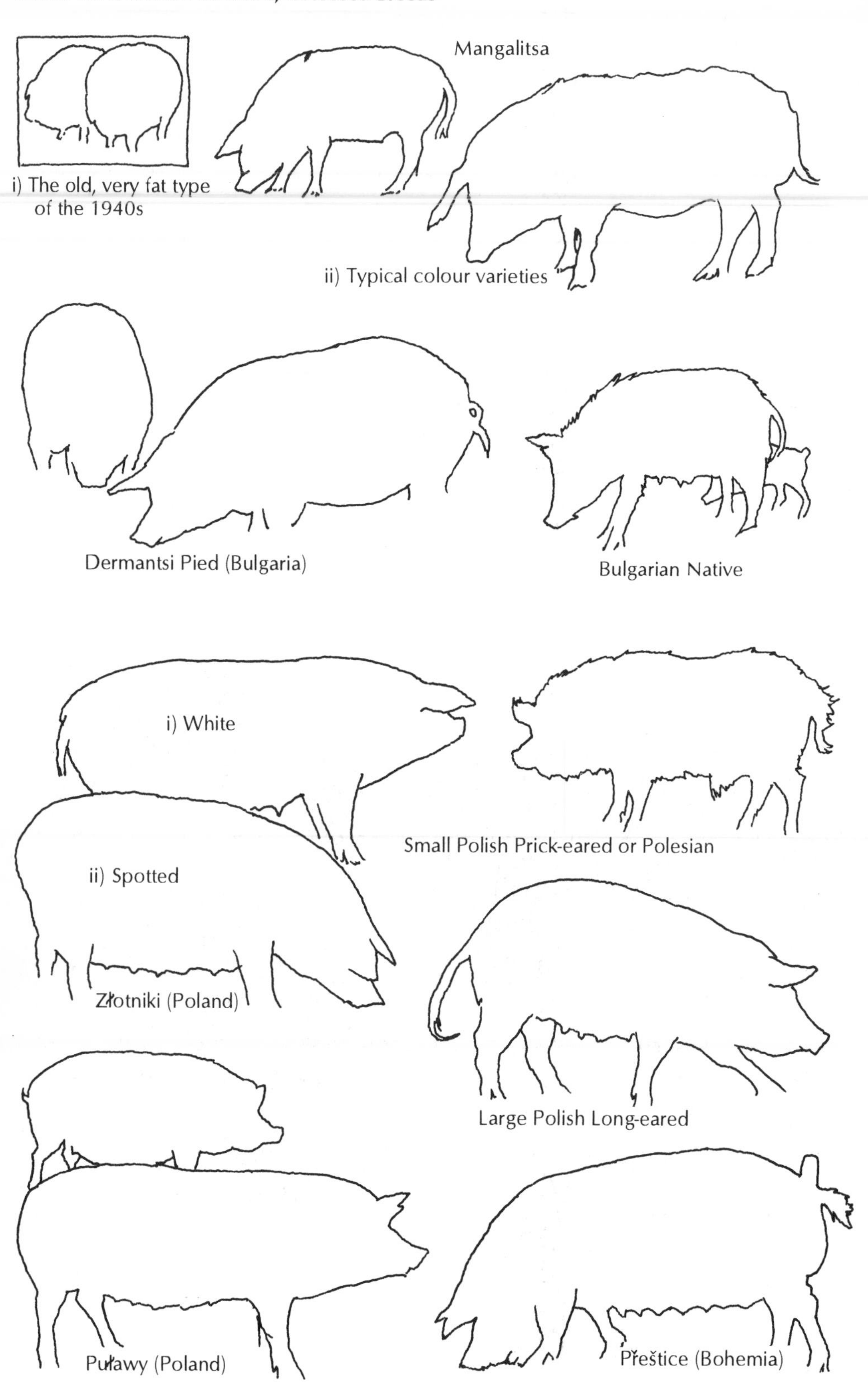

Plate 11 colour-21

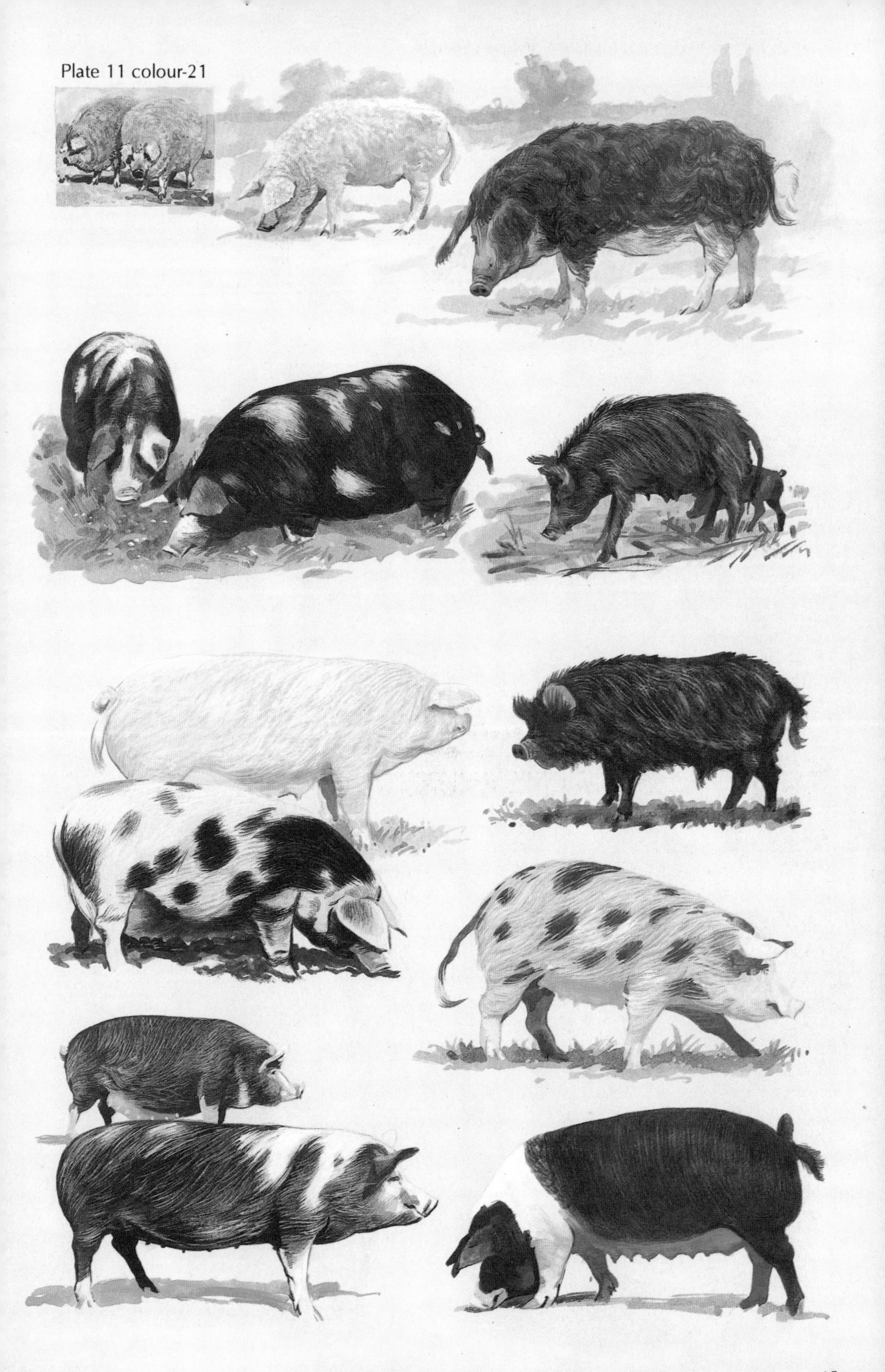

PLATE 12: EASTERN EUROPE, White Breeds

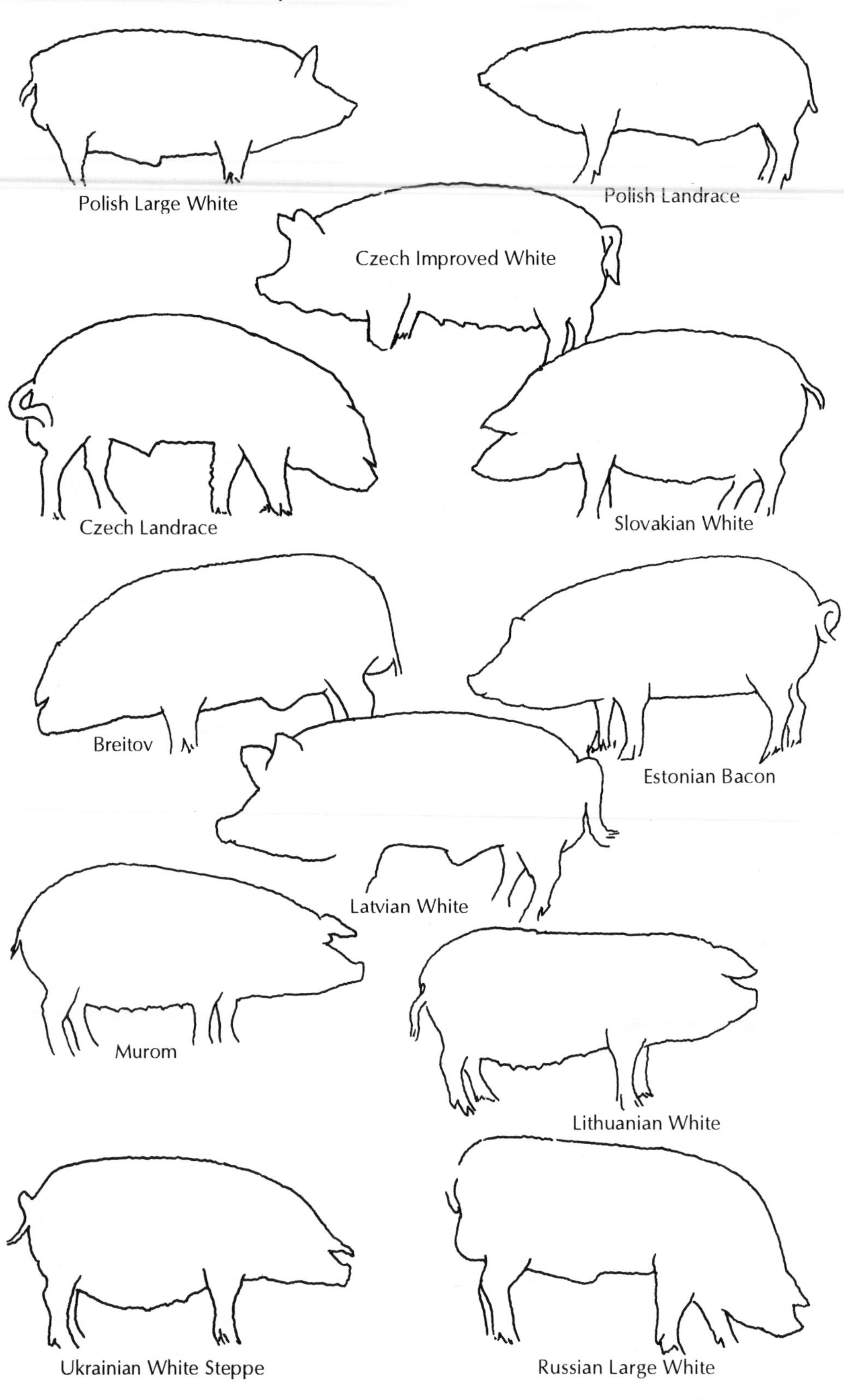

Plate 12 colour-23

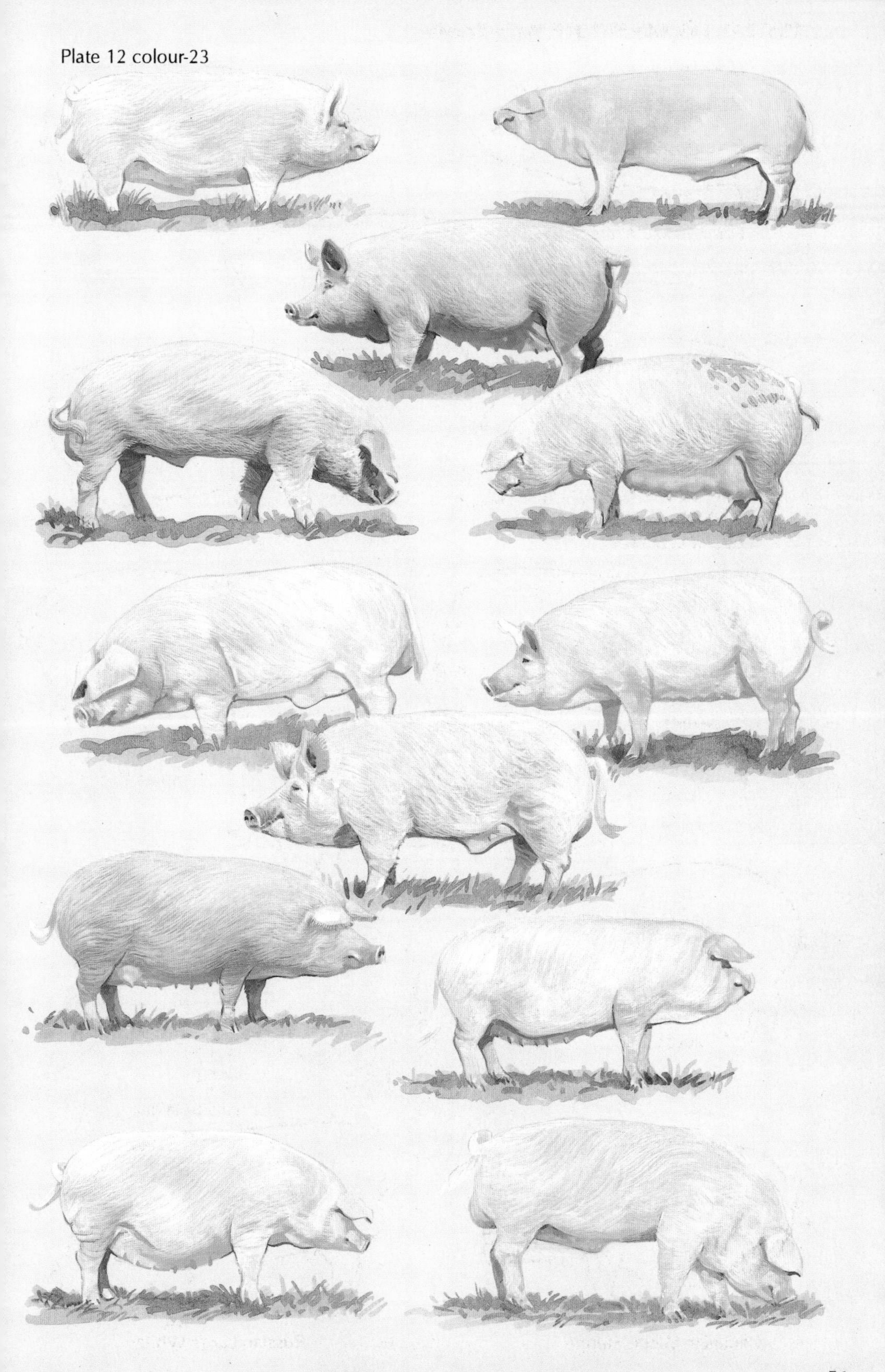

PLATE 13: RUSSIA, UKRAINE AND TRANSCAUCASUS

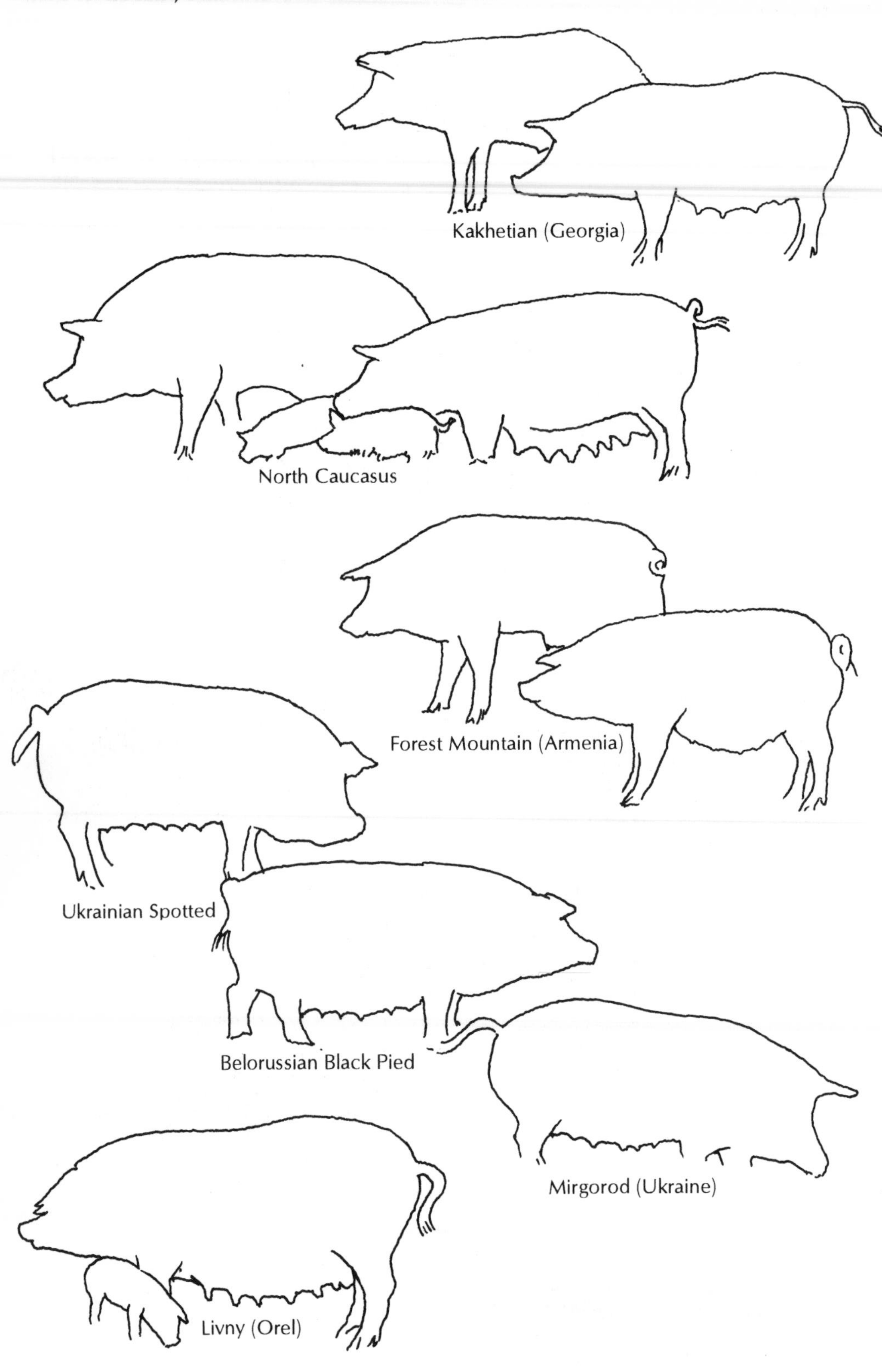

Plate 13 colour-25

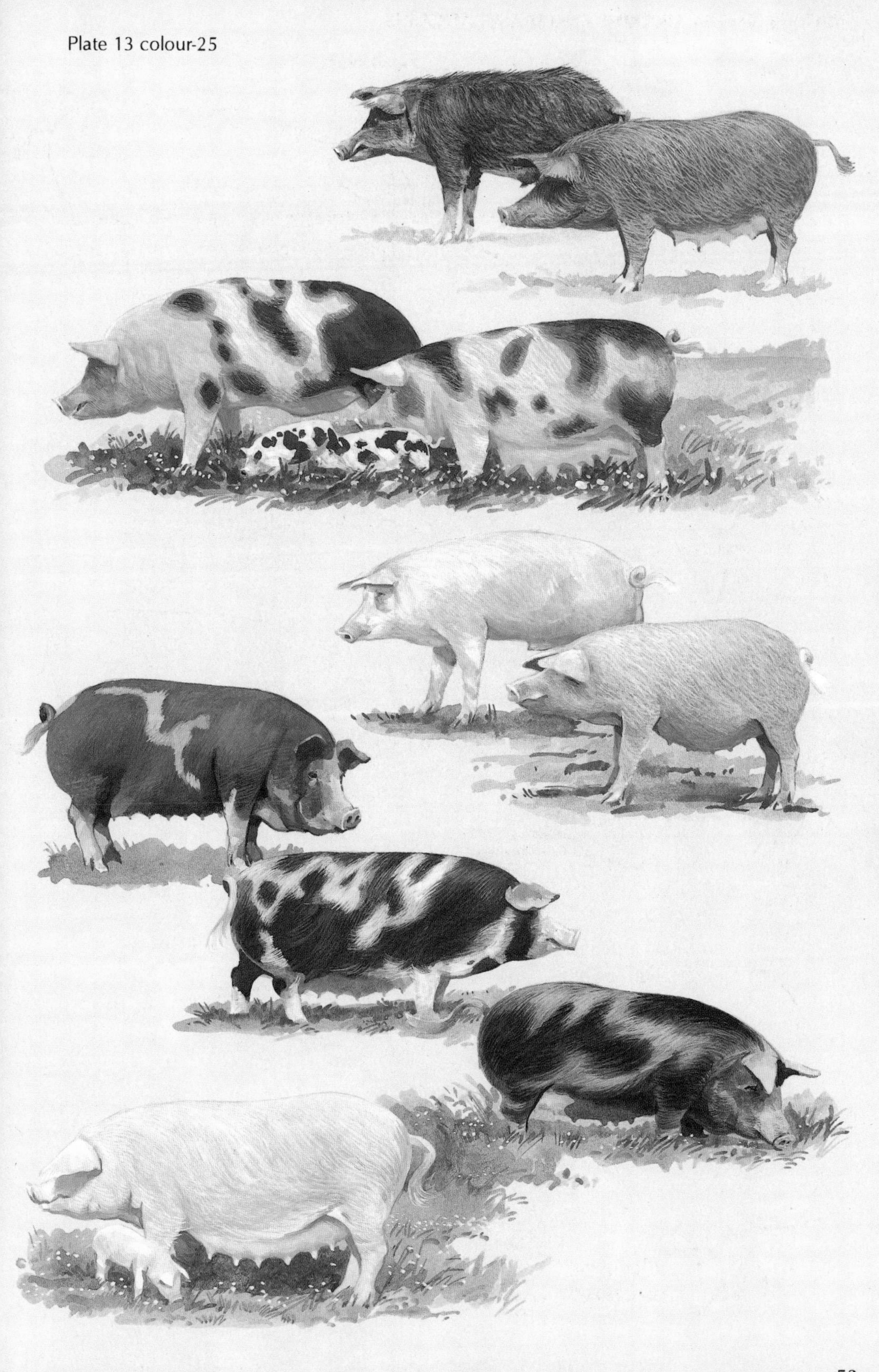

PLATE 14: SIBERIA AND KAZAKHSTAN

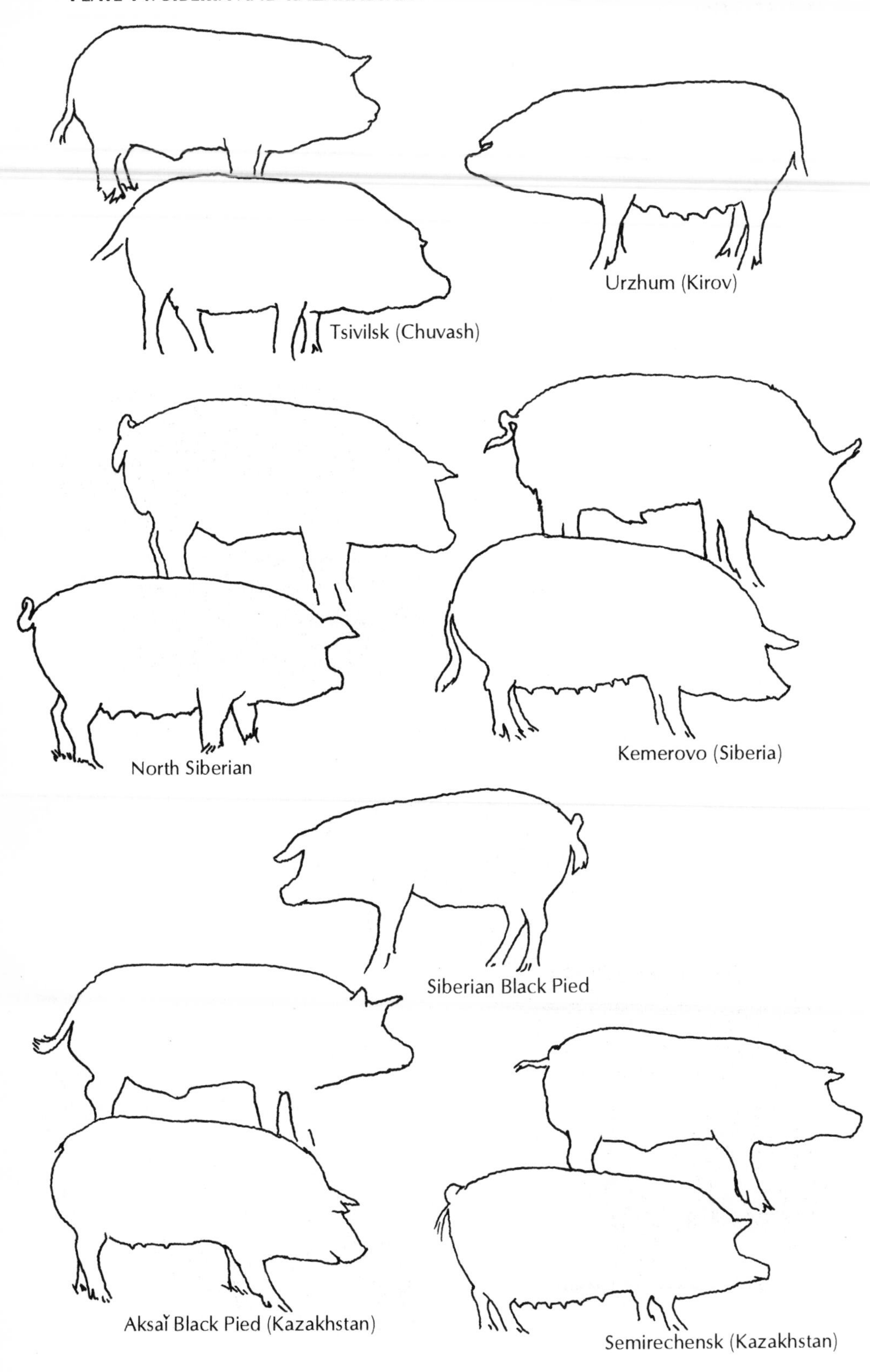

Plate 14 colour-27

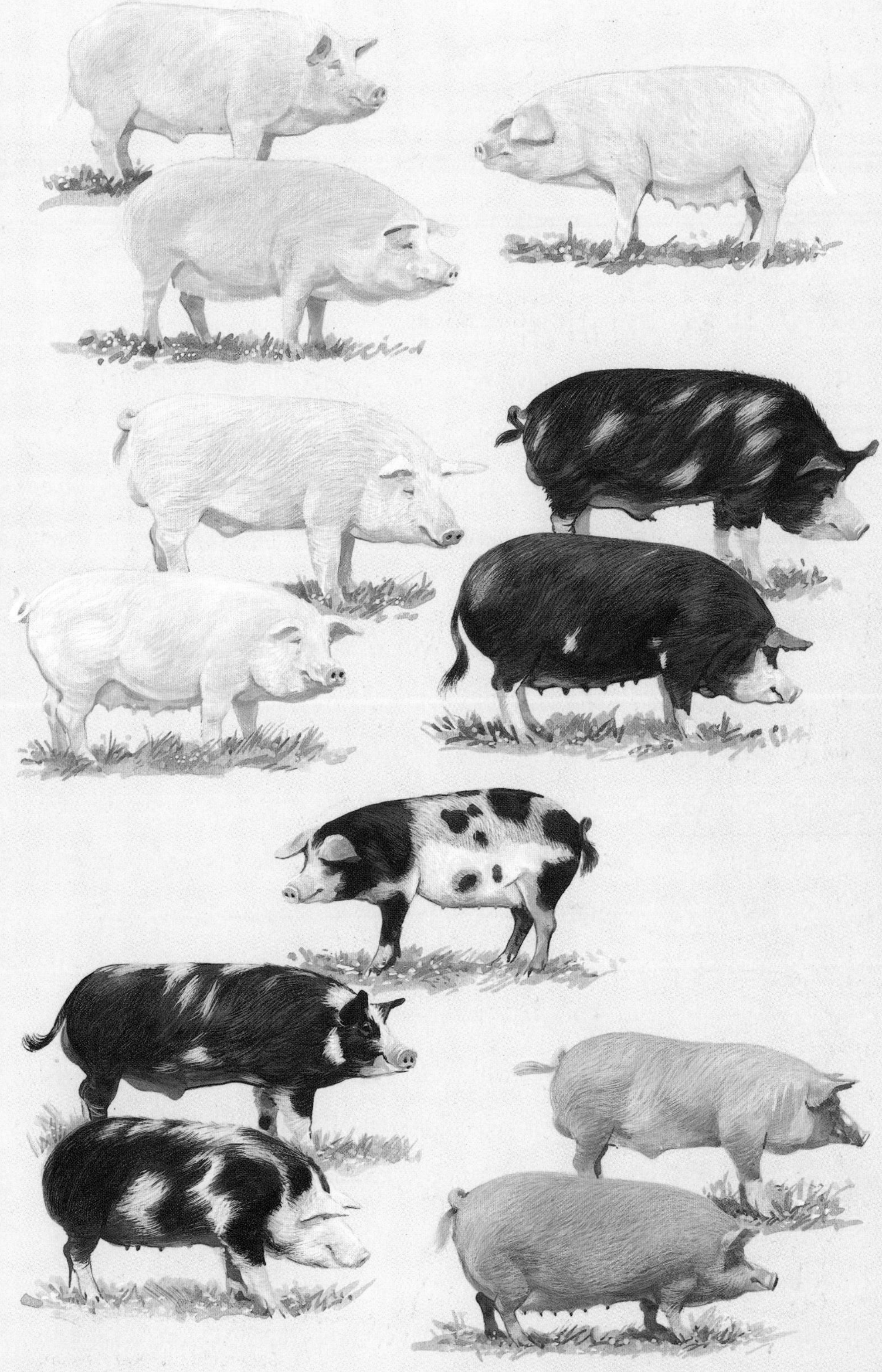

PLATE 15: CHINA, Taihu Group

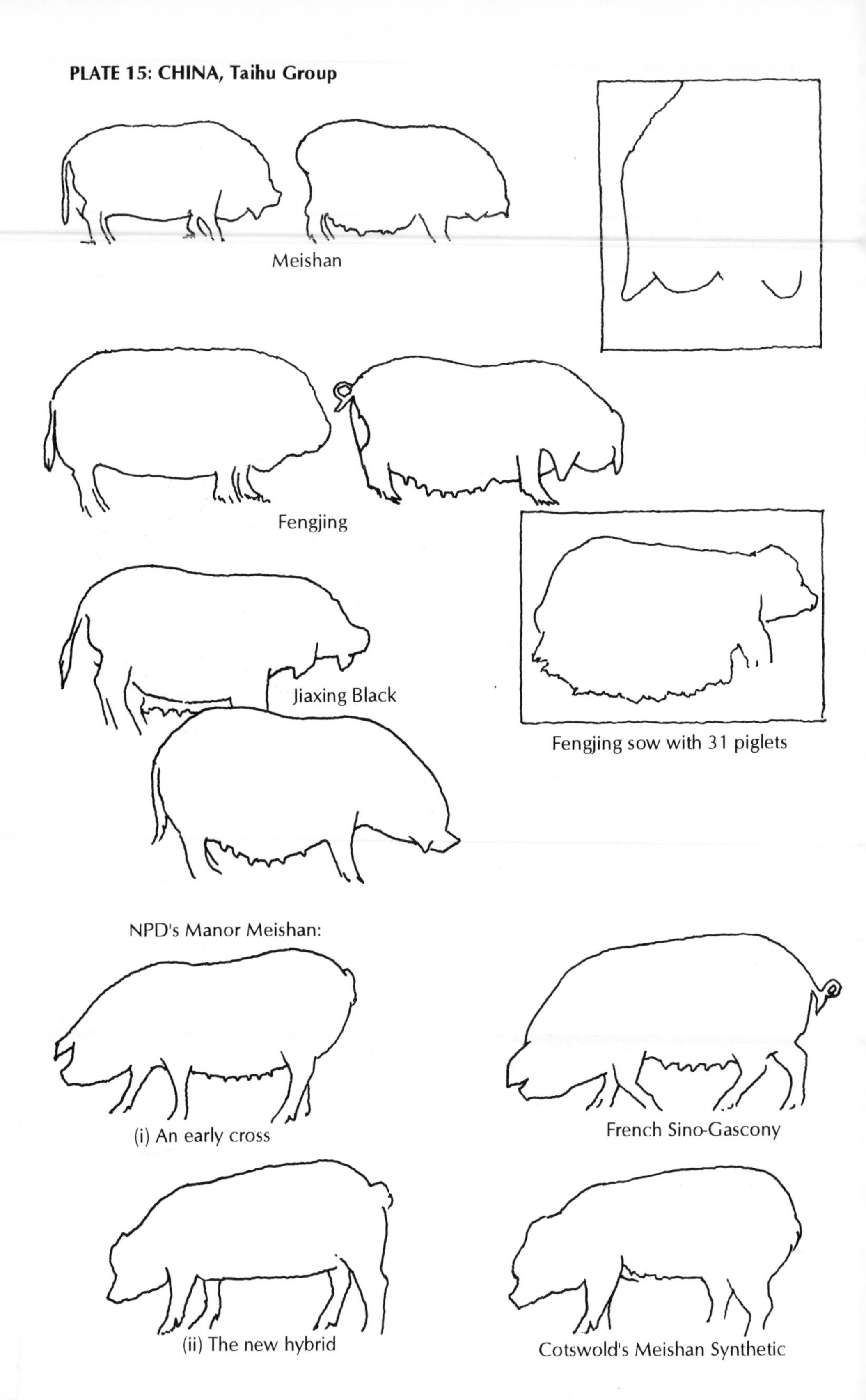

Plate 15 colour-29

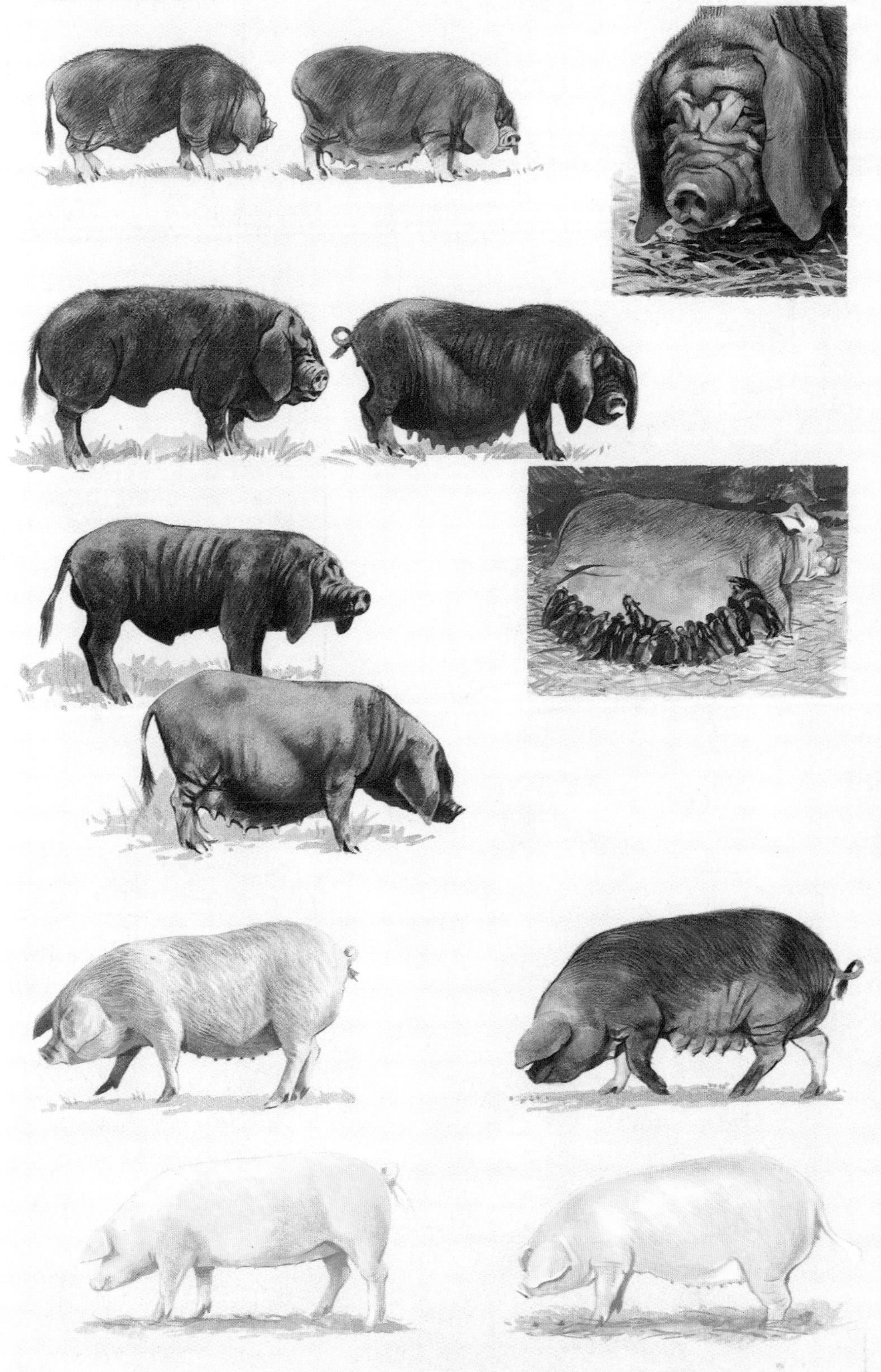

PLATE 16: CENTRAL AND SOUTH WEST CHINA

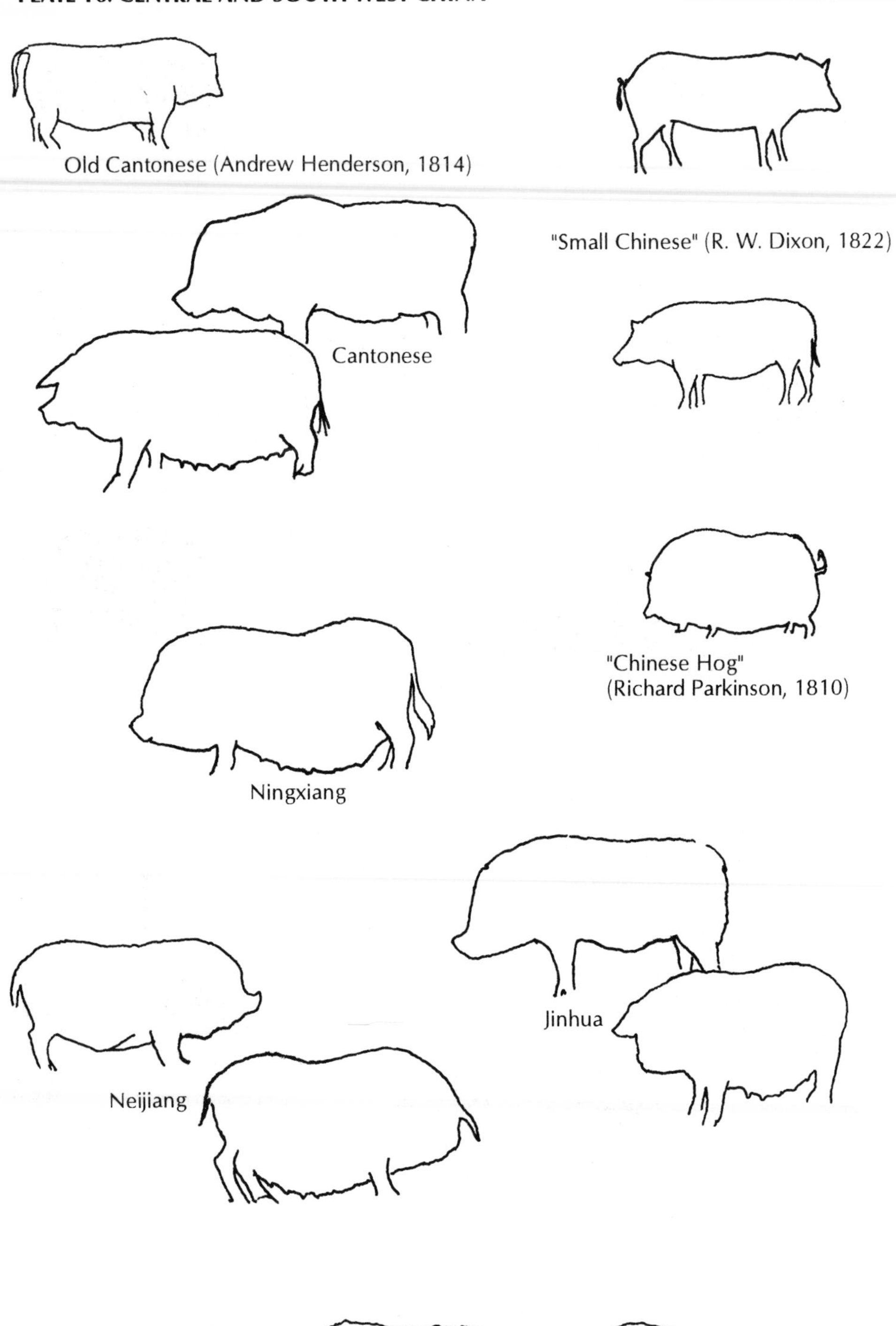

Plate 16 colour-31

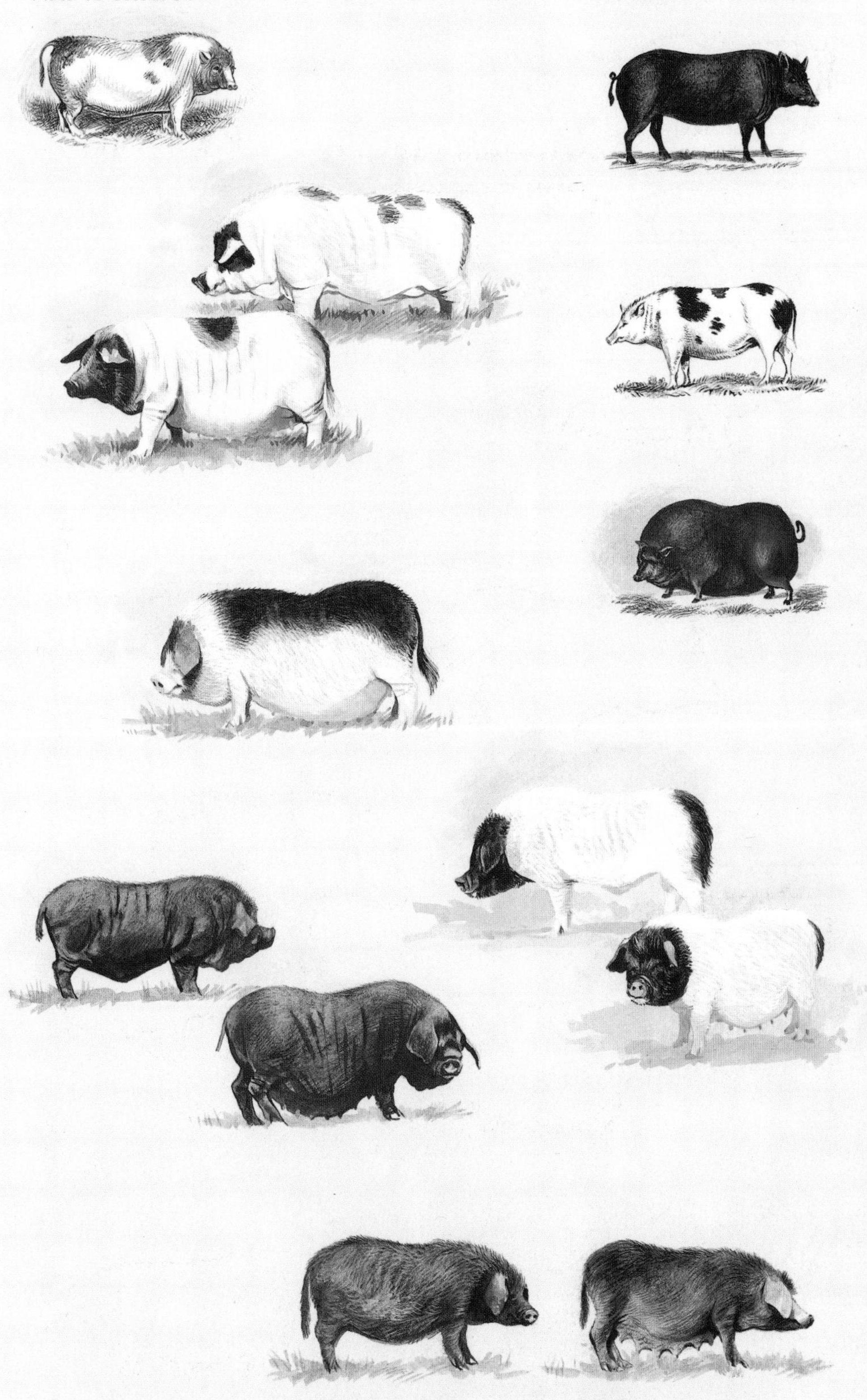

PLATE 17: SOUTH CHINA

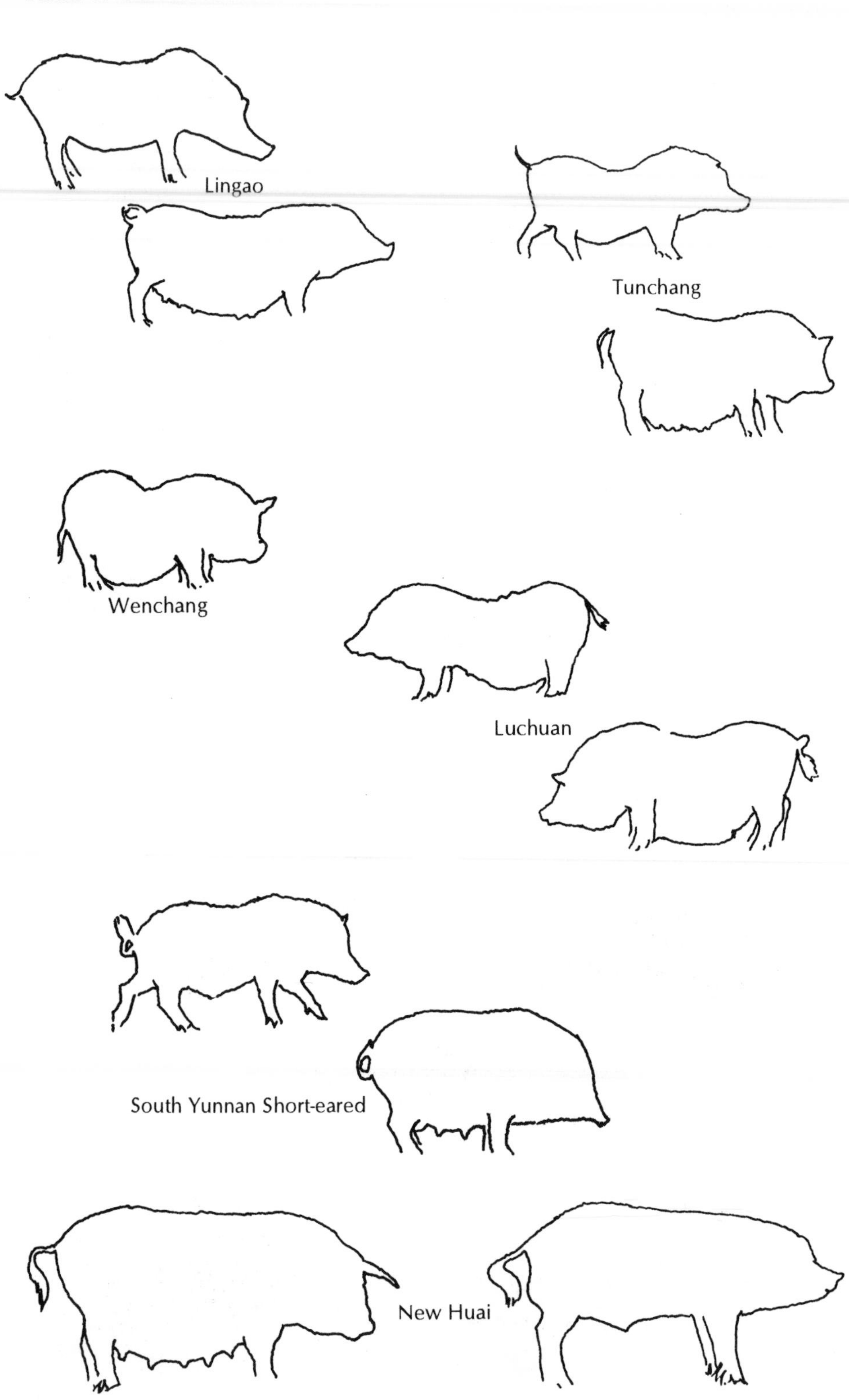

Plate 17 colour-33

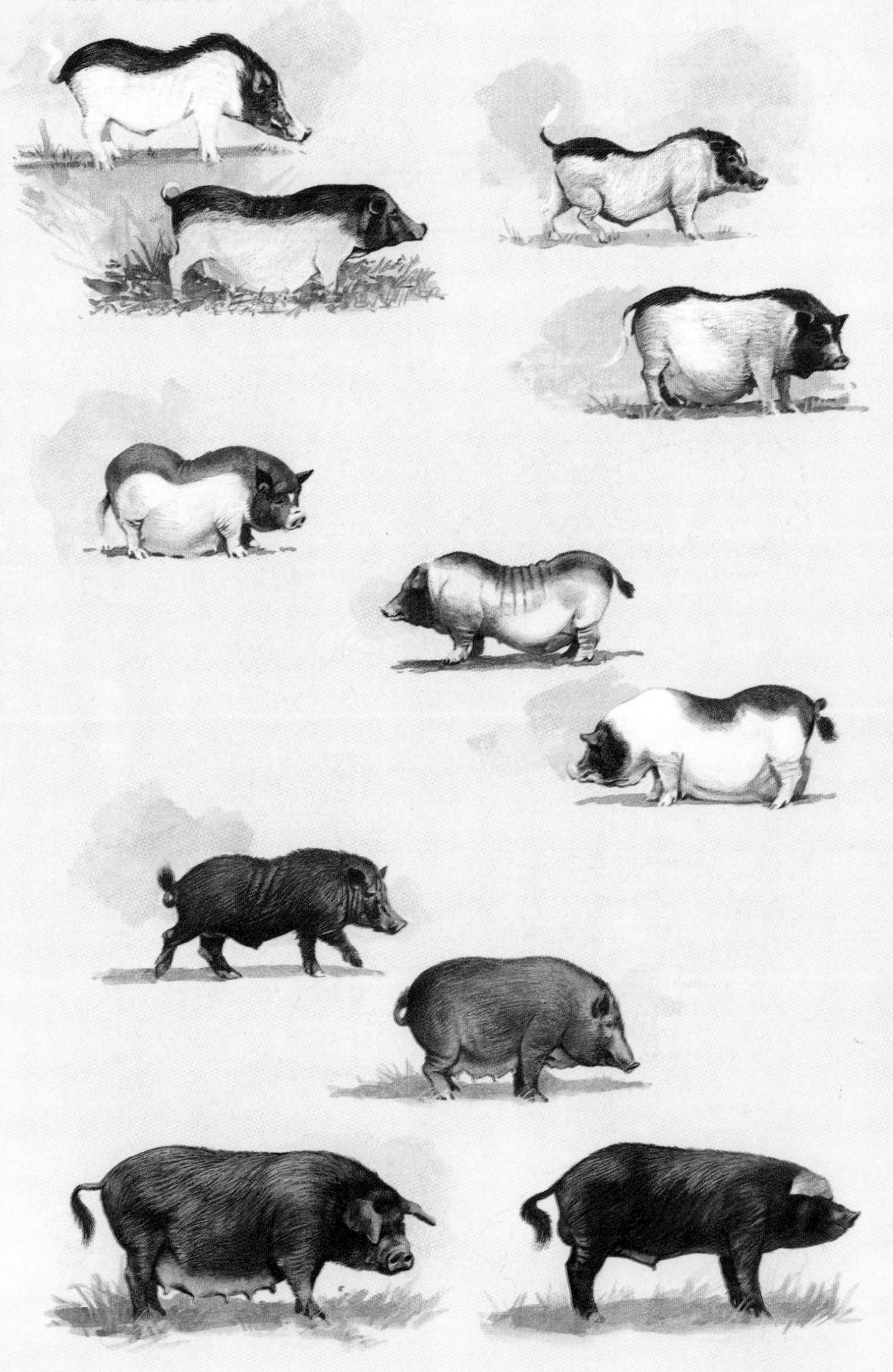

PLATE 18: NORTH CHINA AND PLATEAU TYPES

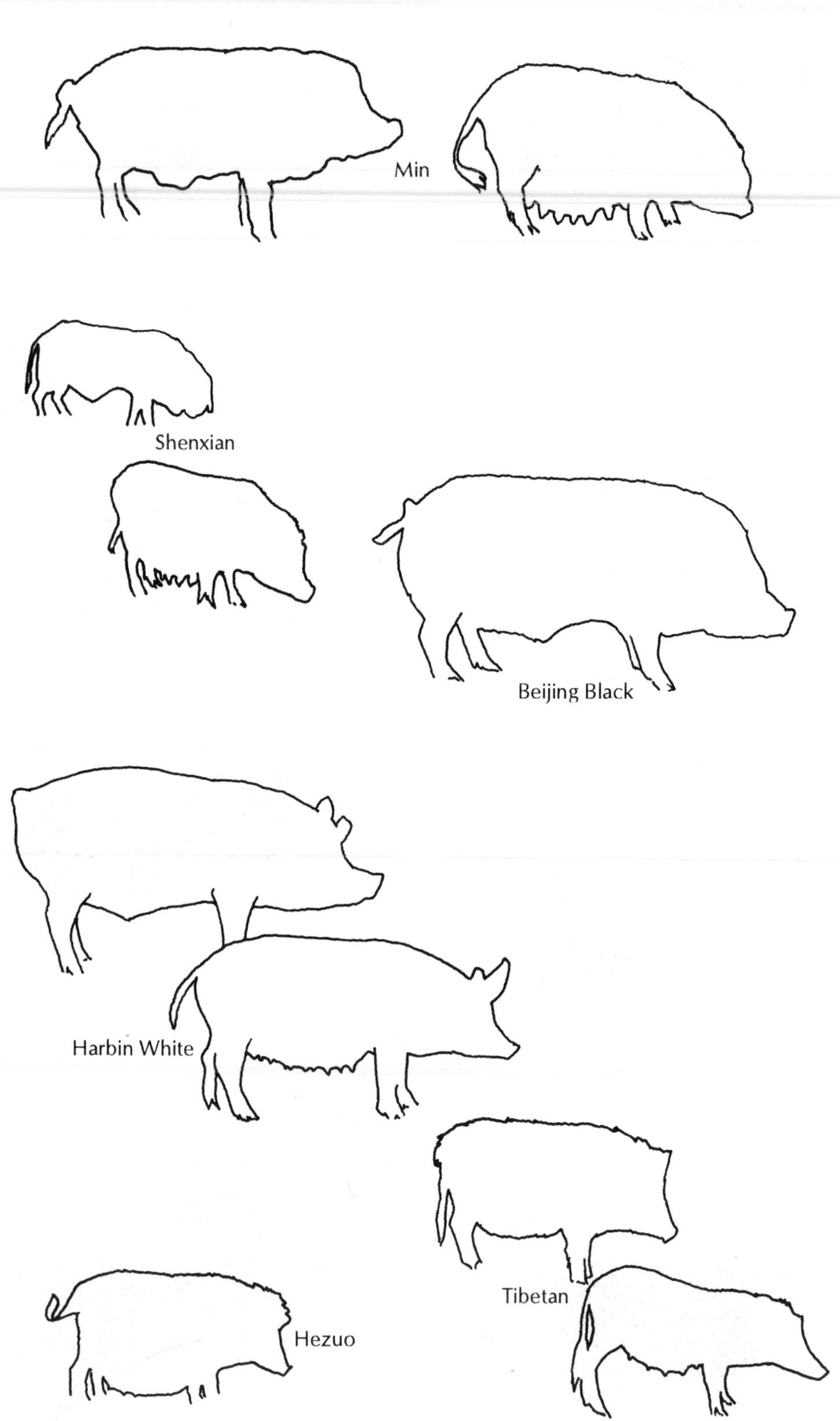

Plate 18 colour-35

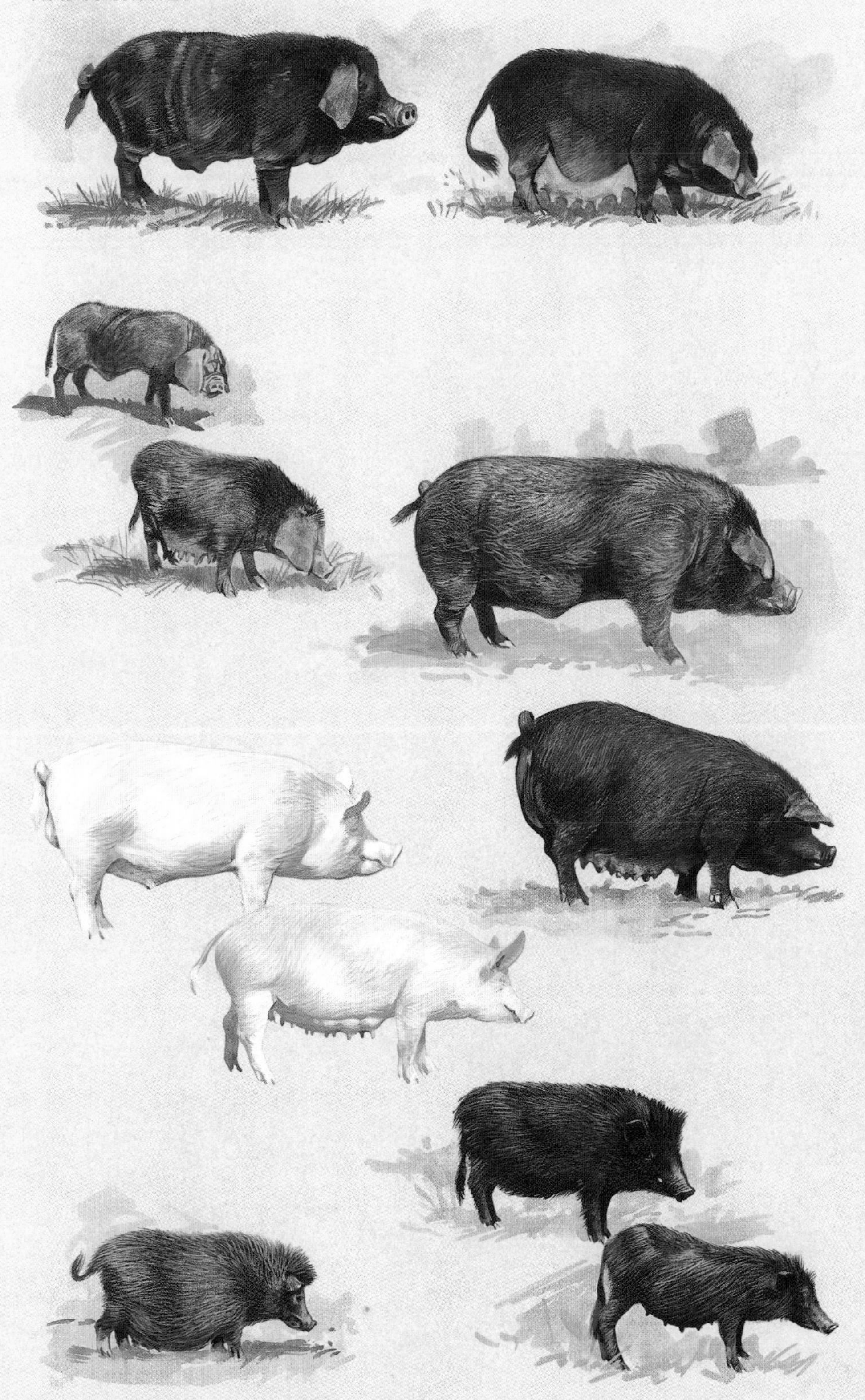

PLATE 19: SOUTH EAST ASIA

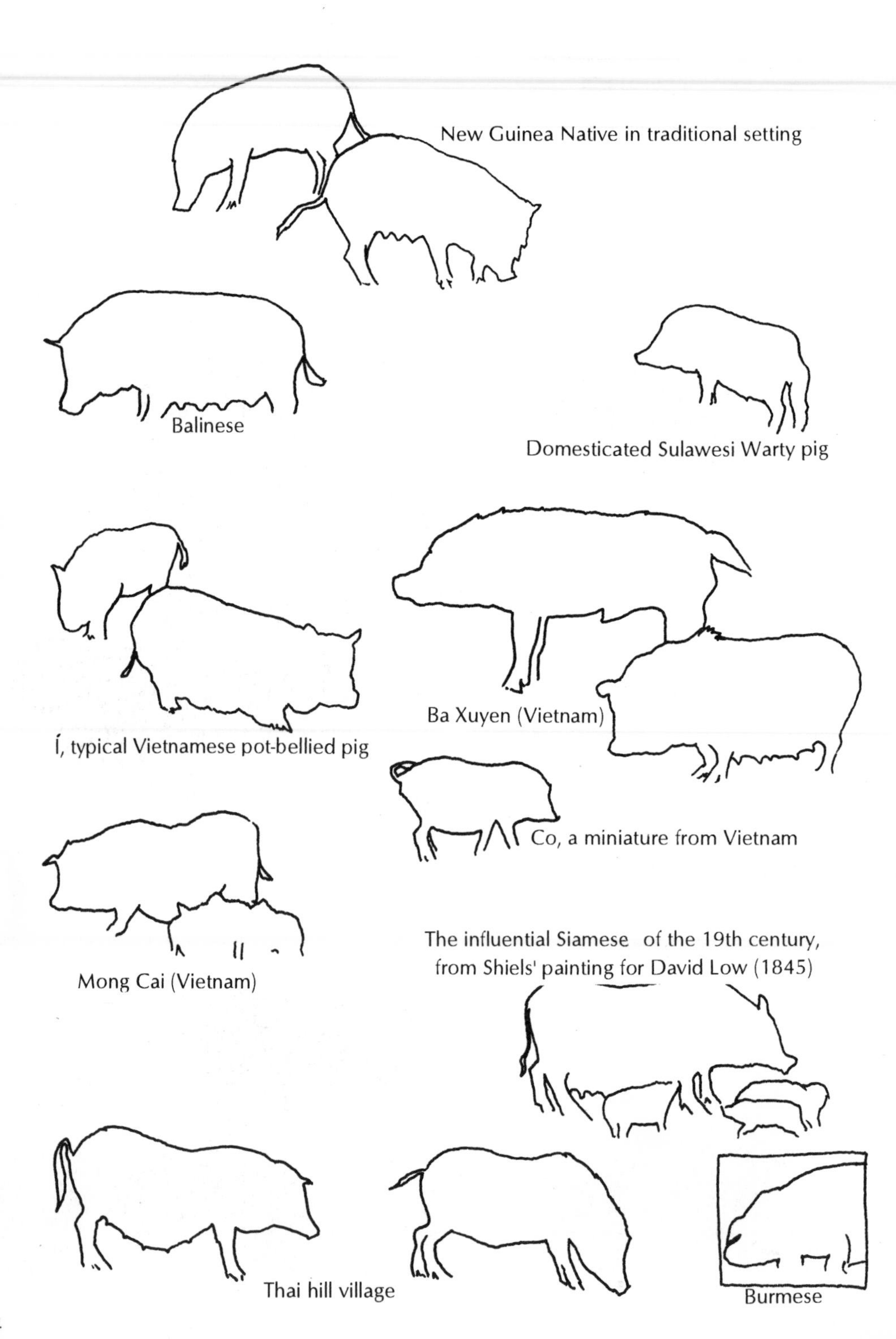
New Guinea Native in traditional setting
Balinese
Domesticated Sulawesi Warty pig
Í, typical Vietnamese pot-bellied pig
Ba Xuyen (Vietnam)
Co, a miniature from Vietnam
Mong Cai (Vietnam)
The influential Siamese of the 19th century, from Shiels' painting for David Low (1845)
Thai hill village
Burmese

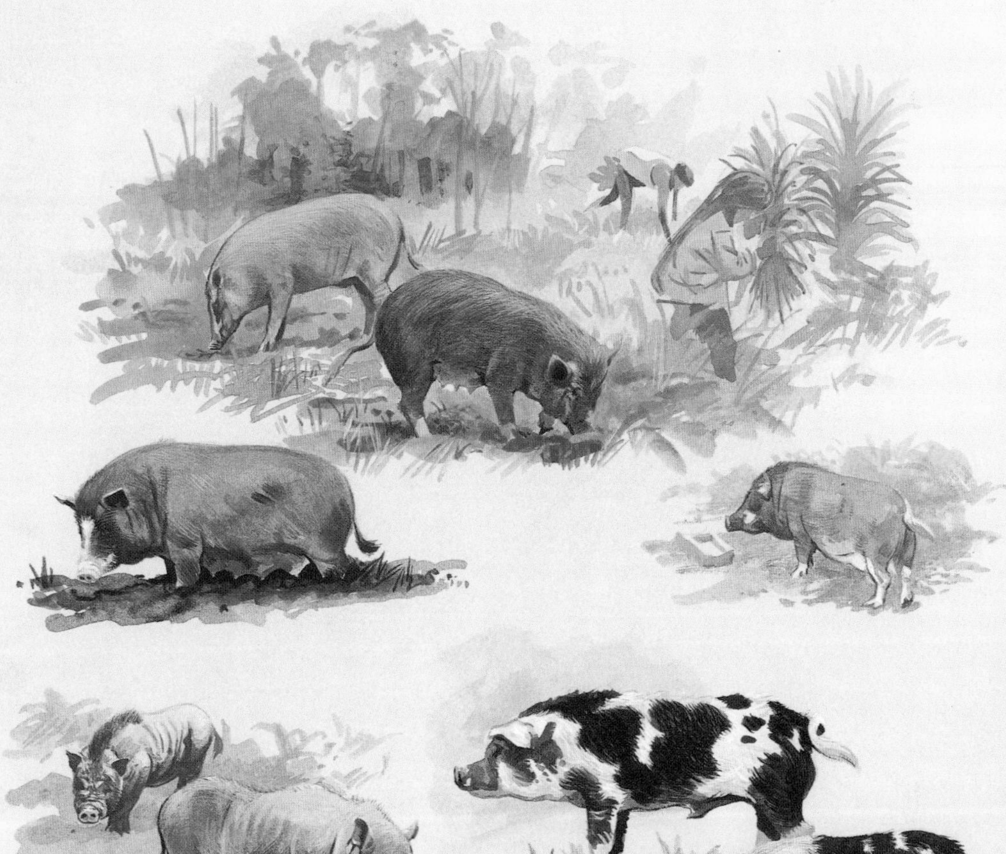

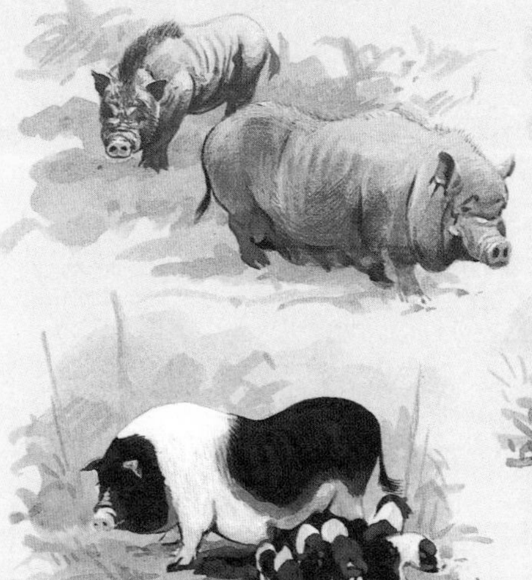

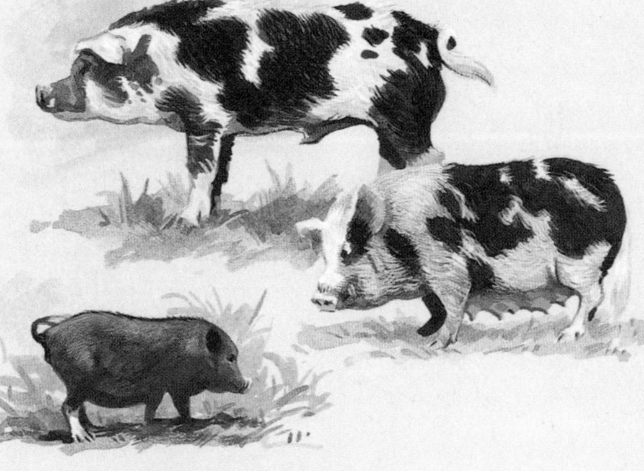

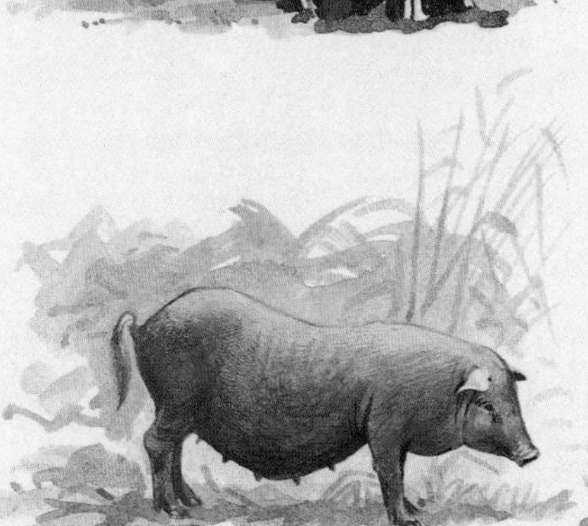

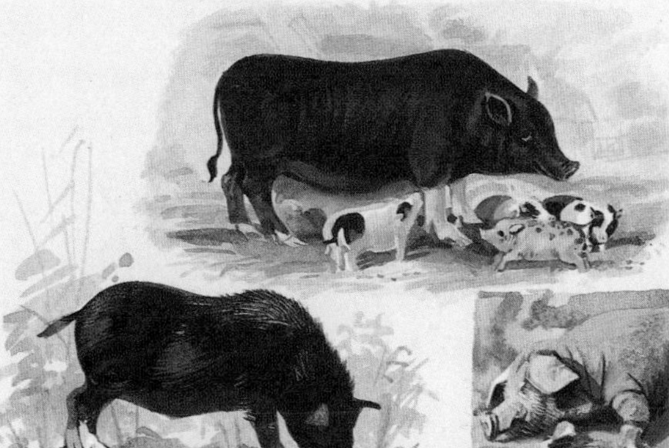

PLATE 20: AUSTRALASIA AND AFRICA

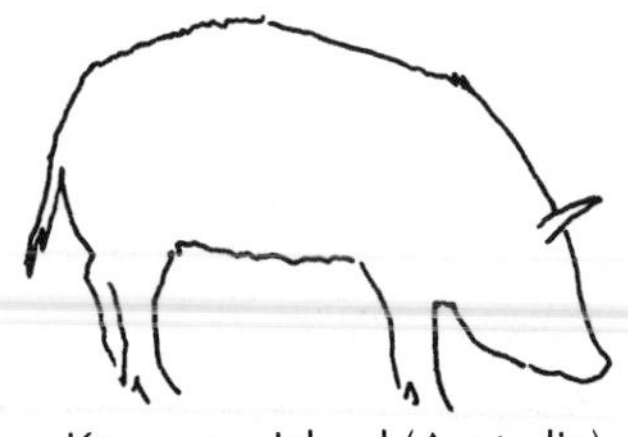

Kangaroo Island (Australia)

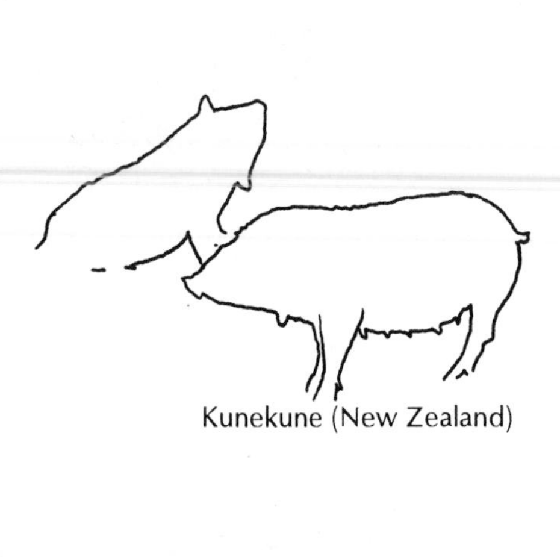

Kunekune (New Zealand)

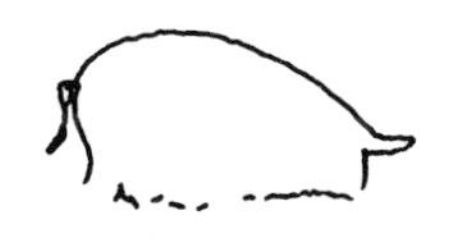

Australian ferals

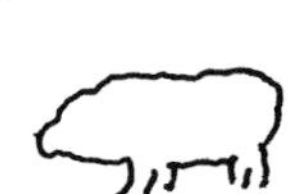

Nigerian Native

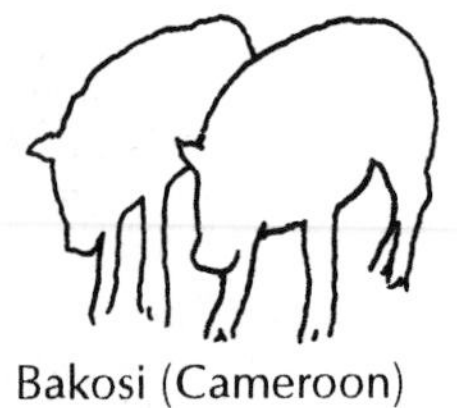

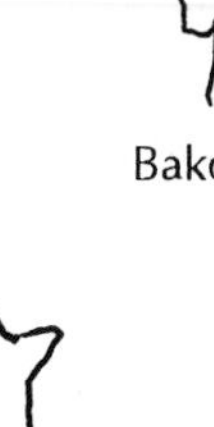

Bakosi (Cameroon)

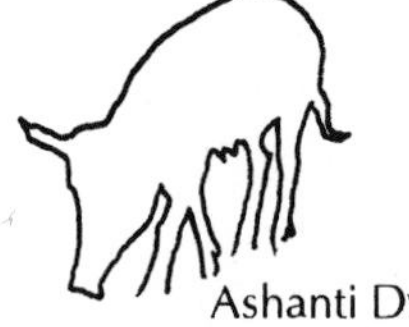

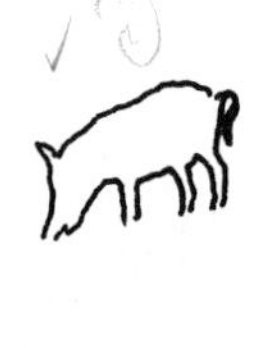

Ashanti Dwarf (Ghana)

West African, typical dwarf of the region

South African Landrace

Windsnyer (South Africa)

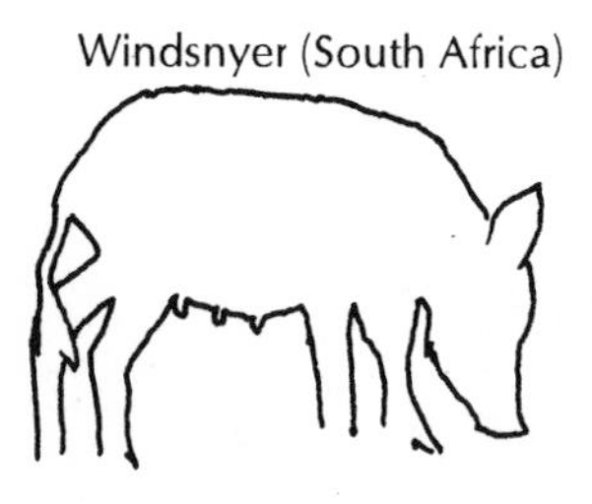

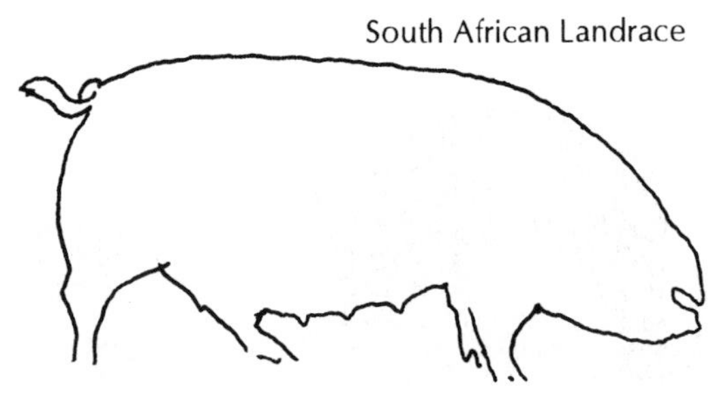

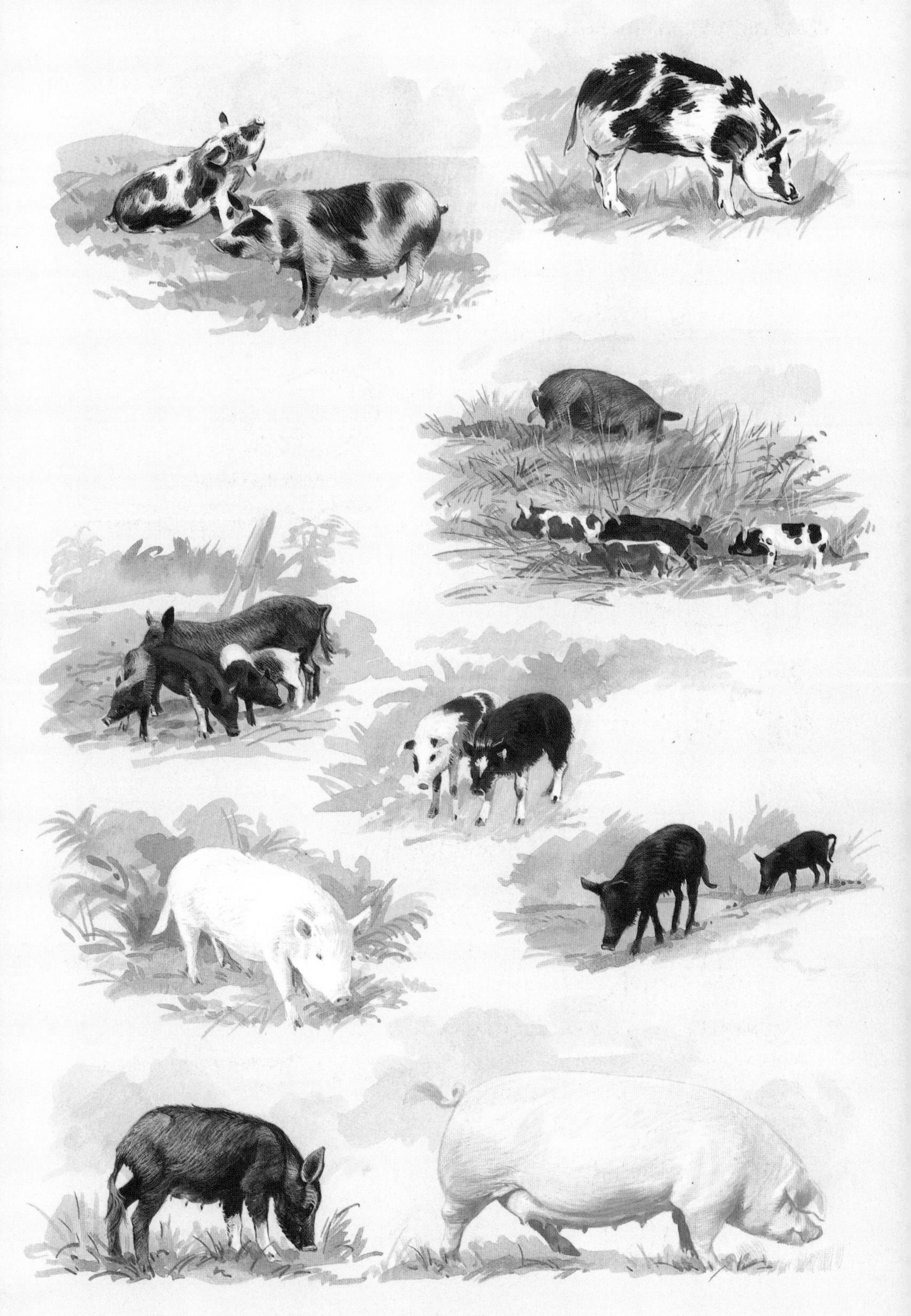

PLATE 21: NORTH AMERICA, Major Breeds

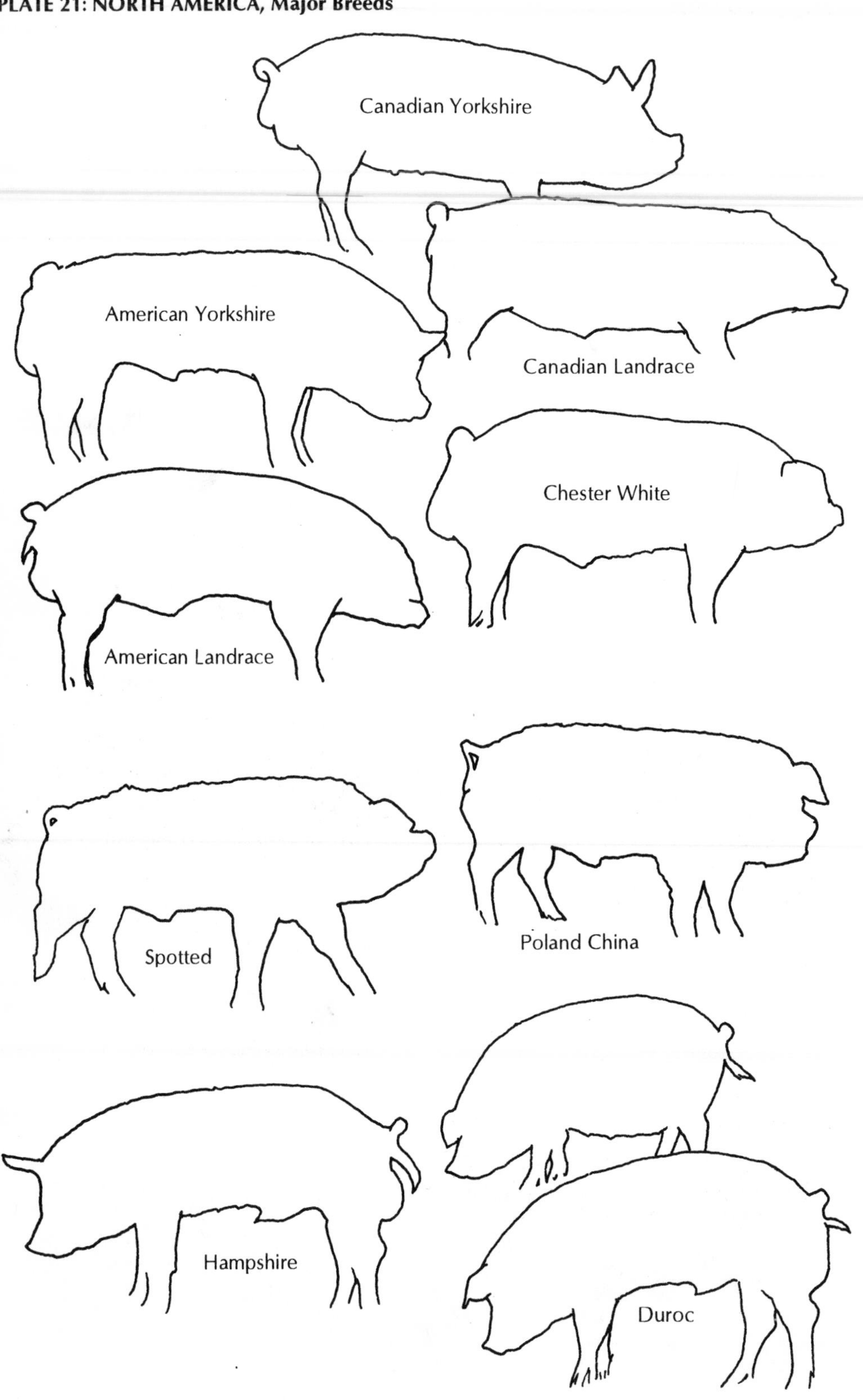

Plate 21 colour-41

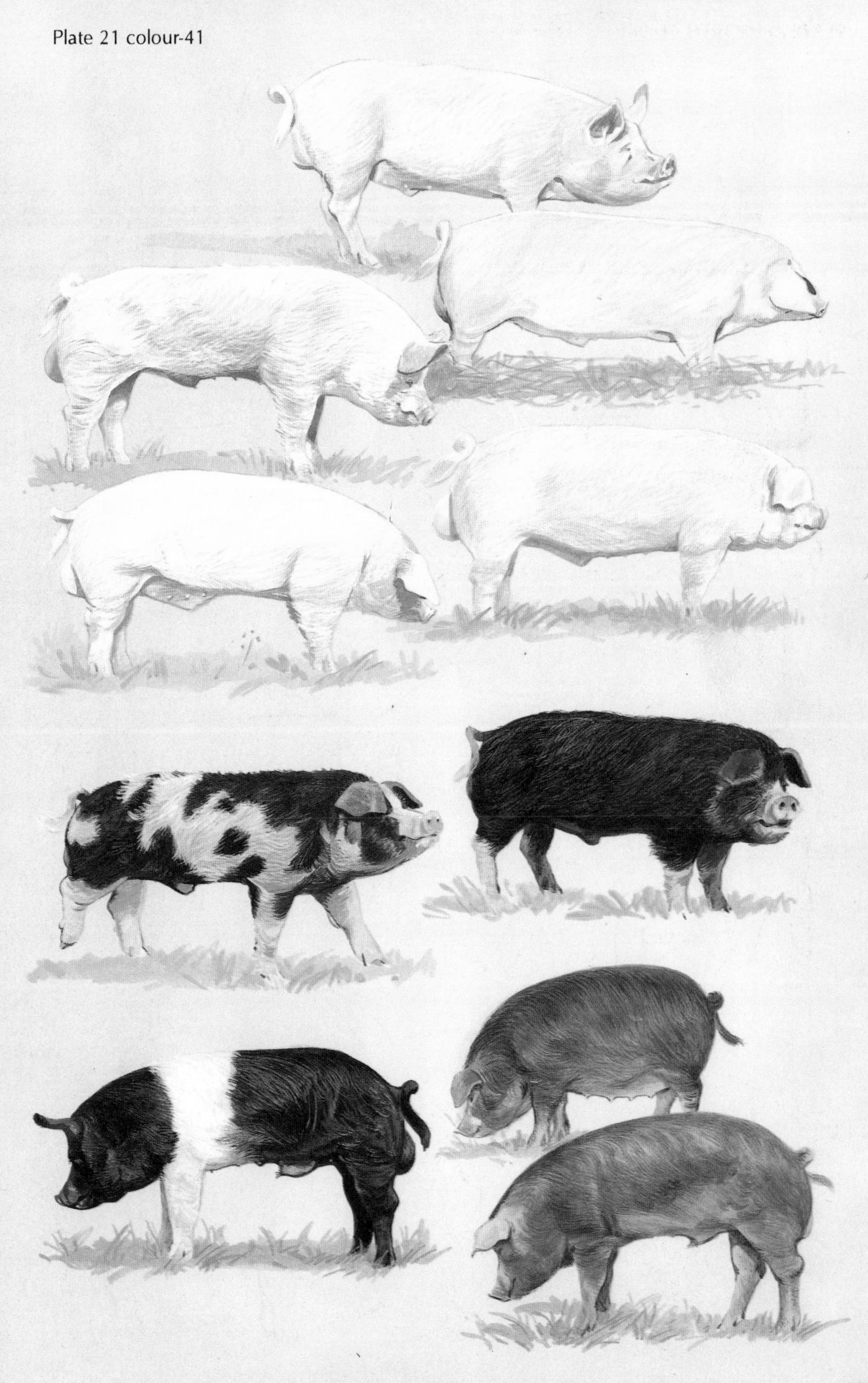

PLATE 22: NORTH AMERICA, Minor Breeds

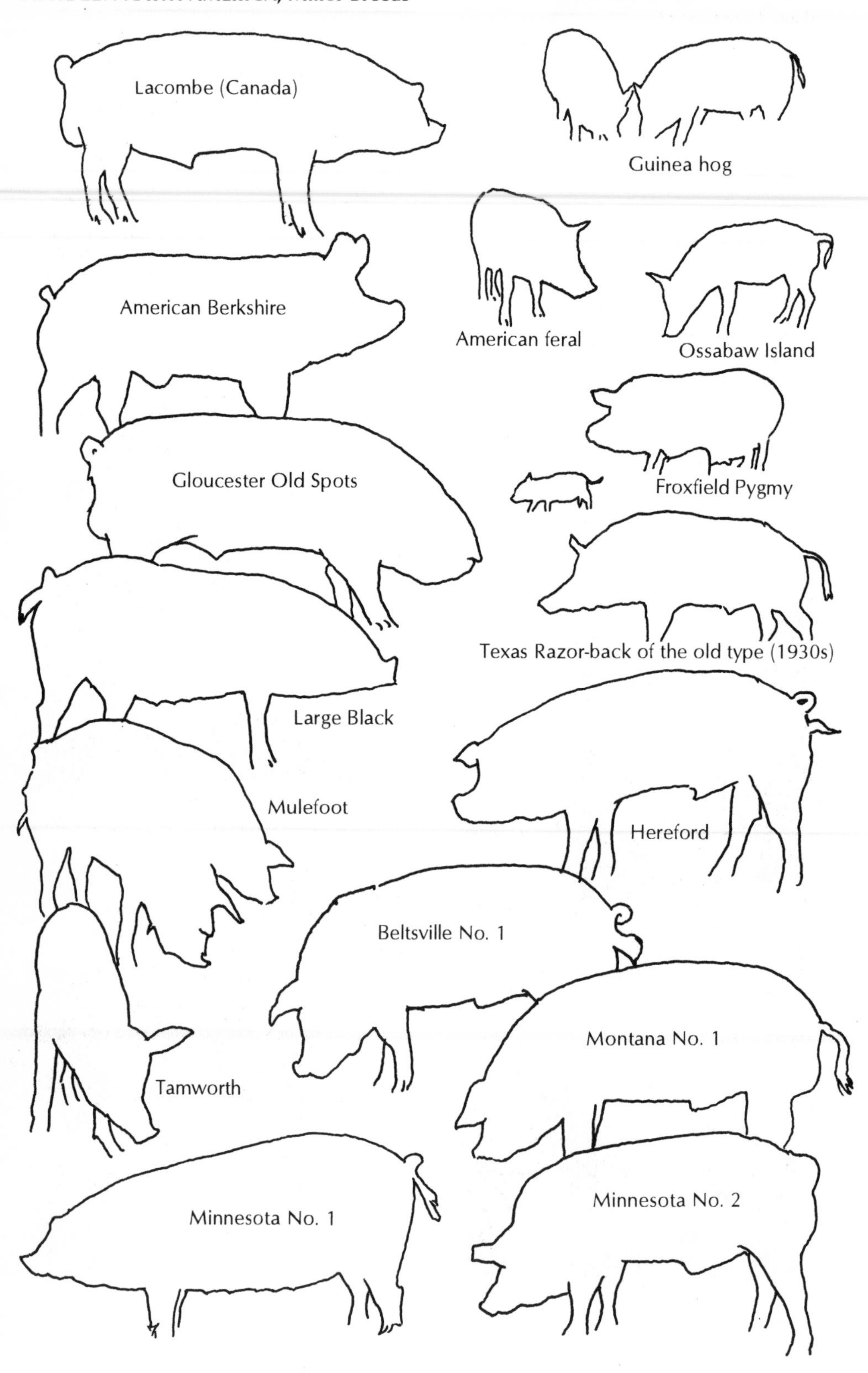

Plate 22 colour-43

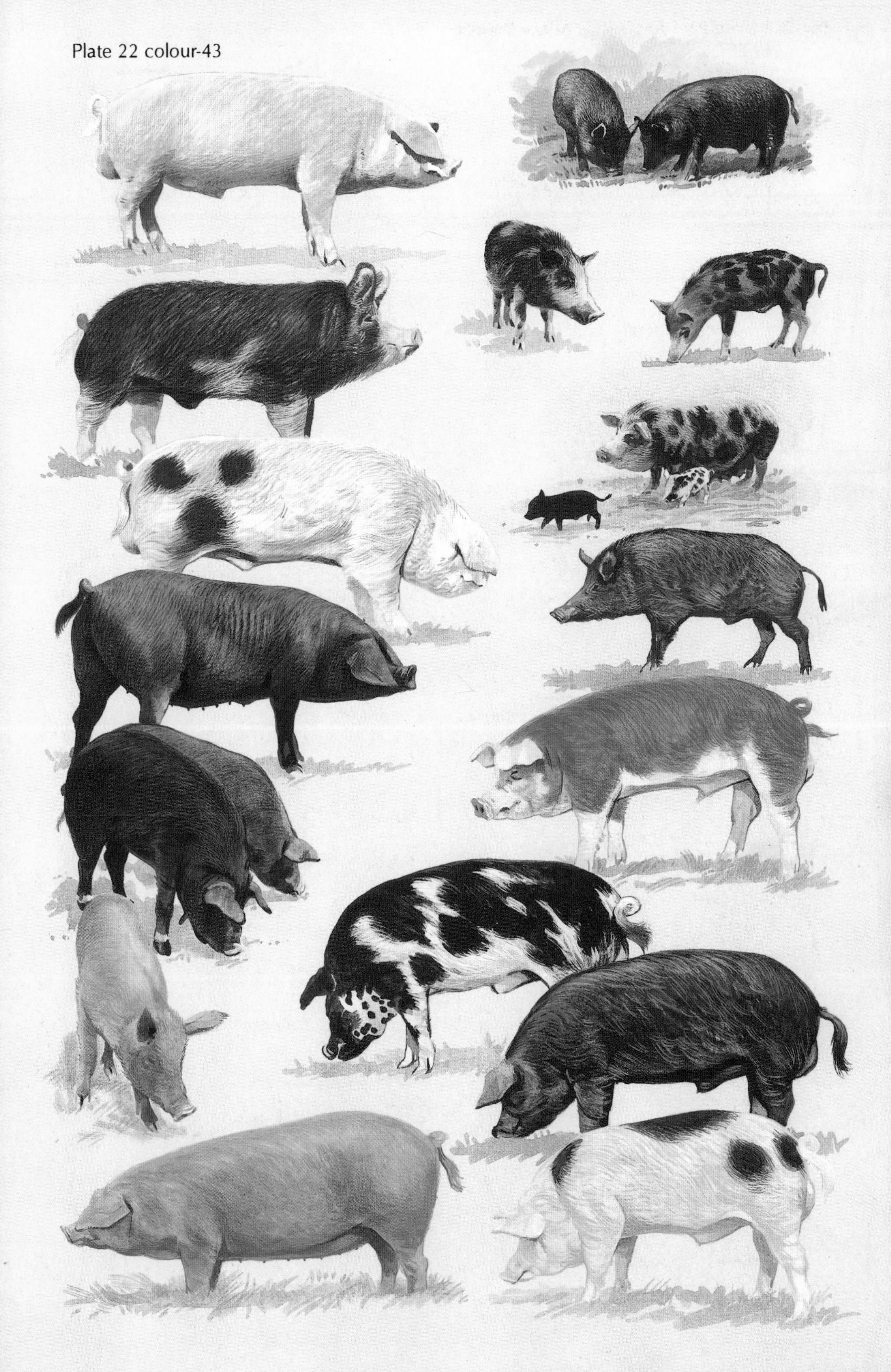

PLATE 23: BRAZIL

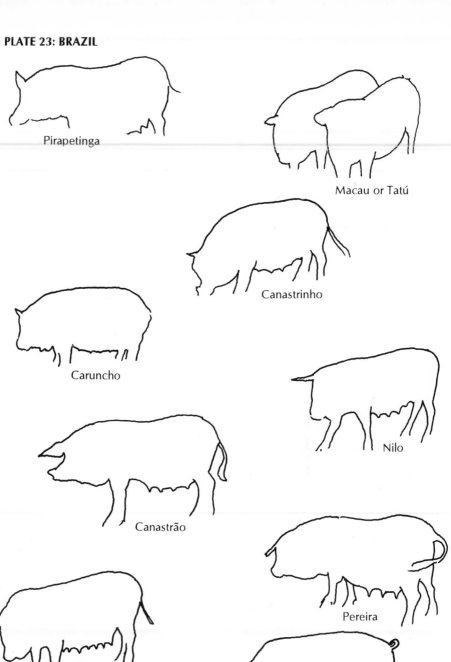

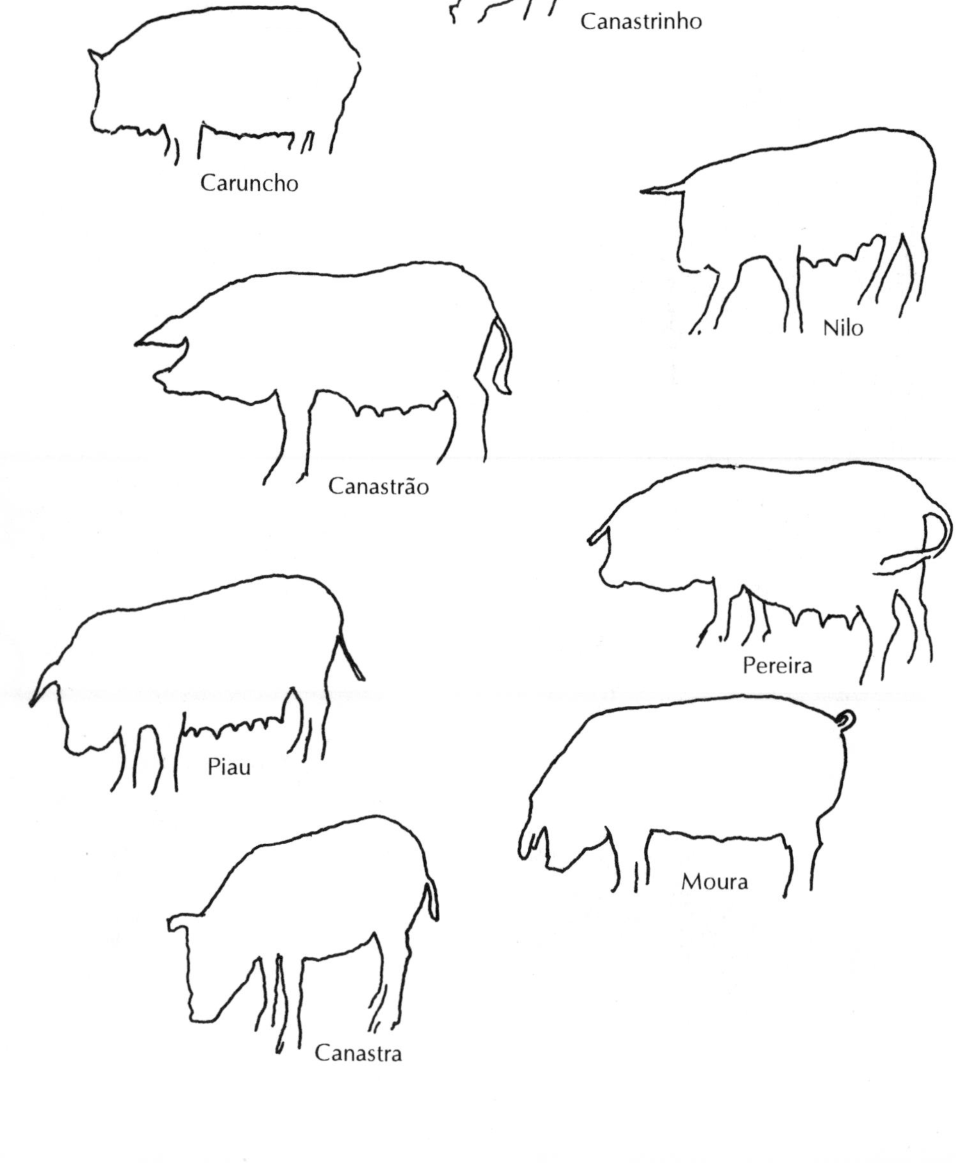

Plate 23 colour-45

PLATE 24: LATIN AMERICA

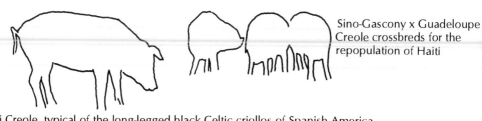

Sino-Gascony x Guadeloupe Creole crossbreds for the repopulation of Haiti

Haiti Creole, typical of the long-legged black Celtic criollos of Spanish America

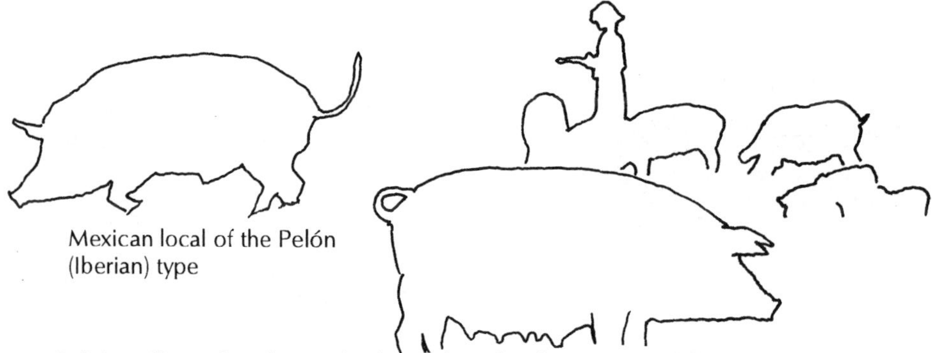

Mexican local of the Pelón (Iberian) type

Bolivian village pigs, the result of cross-breeding between local black criollo and European imports

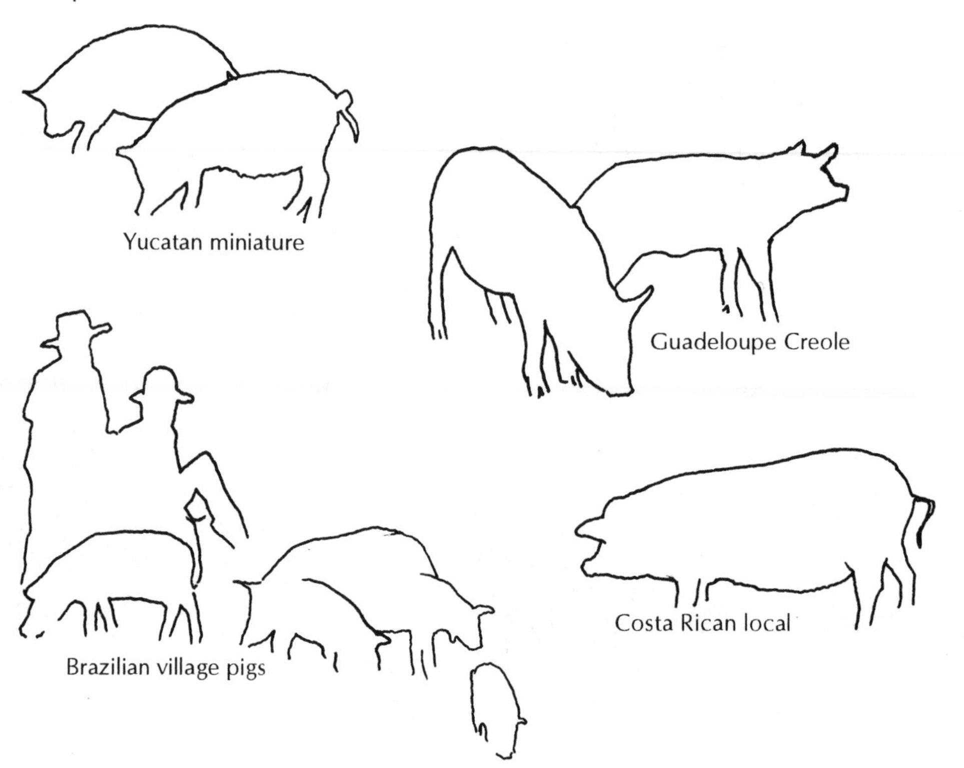

Yucatan miniature

Guadeloupe Creole

Brazilian village pigs

Costa Rican local

Plate 24 colour-47

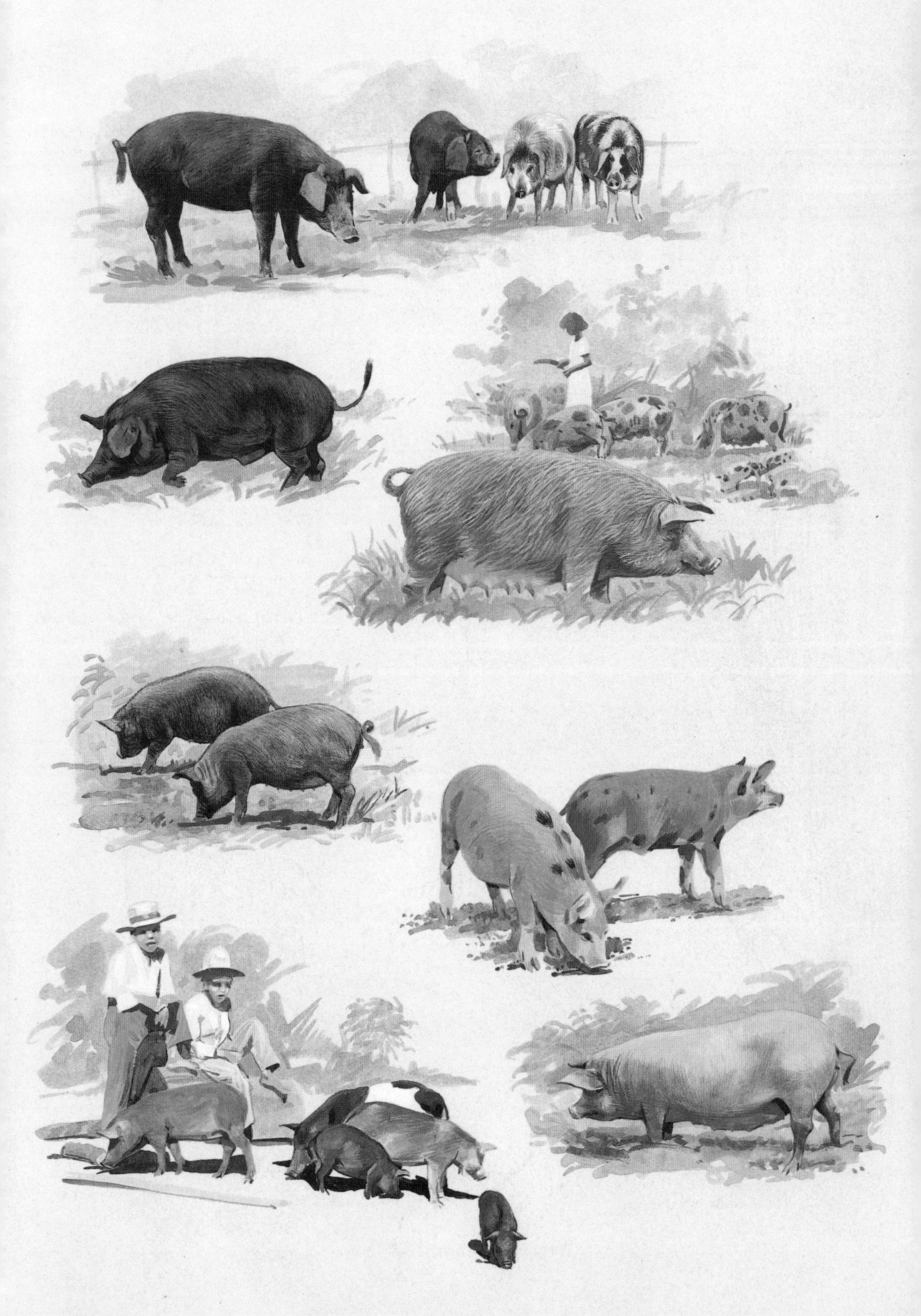

EUROPE

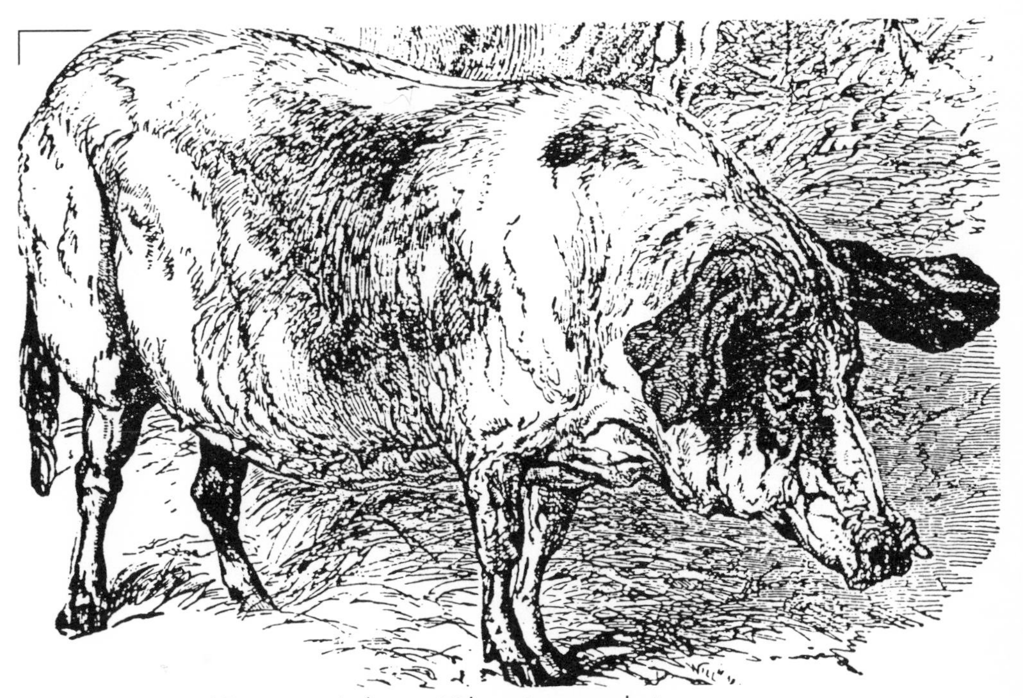

Fig. 8. Unimproved European pig from a 19th century woodcut.

MAP 2. Pig Breeds of Europe

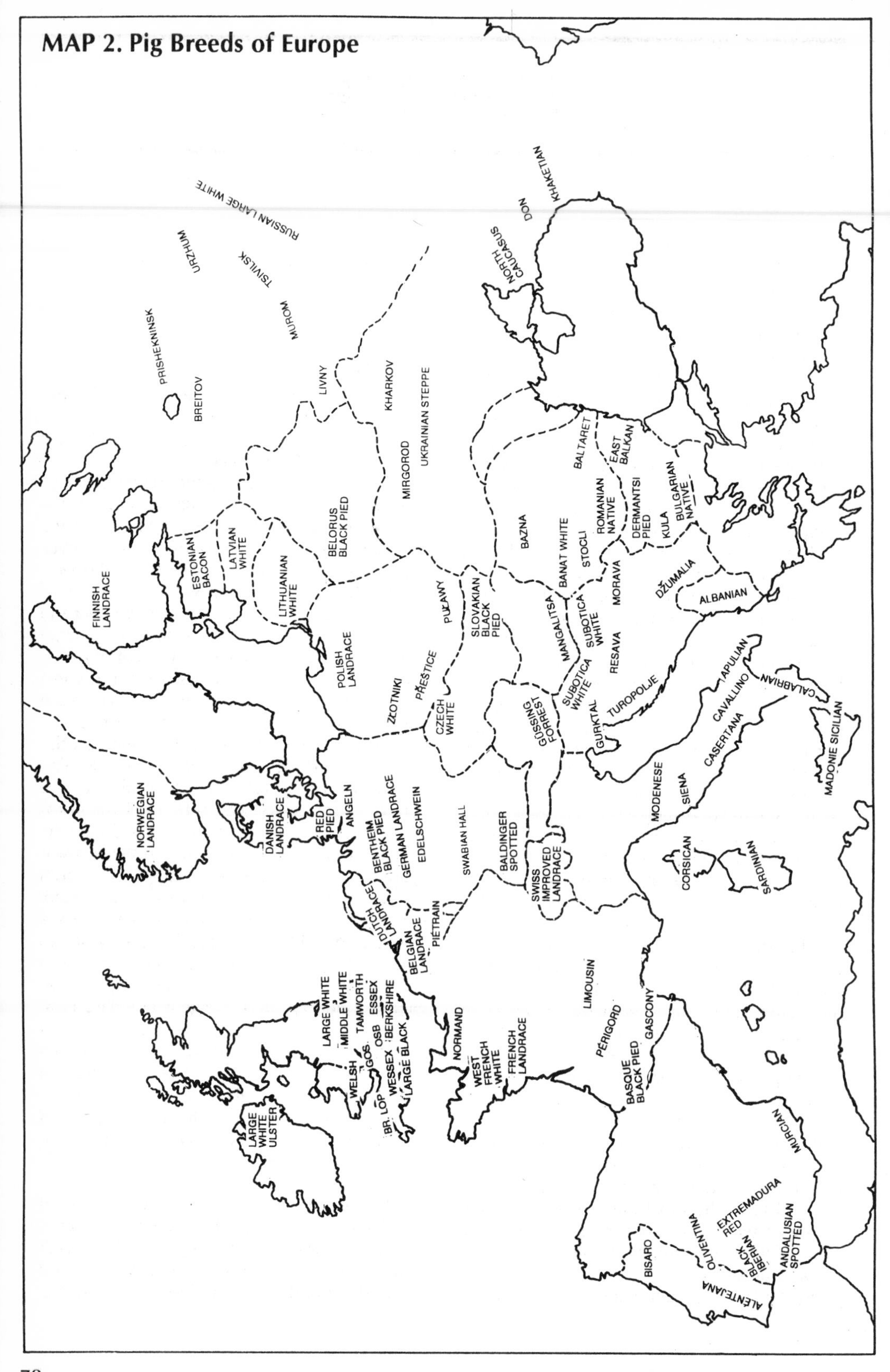

EUROPE

Until the present century, the majority of Europe's pigs were coloured animals. The development of the white Yorkshire pigs, and later the Landrace, heralded something of a revolution in pig-farming which gathered speed as what had long been either a backyard sty or a pasture-and-pannage herd system became instead an industry. The biggest change of all came when that industry switched from coloured sows rearing their litters in the open to housed white sows in intensive systems for maximum efficiency and production, whether on the commercial farms of the western nations or in the state farms and co-operatives of eastern Europe.

There are several ways of grouping the pig breeds of Europe, each of them oversimplified in that there has inevitably been considerable mixing of types, especially since the concept of "breeds" was clarified towards the end of the 19th century. At that time the British pigs were being widely exported and were highly influential in improving other regional types, or in encouraging other countries to pay more attention to the idea of breeds and their classification. In fact the British had really been encouraged into establishing formal breed standards by the Americans, who complained that they never quite knew what to expect of the pigs they imported. The Berkshire of the late 18th and most of the 19th century, for example, lent its name to all sorts of pigs that had no right to it at all.

The British system by the beginning of the 20th century was based on production goals, so that the breeds were classified as pork (smaller and fatter, and usually with plenty of Asian blood) or bacon types (longer and leaner). In the rest of Europe pig farmers were not yet dominated by market specifications and their breeds were grouped by, say, the shape of the face and head, the type and size of ears, the rate of maturity, the colour and coat pattern and, where possible, the origins or alleged origins of the breed, especially the degree of oriental influence. One of the most basic divisions in the European type is between the so-called Celtic races of the north and the Iberian races of the Mediterranean.

By the 1960s the tendency was to classify all the European breeds into three groups: the multipurpose meat types, the highly specialised breeds, and a wide variety of increasingly rare local breeds or types. At that time the groups included the following:

(1) White meat types:

* Prick-eared, dominated by the **Large White** of England.
* Lop-eared landraces, dominated by the **Danish Landrace**.

This commercially very important group represented perhaps half the pigs in Europe in the 1960s, and an even larger proportion of the pedigree breeding stock. Many countries developed their own national versions of the two. Before the Second World War, the sources of pedigree Large Whites were mainly either the United Kingdom or Germany (where the Large White or Yorkshire type was the **Edelschwein**), while the lop-eared breeding stock came mainly from Denmark or from Germany, which each produced a different extreme in conformation: the Danish Landrace was very long and lean, the German Landrace stockier and more muscular.

The war brought about considerable changes. Denmark restricted its export of pedigree stock. Germany's population of prick-eared pigs declined, and Sweden stepped into the postwar gap to become substantial suppliers of both prick-eared and lop-eared whites. Most European countries were by then experiencing a change in public taste: pig fat, previously an essential part of the popular diet, ceded to a demand for greater quantities of lean pig meat, and this led to a rapid change in breeding aims. In due course purebreds became less important as breeders experimented with crosses or developed special lines within a breed to meet the new criteria. There began to be greater performance differences between the new strains and hybrids than between the main pure breeds. In the mid 1960s, the whites dominated nearly every country in Europe.

In most countries the white sows were based on the prick-eared Yorkshires and the lop-eared national Landraces. The sequel, building with gathering speed from the 1960s, was a trend towards hybridisation, at first by mating between the two white breeds to gain hybrid vigour in offspring designed for intensive units. Then in the 1980s came the three-breed crosses, with the hybrid white sows put to meaty boars with a continental accent, such as Piétrain, or to those with the Transatlantic twang of Hampshire and Duroc.

(2) Highly specialised pigs

There was a time when this second group included specialist porkers like the Middle White of Britain. By the 1960s, however, there were really only two specialised European breeds on any scale and they represented two extremes. They were the **Piétrain** of Belgium, with its extreme leanness and extraordinary musculature, and the **Mangalitsa** of eastern Europe, with very thick backfat and high quality sausage meat.

(3) Local breeds

The breeds in this third category were often restricted to very local areas, meeting traditional local needs. Some, however, had originally been local, and were given regional breed names, but had subsequently enjoyed a period of more widespread popularity. The local breeds fell out of fashion as the lean whites took over, especially when pig industries began to use more intensive management on a large scale. The local breeds were usually better suited to less intensive outdoor herding. Breeders have reacted too late to save many of the local breeds from extinction and their potentially valuable traits have been lost from the genetic pool.

The demise of the hardy local was rapid. Many have become extinct or are so rare (and consequently inbred) that their extinction cannot be long in coming. In France for example: in 1934, local breeds formed 94.5% of the national herd; in 1953 the proportion was 66.4% and by 1965 it had fallen to 31.3%. In West Germany the proportion fell from 26.2% in 1953 to only 5% in 1965, though in Spain 75% were still of local breeds in the mid 1960s. The situation was so alarming by then that a group of countries convened to discuss the problem at an international symposium, and a census revealed the details shown in Table 2.

Since then, several European countries have established private or, occasionally, state-supported organisations which seek to conserve what is left of the local breeds and to increase their numbers to more healthy proportions. Notable among them is the Rare Breeds Survival Trust (RBST) in the United Kingdom, established two decades ago, which is concerned about almost all the British native pig breeds, most of which are categorised as rare. Hungary is another country which is very actively interested in its vanishing native breeds; likewise France, Italy, Spain and others. It is perhaps ironic that some of the major pig breeding companies, whose highly efficient development of commercial lines and hybrids sharply accelerated the decline of so many traditional breeds, are now

TABLE 2: EUROPE'S ENDANGERED BREEDS

In 1980, the EAAP's Commission on Animal Genetics established a working party to consider the conclusions of an FAO/UNEP consultation on animal genetic resources, held in Rome earlier that year. The working party surveyed European countries to discover the populations of different breeds of livestock so that conservation measures could be considered where necessary. The following is a list of the pig breeds it considered to be endangered, with fewer than 200 breeding sows, or with fewer than 500 sows but reducing, or fewer than 20 breeding boars.

CYPRUS
Berkshire
FRANCE
Basque Black Pied
Corsican
Créole
Gascony
Limousin
Normand
GERMANY
Angeln Saddleback
Swabian-Hall
GREECE
Greek Local
HUNGARY
Mangalitsa
ICELAND
Icelandic
ITALY
Casertana
Madonie-Sicilian
Mora Romagnola
Sardinian
Sicilian
POLAND
Ziotniki Spotted
Zlotniki White
UNITED KINGDOM
Berkshire
British Lop
Gloucester Old Spots
Large Black
Middle White
Oxford Sandy-and-Black
Saddleback
Tamworth
YUGOSLAVIA
Black Slavonian
Krškopolje
Šiška
Šumadija
Turopolje

scouring the world for genetic qualities so often found in the very breeds which have become extinct in their own back yards.

Those old breeds have, or had, much to offer and not only in local situations, though they were evolved for local environments and markets. Most were hardy, disease resistant, easy to breed and rear, able to make use of cheap local feedstuffs and to produce what local people required, and it is as well to remember that even such influential breeds as the Large White and the Piétrain, say, were originally local breeds. They were simply lucky enough either to be developed rapidly by breeders with their fingers on the pulse of the wider markets, or to have the support of particularly active breed societies with a sharp sense of promotion, or both.

The unlucky ones were not necessarily any less potentially useful but were not (or were not considered to be) able to adapt to the development of intensive agriculture in many European countries and to the rapidly changing demands of a market that required uniformity, size and large numbers, increasingly so as supermarkets began to drive small specialist butchers out of business.

It was a *Catch-22* situation for many local breeds. There were already too few within the breed to produce marketable slaughter pigs on a large scale, and there were also too few for the intensive degree of selection within the breed that was necessary to keep up with the speed of changing demands for improved pigs. Inevitably, therefore, their numbers dwindled further as many local herds were upgraded to the white meat breeds, contributing their local genes to the white industry as a whole but at the expense of their individuality, until the contributing breed no longer had a separate identity.

This leads ultimately to a dangerously shrinking gene pool. The modern hybrid depends upon the greatest possible divergence between its parents in order to precipitate maximum hybrid vigour. It also needs a reservoir of genetic traits at present unfashionable but which might well be needed in the future in a volatile market, whether in terms of carcass quality, welfare, disease, efficient use of non-concentrates or some other area which might not at present be foremost. This is quite apart from producers' economic and practical concerns such as general feed conversion efficiency, good growth rates, fecundity, ease of parturition, adaptability to difficult situations and so on.

Much of the genetic make-up of traditional breeds is unknown, though there are now major projects to determine them. It could be that they might offer valuable genes for a fast-changing world. Who knows, for example, what climatic shifts, depletions of non-renewable energy resources, new diseases and other factors may be lying in wait to bring the collapse of the present commercial types? The worry must be whether enough genetic diversity has been retained to meet the changing needs of future generations.

Today the remaining European breeds, already overwhelmed, are facing threats from further afield as the fashion swings to the use of American breeds like the Duroc and the highly prolific Chinese breeds to "improve" the national herds. Yet the American breeds virtually make the case for the resuscitation of European local breeds: they have been introduced to improve meat quality (restoring taste and succulence, for example) and to meet the growing return to less expensive outdoor systems. The old Wessex Saddleback, as the probable ancestor of the American Hampshire, might look askance at the use of the latter in the Wessex's "rightful place", while the old red Iberian pigs of Spain and Portugal might have similar thoughts on the Duroc.

The Celtic Type

The ancient Celtic peoples had much use for the pig. It was their most numerous species of domesticated livestock and there have been many finds not only of pig bones but also little statuettes of a type of pig with a long head, large tusks, a narrow body, long legs, curly tail and a "carp's back" with a thick crest of erect bristles along its length. The type persisted in much of north west Europe for many centuries and became the basis of many landraces.

The term Celtic is now generally used to distinguish the lop-eared pigs of the northern regions of Spain, Portugal, France and Italy, where they are usually white, or spotted or saddlebacked, from the so-called Iberians - coloured pigs with semi-erect ears in the Mediterranean regions of those countries. However, the Celtic umbrella also embraces nearly all of northern Europe's indigenous lop-eared pigs. The Celtic was a large, coarse, late-maturing meat type with those long lop ears, long legs, flat sides, and was a dirty or yellowish white colour with or without varying degrees of spotting or belting. Or at least, that is what it was like before it was refined with Asian blood.

The Landraces

The Celtic type was found all over the northern countries of Europe, the linking characteristic being the lop ears hanging over its eyes. The story of the Landrace as a breed begins before the turn of the century, in Denmark, almost as a reaction to the already huge influence of Britain's prick-eared Large White pigs which had spread from their original breeding area in Yorkshire and had come to dominate the pig industry in several countries, often being used to upgrade local stock with the help of the other British improving breeds such as Berkshire and Middle White.

It is claimed by some that the Danish Landrace originated from crossing the Large White with local Celtic types but the Danes make out a reasonable case for denying the Large White influence on the famous Danish Landrace. Whatever its background, the breed that emerged from Denmark was designed as a baconer to meet the lucrative market in Britain for Wiltshire-cure meat, a process which needed length and leanness in the pig. Continental pigs of the period were too short for that special market and the Danes set about stretching their pigs to fill this promising niche. Their fine-boned, lop-eared Landrace became exceptionally long in the body, yielding ample bacon cuts for the market the Danes had so unerringly targeted and then exploited with great efficiency and flair. The breed was soon being exported and, directly or indirectly, it became the basis of all the developed Landraces.

In Germany, a different type of Landrace began to emerge. It was much meatier (like many German pigs), which suited the German market for pork and sausage meat. It was derived from the indigenous German land pig with plenty of Large White (Edelschwein) to influence it and produce a shorter and more compact pig of medium length and heavy bones. This meaty type was developed to an even greater extreme of muscularity in Belgium, where it displayed the Piétrain's characteristic double-muscling and was short in the body.

During the first half of the 20th century, other countries were developing their own national Landraces, largely by using the Danish Landrace on their native land pigs. These were mostly intermediate in type between the Danish and Belgian extremes. Gradually the newly improved Landraces of various different countries were used at different stages in each national breeding programme, so that it became quite a complex breeding web, with several national Landraces owing their origins to more than one foreign Landrace. The Landrace chart attempts to show how the web developed.

Despite so much sharing of breeding stock, there are still noticeable differences between the various Landraces today. The extreme Danish bacon type, which was virtually the only breed in Denmark in the 1960s, has almost disappeared as it has proved uneconomical; the Danes selected for length and bacon carcass but lost productivity until they introduced Large White blood during the early 1970s. The other Scandinavian Landraces in Norway, Sweden and Finland are still baconers, though not extreme: they have all evolved over the years, as breeds always do, and have been an integral part of pig breeding companies' programmes. The Scandinavian Landraces tend to be favoured as breeding sows with good maternal

Landraces: Their Influences on Each Other

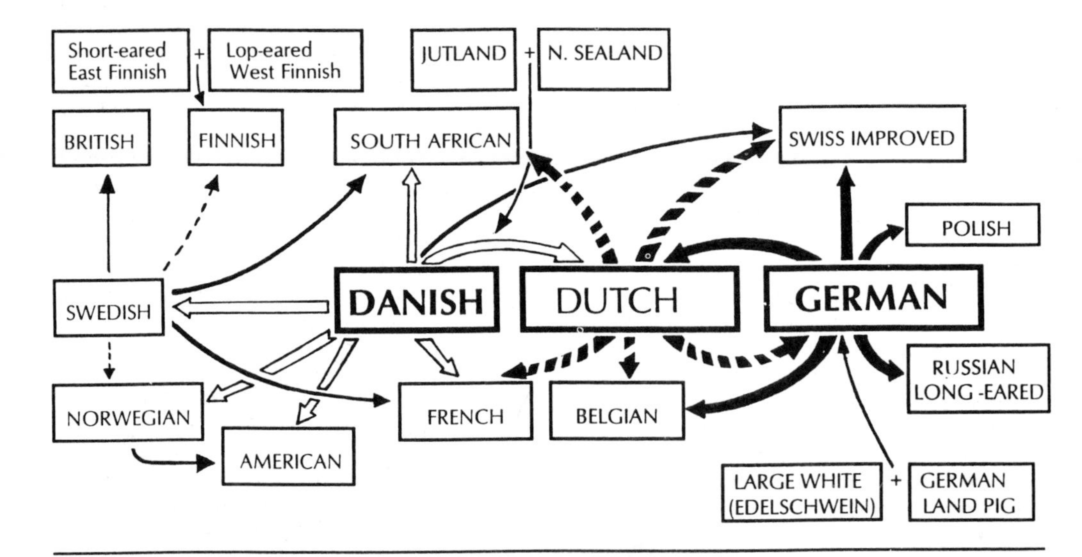

traits; the Belgian, on the other hand, is more often used as a terminal sire to "beef up" the carcass of his progeny.

By the late 1970s and early 1980s, a problem was becoming noticeable among the more compact and muscular Landraces, especially the Belgian, which shared the problem and its cause with Belgium's other important breed, the Piétrain. The problem, susceptibility to stress, was finally shown to be linked to the halothane gene which, in turn, was linked to the double muscling that characterises the two Belgian breeds (see Genetics section).

Since then, many breeders have introduced rigorous testing for the halothane gene and have selected accordingly - but not necessarily to eliminate the gene entirely in all cases, as it does offer advantages as well as disadvantages.

The Iberian Pigs

The "Iberian" or Mediterranean types of southern Europe have for the most part given way to the improved Celtic meat breeds but they linger here and there, usually as rare and very local types but sometimes in healthy numbers - for example the black and red Iberian pigs in Spain.

The Iberians, which tend to be lard pigs, are long-snouted, with sub-concave profiles, elongated heads, small or medium-sized ears which are semi-erect, leaning forwards but not flopping over the eyes, and a generally compact conformation. Their skin and bristles are usually black or reddish-brown; some animals are pied. The colour gives useful heat protection in the warm climates of their native regions.

They received quite early infusions of Asian blood. Indeed the **Neapolitan**, with a goodly proportion of IndoChinese genes, was eventually used in the United Kingdom to improve the Old English types and helped to start the whole British trend towards improvement, breed fixing and widescale export. However, the Iberian pigs of Spain and Portugal had spread their genes overseas long, long before the improvement of the Berkshires and Yorkshires: they naturally accompanied explorers and settlers sailing for the Americas from the late 15th century onwards and also accompanied the Portuguese to West Africa - they are probably the ancestors of that region's dwarf village pigs and, in the guise of the Red Guinea pig, came over in slave ships to the Americas and possibly contributed to the now popular Duroc.

In the mid 1960s the Iberian type still formed 50% of Italy's pig population as primitive pasture pigs, usually with black skin and virtually erect ears, with the characteristic long head, pointed snout and more or less straight profile. They were late-maturing and are rarely used commercially today. In France the Iberian type was represented by the **Gascony**, the **Basque Black Pied** and the **Limousin** - all with long snouts, medium-sized semi-erect ears, compact bodies and black or reddish colouring. They are the rare breeds of France today.

The Asian Influence

The pigs of east Asia are markedly different from those of Europe, especially in the Chinese tendency for wrinkled skin, straight rather than curled tails, short legs, short dished faces, prick ears and often a drooping belly and dipping back. They have been in Europe for several centuries, however, and were mixed originally with the Mediterranean pigs, accounting to some extent for the differences between Iberian and Celtic types. They also came to England in the late 18th and early 19th centuries and were deliberately bred with local types for their ability to fatten early, to pass on their fine bone structure and general air of refinement in contrast to the coarse Celtic pigs, and to improve prolificacy and early maturity. They were much smaller than the Celtic and they left their traces quite strongly.

The Melting Pot

Thus the European pigs mingled with each other and mingled also with imported exotics. In Europe today, trade barriers are falling rapidly and there is increasing competition but also cooperation between its nations. In the wake of huge political upheavals that are changing the map of Europe almost daily, and shifting the focus of what used to be tightly bound trading groups, there is a trend for countries in eastern Europe in particular (traditionally dependent on pigs) to seek pig meat markets in the west on a much larger scale than before, and for western commercial breeding and marketing companies to set up bases in the eastern countries, helping the latter to modernise their breeding stock, management techniques and processing plants where necessary - partly to protect themselves against the possible decline of western pig industries in the face of large quantities of cheap pig meat imported from the east.

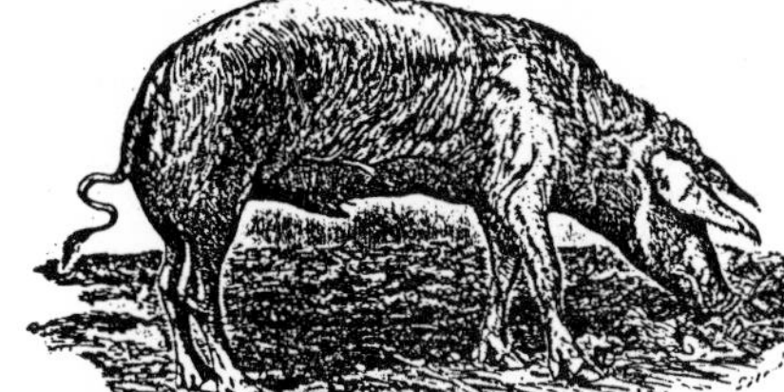

Fig. 9. Common pig of Europe [Long, *Book of the Pig*, 1842]

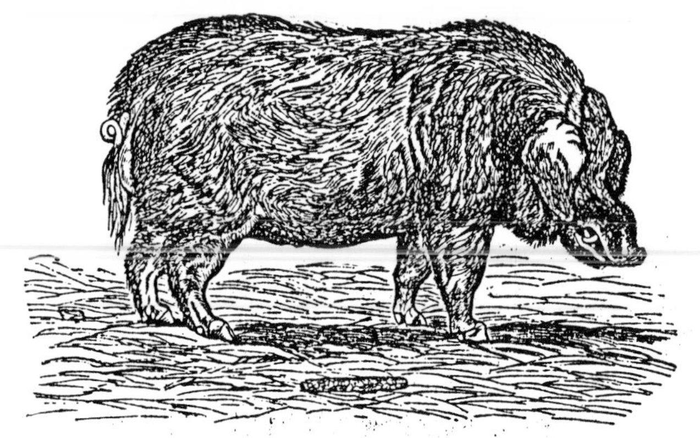

Fig. 10. Original Old English pig [*Harris on the Pig*,1881]

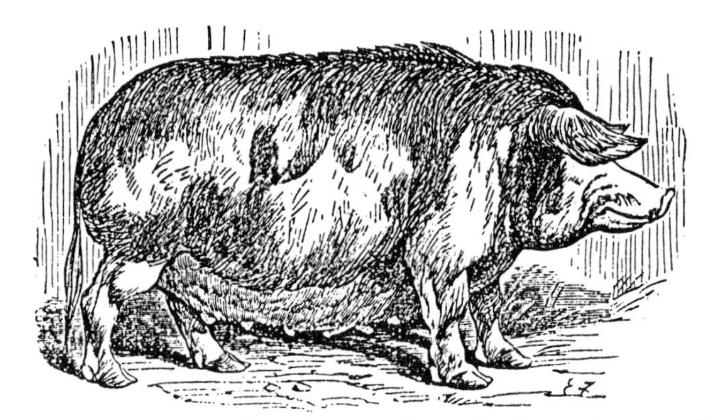

Fig. 11. Hampshire pig [London, *Encyclopaedia of Agriculture*,1825]

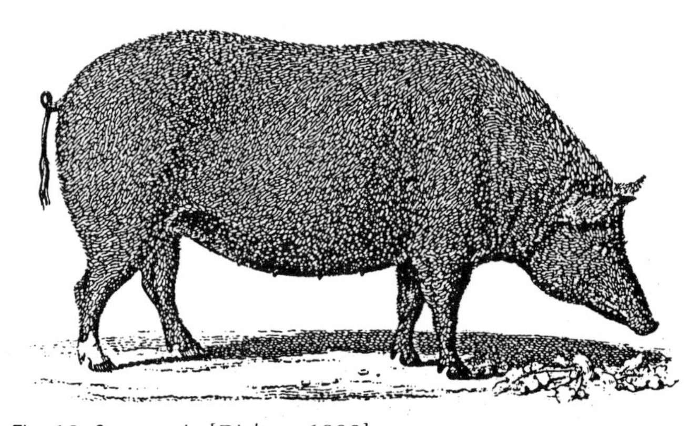

Fig. 12. Sussex pig [*Dickson*,1822]

UNITED KINGDOM AND IRELAND

ENGLAND

The Smithfield Show - England's major centre for the exhibition of its prime livestock - admitted pigs for the first time in 1801. There was only one class: for fat pigs up to six months old. The pigs of Britain were only just beginning to form into more or less recognisable breeds, or rather types, based on the widespread Old English pig - a large, gaunt, bristly animal with hanging ears. Such developed types as there were tended to be known only very locally, but even in those early years of the 19th century there was a relatively stable type worthy of comment and already widespread far beyond the county from which it took its name: the **Berkshire** <Plate 2>.

Smithfield created a class for "Berkshire breeds" (note the plural) in 1878; two years later a separate class was added for the Large White, the Small White, the "Black breed" and any other distinct breed or crossbreed, and the Tamworth was allowed its own class rather than continuing to be considered as a Berkshire. In 1884 the National Pig Breeders Association was founded, originally recording the pedigrees of only Large White, Middle White and Tamworth, and by that year the white entries at Smithfield were expanding so fast that they were subdivided into Small, Middle and Large. Thus the classes remained for more than thirty years, with the addition of the Lincolnshire Curly-coated and, eventually, the Saddleback. The breeds of Britain had sorted themselves out into some sort of order at last by 1914.

In those 120 years or so, countless local types vanished or were "improved" beyond recognition to form new breeds, or were graded up and swallowed by dominant breeds like the Berkshire, the Small Black and the whites from Yorkshire. Numerous new breeds proved to be but passing fashions that disappeared almost as soon as they had been conceived; others changed their name so frequently that it was difficult to trace their origins at all; others simply adopted the name of the most popular, with no right to it at all; and some old favourites lingered on for many years, fighting a losing battle against the fat that had once been their breeders' pride and joy but which later greased the slippery slope to the pigs' extinction.

Gradually, though, the business of pig breeding became more methodical. By the 1920s pigs were moving out of the show ring and the cottager's back garden and on to the farms. This change accounted for a huge increase in pig numbers nationwide: pig breeding and pig raising was becoming an industry. Yet the whites had still not taken over - and it would not be until the 1950s that the Landrace would be seen in Britain, introduced from Sweden and released to farmers in 1953. The Large White was already widely used as a sire, and the swing to the whites was now unstoppable. Then in 1966 the curse of swine fever was lifted from the UK and the way was clear for the development of large-scale intensive units, to which the whites proved admirably suited. The reliable old coloured outdoor breeds were cast aside.

Today, the whites are dominant and most of the breeding sows are hybrids and crossbreds. Britain's pig industry is substantial and has become increasingly specialised, scientific, professional and intensive. In 1990, some 80% of all breeding sows in the country were on only 2,500 units - about 620,000 animals, an average of 247 sows per unit. In 1992, when the average herd size overall was 60 sows per farm, there were fewer than 13,000 farms with breeding pigs, which was a huge drop from the 110,000 in 1962, a year in which about 750,000 breeding sows were on 90,000 units and the average was 8 per herd. In the last thirty years, an average of 90 farmers a week have gone out of pig production.

In 1990, some 14 million pigs were slaughtered, producing some 943,000 tonnes of pig meat. Home consumption has remained remarkably stable during the last 30 years, at about 21kg per capita per annum, but the type of carcass has altered dramatically: backfat levels, for example, have halved to 12mm in the last thirty years. There have also been substantial advances in all aspects of production efficiency.

Many breeders now use artificial insemination to improve commercial performance. The history of AI is a recent one: it was first advocated in Russia in 1932 but did not become a practical reality until 1948, after considerable work in Japan. It was first used in the United Kingdom in 1956 - two years before Norway and Sweden, who were followed in the early 1960s by West Germany, France, Finland, Belgium and Denmark, and in the early 1970s by Austria and Switzerland.

One of the major factors in the national herd's improved performance has been the effect of the pig breeding companies which have developed during the last thirty years, and by 1987 more than 80% of pig farms were buying at least 60% of their boars from the companies, while 63% bought at least 75% of their replacement gilts from the same sources. And, in a huge change over that period, 91% of producers keep 75% of their herds as hybrid sows. Hybridisation has been the key to productivity.

But there is a backlash and in the 1990s the public increasingly voices its concern for animal welfare, which it perceives as being neglected in intensive systems. There is now a gentle swing towards outdoor rearing systems, or at least more extensive systems on straw. The Meat & Livestock Commission's 1991 *Pig Year Book* noted that the sample of herds with more than 300 sows showed a high proportion of outdoor herds and stated that it was believed the number of outdoor sows would continue to rise at the expense of more intensive systems. This has encouraged the pig breeding companies to alter some of their programmes and create types which will thrive in less intensive systems. It is perhaps ironic that just such a return to "open-air pig-keeping" was noted in about 1920.

History of British Breeds

The Old English hog gleaned what it could from medieval pasture and pannage, and needed a strong constitution and good long legs for its ranging. Self-sufficiency was more important than looks and it had flat sides, low shoulders, a narrow back, long snout, coarse bristles and coarse bones, and big slouch ears flopping down over its eyes. It was widespread, especially where there was still plenty of woodland for its foraging. It became the cottager's walking larder after the middle ages, recycling household scraps and other gleanings into fat bacon and dripping above all, and also ham and sausage meat, though being late maturing it could take a long time to do so. The emphasis on fat bacon and lard would be of great importance in shaping the breeds that developed from the 18th century onwards.

Even in the early decades of the 18th century there was plenty of regional variation in the pigs, their characteristics determined by a combination of environment, management and personal preferences. Some were half-wild scavengers in the forests and on the commons, often herded communally; others were cottage pigs; and others, the most favoured, fared well on byproducts from local dairy and arable farms. Every county had its own type and there were lop ears and prick ears, long bodies and short bodies, long legs and short legs, and colours ranging from the common isabelline yellowish-white to red and black, with a lot of mixtures and splodges and belts and spots in between. A thorough comb through the literature and the illustrations of the period merely confuses with its variety.

The Old English type illustrated in about 1780 was long in the head with a light jowl, a straight underline to the jaw, a slight brisket, and a hint of a crest of strong hairs along its back. It was a large and reasonably uniform animal with a straight facial profile, a long tapering snout, ears forward like horizontal blinkers, partly over the eyes, the back only slightly arched or even slightly dipped, quite reasonable hams, a good covering of hair and good, strong legs. In Professor Low's illustrations of domestic livestock (published 1842) this type was shown as black with a white belt, and many were black spotted or merely dirty white.

It is very tempting to classify breeds by their colours but that can be misleading, as the history of British breeds demonstrates - especially that of the Berkshire, which Low illustrated as a basically sandy red pig with random dark splodges, and white socks and tail tassel. It had all the elements of colour in the pig and could have been developed in almost any direction.

Colour is a superficial trait but it is one of the most obvious badges by which a breed is identified. As the 19th century progressed, there was a noticeable colour prejudice on a geographical basis: the counties in the northern half of England were largely populated with white pigs; the south seemed to prefer black or black-and-white; and in between there were regions where coloured pigs were common, in red-and-black, or black-and-white-and-sand, or variously spotted. The divisions were not hard and fast but the trends were marked and were still evident to some degree at the turn of the century.

The Old English lop-eared pig was typical of the Celtic type found all over northern Europe and offered the advantages of a large frame (useful for a bacon pig), hardiness and a certain prolificacy but it took 16 months or so to fatten. That might be tolerable for the self-sufficient cottager but the 18th and especially the 19th centuries saw a huge growth in the human population and a great surge into urban areas, where backyard pig keeping was not practical. These masses needed to be fed, and the Old English pig was much too slow for the job.

The Asian Influence

During the 18th century it was found that the introduction of Asian blood could reduce the age at slaughter to a mere 9 months or less, producing a much smaller carcass with delicate pork: early maturity was one of the great advantages of the Chinese and Siamese pigs. The other main influence was the Neapolitan, an Italian pig of the Iberian type with Asian blood, which contributed symmetry, good flavour, excellent mothering, an aptitude to fatten and a moderate size to counteract the extreme smallness of the Chinese. The general effect of these exotic introductions was to bring earlier maturity and quicker fattening (with plenty of fat and good pork), finer bones, finer skin and hair, smaller shorter carcasses, shorter heads, smaller prick ears and often dished faces, and a general air of refinement. James Long pinpointed the difference by saying that "high bred" pigs in his time had small ears (usually erect) and short heads, whereas the "common" pigs had very coarse and usually flopping ears and very long heads. The Asian brush, then, changed the whole appearance of what were called the "improved" pigs - such a "Chinese fever" developed that the Asian pigs (whether Chinese, Siamese or Neapolitan) found their way into most of the country's breeds, though they were less welcome in Cornwall and Wales, for example, and seem to have made little if any impression on the Tamworth of the midlands. Elsewhere, however, they certainly did make their mark, especially on some of the northern whites and on the Berkshire.

This was the first radical change in British pig breeding. The next would be the overwhelming influence of the Large White and the Landrace, and the third would be the development of the pig breeding companies in the 1960s.

Chinese

It is usually said that the first Chinese pigs were imported in the 1770s. In fact there had been much earlier importations on a smaller scale, and in 1732 there was an obscure reference to a "small wild Black, China or West Indian breed".

In his *Breeding and Management of Livestock* (1810), Richard Parkinson described seven varieties of Chinese pig, and he could well have been right - there are many different regional types in that large country. However, most writers settled for two: one larger and black, which was excellent for a bacon cross, and the other small and white for porkers. Usually the pigs imported direct from China were very small and were generally from the Canton region.

Parkinson claimed that the foreigners were delicate and difficult to rear, but at the turn of the century an entry in the *Annals of Agriculture* had said they were very hardy and could live on far less feed than most English pigs, and were rarely seen in poor condition or lean: they fattened well on amounts that could barely have kept other breeds alive. They were always claimed to be particularly docile, and tended to wear their fat like a thick layer of blubber under the skin.

Chinese pigs were often illustrated with varying degrees of exaggeration. Parkinson showed a grossly fat "Chinese hog" which was black, sway-backed, prick-eared, with a long tapering snout and with its belly touching the ground. R.W. Dickson, in his *Management of Livestock Cattle* (1822) illustrated two Chinese pigs: one was black, with a curled tail, and the other was white with black patches and a straight tail; both were prick-eared with tapered muzzles of medium length and only slightly dished profiles, and both were about half the size of an old English type, described as a Hampshire pig, drawn alongside for comparison. Andrew Henderson's *Practical Grazier* (1814) had a little sketch of an almost square white Chinese pig with a very dished and shortened face and short prick ears. Richardson (1846) showed a plump but quite long-bodied black Chinese with a low-slung belly, slightly dipped back, very short dished face, small prick ears, straight tail and very short legs. Other 19th century artists illustrated black-and-white Chinese pigs, typically white with a black head, white blaze down the muzzle, black patches on the rump, straight black tail, and a few black patches on shoulder and sides; they have short prick ears, short dished faces and short legs.

So period illustrations of the Chinese vary wildly. Some show the exaggerated fat, rotund type with a very squashed face. Others show a longer pig with small upright ears and a longish tapering snout and almost straight profile. Colours vary and include black, white, white patched with black, or blue-and-sandy. The blacks are illustrated most often, but the literature refers more often to a white Chinese with only occasional references to black or pied. Most were described as fine-boned, short-legged, sway-backed, light in the ham, with short erect ears. James Long referred to the Chinese in the present tense in *The Book of the Pig* (second revised edition 1906) and said that it was "remarkable for its fertility and for the rapidity with which it lays on flesh without increasing materially in offal or bone." He described it as short-headed with small erect ears, short legs, high and broad chine, wide jowl, very little hair, a pendulous belly, generally dark skin, with flesh "especially delicate and white," and commented: "There is no animal that comes to maturity so rapidly."

Is there a breed in China today which is the likely ancestor of these "improvers"? Consider first the **Cantonese**, as so many were imported from that area. The modern Cantonese <Plate 16> is typical of the Central Chinese type described in the Asian section, a group of black or pied pigs with small lop or semi-lop ears. Given artistic licence, Henderson's illustration looks something like the modern Cantonese except that the ears of his pig are much more erect, rather like those of the sway-backed, pot-bellied South China pigs that are also found all over IndoChina. As for dished faces, the most extreme examples are seen in the **Neijiang** of South West China and in the highly prolific **Taihu** group of the lower Changjiang (Yangtse) river basin.

The Chinese was not known in the UK after about 1860 (James Long had a good memory for his youth) - until it was reintroduced in the 1980s and is set to start another revolution in the pig breeding industry of the 1990s.

Siamese <Plate 19>

A three-year-old Siamese sow, imported from Singapore by Messrs Dugdale of Manchester, was painted by Shiels for Low's illustrations of domestic livestock, with a litter (by a halfbred Chinese boar) of interestingly mixed piglets. One has the colour of the modern Chinese **Jinhua** (a neat round black patch on the rump), others have more random black and white areas, another is wholly white, and the most interesting of all is a sandy piglet with small black spots sprinkled mainly over its back. They seem to be ideal porkers of the early-maturing type.

The sow herself is black, with short white socks on the hindlegs and white to the knees on the forelegs, and her udder is pink. She is long in the snout and slightly convex in profile, with medium-sized prick ears and a typical straight oriental tail. Her skin is wrinkled but her face looks quite clean.

The Siamese was described as quiet and gentle, with a cylindrical body of acceptable length, broad loins, smooth and rounded shoulders, and round, deep, thick hams. The deep body was well "ribbed up" and pleasingly rounded; the belly hung low, as the legs were short and fine; the tail, curled near the rump, was slender; the slender ears were short and erect (very like the modern Berkshire's); the black hair was soft, silky and thin; there were no bristles and the skin was fine and dark (sometimes described as of a rich copper colour, which gave the pig a bronzed look, or sometimes as "slate to plum"); the delicate white flesh was firm and very tender. The breed matured at 12-15 months and was very hardy, able to tolerate cold and heat quite happily.

This delightful pig probably first came to the United Kingdom as early as 1732. It was sometimes known as the Tonkey or Tunkey, after the Tonquin district in Indo-China from which it was imported. It also sneaked into the country during the 18th century in the guise of a Portuguese breed, and its slate skin colour was seen in the Neapolitan as well - some say that the latter was originally a Siamese cross anyway.

The pigs of Thailand (old Siam) seem to be of South China origins, possibly from the prick-eared, smooth-skinned, long-headed **Hainan** type, which today is a small or dwarf black pig with plenty of white markings. In western Malaysia a black type known as the South China Black takes the synonym Cantonese (just to complicate matters) and there is also a South China, which has a black head and back but white belly and legs. Of course, it also possible that the Siamese originated from Vietnam ...

Neapolitan <Plate 9>

There is a painting of "A Bacon Hog weighing 27 stone 3 pounds of Lord Western's Improved Neapolitan. Bred and Fatted by C. Steward. Killed 1848. Painted from Nature by R. Farmer, 1848." It shows a wholly black and possibly hairless curly-tailed animal with short prick ears and a right-angled profile, with a snout of medium length. It is easy to imagine it as a Berkshire, though it lacks the white points and its muzzle is longer.

Professor David Low said that the best Italian hogs were produced in the Duchy of Parma, home of the famous air-cured hams, and were larger than the Neapolitan, with an even greater aptitude for fattening and able to produce pork "equally white and delicate". His illustration of a Neapolitan boar and sow (belonging to the Rt Hon Earl Spencer and imported from Naples by Hon Captain Spencer) shows two light black, well shaped pigs with almost straight topline and underline, fairly large semi-erect ears projected forwards like a dog's, long tapering muzzles and slightly dished profiles. The boar's tusks are short but apparent; the sow seems to have only four pairs of teats, which suggests low prolificacy. There is something about the pair that reminds one of the Tamworth.

Long's engraving of a Neapolitan sow (2nd edition 1906) also shows only four pairs of teats. She is a wholly black animal with a long, tapering snout, fine ears carried horizontally forwards, a convex profile, strong-boned legs, and a straight topline. He says the breed was used with particular success to improve the old Black Essex and obliterated the latter's originally parti-coloured markings. His description of the Neapolitan is "entirely black, almost without hair, tolerably short in the face, and with small, erect ears, carried a little more forward than those of the Chinese. It is also short in the legs, long in the body, tolerably wide, and a remarkably easy animal to fatten, but it is not so prolific as the Chinese, and its constitution is much more delicate."

Richardson's picture of a Neapolitan (c1850) is of a barrel-shaped pig with a slightly dished face, a tapering snout of medium length, a short and wavy tail, strong-boned legs, and prick ears of medium size.

It was usually said that the Neapolitan, though not unlike the Siamese, had better hams and back; it was always black, completely free from bristles and almost hairless. The fine skin felt something like silk. The claim was made that the Neapolitan was directly descended from the ancient Roman type of pig and had been given a late 17th century boost by a black Chinese imported by the Italians to give local pigs better resistance to sunlight and heat.

Much of the credit for introducing the Neapolitan to English breeders goes to Lord Western (1767-1844) of Rivenhall, Essex. A life-long bachelor, he entered Parliament in 1790 and was MP for Malden; he became a leading promoter of the 1815 Corn Bill and saw himself as representing agricultural interests in the House. He was created Baron Western of Rivenhall in 1833, when he retired to improve his farms. A great traveller, he had a special interest in classical Rome and loved to collect marble busts, urns and other knick-knacks. It was during his Italian travels that he saw the black pigs and decided they were just what he needed for improving his Essex breed.

Writing to Earl Spencer, Lord Western said that the Neapolitan was "a breed of very peculiar and valuable qualities, the flavour of the meat being excellent, and the disposition to fatten on the smallest quantity of food unrivalled." He acquired a thoroughbred pair.

Actually they should never have been called Neapolitans. They were probably **Casertana** pigs which happened to have been purchased in Naples, erroneously described as the principal breeding centre for the Casertana. In the craze for Italian pigs that followed Lord Western's experiments, Casertana pigs were imported by many others in England: Lord Harborough crossed them with a Siena pig, Buckley of Normanton with a Warwick sow, Druce and Smallbones with Berkshires and so on. A similar type was brought in from Malta at one stage.

The modern Casertana has slate-black skin with no bristles but perhaps just a little hair on the head and neck; it has a straight profile, fairly short ears growing forwards, and, like several Italian pigs, it often has a pair of wattles dangling from the angle of the jaw. Many theories are given about its origins and most agree that it has Asian blood of some kind at some stage. It is now very rare.

The British Breeds

In the early 1970s Professor J.C. Bowman, then at the University of Reading, published a survey of current breeds in response to concerns which had been expressed about the rapid decrease in the number of UK breeds. It was the period in which the Rare Breeds Survival Trust was being formed to protect breeds in danger of extinction. Breeding nuclei of some of these had been established at Whipsnade Park several years earlier and transferred to the Royal Agricultural Society of England show ground at Stoneleigh and to the university's Sonning farm in 1969.

The survey, commenced in 1970, revealed that four pig breeds had become extinct in recent years and five other breeds were very low in total population, though it was likely that the survey had not located all that existed. No more have been lost since then, thanks to the co-ordinating efforts of the RBST, but today the majority of the British pig breeds remain rare and in need of conservation efforts. The indigenous breeds which exist today are as follows

Rare breeds:
- Berkshire
- British Lop
- Gloucestershire Old Spots
- Large Black
- Middle White
- Oxford Sandy-and-Black
- Tamworth

Other breeds:
- British Landrace
- British Saddleback
- Large White
- Welsh

Towards the end of the 18th century the Board of Agriculture instituted an ambitious and detailed county-by-county survey, each filling a large volume and describing rural life in general and agriculture in particular. Some authors dismissed their county's pigs in half a dozen lines as cottagers' animals not worthy of notice, but others gave descriptions of local types, some briefly generalised and others with much more interest in the subject. Pulling together these and many other sources, the following section attempts to be a resumé of English pigs in the late 18th and most of the 19th centuries. It should be noted, however, that breeds have frequently changed name, with different names for the same breed and also the same name for different breeds, as well as changing shape, colour and just about everything else.

The Coloured Pigs of the Midlands

The typical pig in the heart of England in the early 18th century was the coarse, large, lop-eared, fairly long bacon type. It was often parti-coloured - a spotted or patched mixture of sandy red, black and white, or simply "dark", like the smaller, more primitive types that had by then receded well away from cultivated areas.

In Warwickshire, for example, there was an old-fashioned and coarse-boned farmyard pig with heavy slouch ears, thick skin and coarse curly hair or stiff bristles forming its spotted coat. It was a hardy, very prolific and very large beast which, given plenty of time and adequate feeding, could produce a heavy carcass. It was still doing so to feed the growing urban population of Birmingham long after other pigs had been refined and improved into breeds rather than general types.

In Shropshire the pigs were sometimes white but more often a dark mixture of red and black, or occasionally brindled. They had very long slouch ears hanging over the cheeks, exceptionally long bodies, long snouts, short legs, and coarse, wiry coats. The Shropshire pigs, especially the whites, were of considerable renown: they were taken in large numbers to the dairying county of Cheshire, for example, by travelling pig jobbers (who also drove Welsh pigs) and were popular with distillers, as they could turn brewers' waste into pig meat. They were so favoured that any good, lop-eared white pig, wherever it might have been bred, came to be called a Shropshire. By the end of the 18th century, these pigs were being crossed with the major pig of the midlands - the Berkshire - and became increasingly a spotted type. An undated painting by W. Gwynn shows a piebald Shropshire with forward lop ears and a wavy coat.

Cheshire lies on Shropshire's northern border and here they bought large numbers of black, black-spotted and red-and-black animals from Shropshire and Wales (where most of the pigs were yellowish or black-and-white spotted). So far as Cheshire had a pig of its own, it was very large, loose-skinned, big-headed with long hanging ears, long in the body with deep flat sides, and was blue-and-white, black-and-white or white. By the mid 19th century they were crossing them with the Berkshire or with "Manchester" (Yorkshire) boars: eventually Cheshire had no breed it could call its own but a lot of crossbreds. The pigs of Herefordshire, south of Shropshire, were a variety of the Shropshire type but short, with less bone, lighter head, and with slightly smaller, thinner, more pointed lop ears. Their colour was described vaguely as "light", and by 1825 some of them were a patchy red-and-white. The Herefordshire was illustrated in Loudon's *Encyclopaedia of Agriculture* published that year.

To the east of Shropshire is Staffordshire, and Pitt's county report to the Board of Agriculture in 1796 said that the local pigs were whole coloured or spotted, either prick-eared or lop-eared, and generally divided into two simple types: a large slouch-eared and a smaller or dwarf, with most pigs a cross between the two. An engraving in Pitt's report was taken from an anonymous painting of a spherical pig with forward lop ears over its eyes, a straight snout of medium length, and a dark coat - more black (or perhaps red) with lighter areas of sand or white (the paint has probably discoloured over the year). The pig belonged to Mr Dyott of Freeford Manor, Lichfield, and weighed more than 800 pounds at 2½ years old. The most interesting pig in Staffordshire was the Tamworth, at that stage a red-and-black animal well suited to the areas of woodland that were still widespread, but more of this later.

The old **Berkshire** was a variable type of pig, especially in colour, but it had long been the best in England, though it did not become uniform enough to be called a breed until the mid 19th century. Marshall (1780), surveying several counties, said that a black-and-white Berkshire was widespread and one of the commonest pigs in Devon, Gloucestershire and Norfolk, while a black-and-sandy Berkshire was popular in Yorkshire's Pickering Vale. Young claimed that it was also in Ireland before 1780, by which time it had already become finer boned and shorter bodied, with excellent streaky bacon. The type, originally bred around Wantage, was widespread before the end of the century. Culley (1794) described it as "reddish-brown with black spots", and said the pigs had "large ears hanging down over their eyes", were "short-legged, small-boned" and "exceedingly inclined to make rapidly fat." There were Berkshires, he said, in every shire and also in Scotland. Parkinson

(1810) illustrated a piebald Berkshire with a straight profile and prick ears; Henderson (1814) showed it with ears over the eyes; Dickson (1822) showed a prick-eared, long-snouted black Berkshire splattered with white.

In 1825 it was described as: "Long and crooked snouted, the muzzle turning upwards; the ears large, heavy, and inclined to be pendulous; the body long and thick, but not deep; the legs short, the bone large, and the size very great."

Lord Barrington was one of the major improvers in the 1820s and 1830s, and his pigs (like many other improved Berkshires) became smaller as the process continued, until the Improved Berkshire was no longer a large long lop but a shorter, medium-length, prick-eared pig. The improvements caused a Berkshire fever, especially in the midlands and the south, and in 1832 the fever spread across the Atlantic with the first export of the breed to the United States. In fact the old unimproved Berkshires had been imported there before 1800.

Harris, in his *Book of the Pig* (1870), produced four engravings to show how the Berkshire began to change under the Asian influence. Youatt (1847) called it a large breed and gave the colouring as "black-and-white and sandy-spotted", or "sandy or whitish-brown, spotted regularly with dark brown or black spots" and with no bristles. Low (1842) published Shiels's painting of a reddish-tawny Berkshire with a few black splodges (almost like tiger-striping), white socks and tail tassel, erect ears and straight profile, which had been bred by a Mr Loud of Warwickshire. It had changed a lot since the old type with large pendulous ears hanging over the eyes but it still had the sandy-red and black colouring, though its famous "white points" were emerging. It would continue to throw frequent examples of black with red or sandy areas in its litters even when the improved Berkshire's colour had been fixed as black with white points; and rusty-coloured spots were still seen during the 1920s. In America a Red Berkshire was deliberately developed.

Most of the 19th century pictures show the Berkshire with upright ears and a fairly straight profile. The shape of the Berkshire's face has been subjected to changing tastes over the years and it became very dished at certain stages. Fanciers, with the show ring in mind, liked the snub-nosed, dish-faced look and thought it reflected high breeding, and it was the fanciers who developed those six white points as well.

The facial dishing was the result of Asian blood from one source or another. There have been arguments about whether the already well known Berkshire was subsequently improved with the Chinese, or with the Siamese, or with the Neapolitan. An interesting case was made in favour of the Siamese because of the shared characteristic of white socks and because of the overall slate-to-plum colour (rich plum was favoured by many Berkshire breeders in the 19th century) and similarity to the Berkshire's new prick ears.

The Americans were the first to have a breed society for the Berkshire, in 1875. They did not mind a touch of white on an ear or a spot of copper or bronze elsewhere: they did not think these implied any impurity but, rather, reflected the breed's original colours. In fact some of the old Berkshires made a valuable contribution to the development of some of America's early red hogs. Some of the English breeders, however, became very agitated about colour. Some did not object to a few red or white hairs; others deliberately blackened their pigs before they dared to put them into the show ring. Too many discarded any animal that showed even a hint of red or did not have the trademark white points (face, tail tassel and four feet), which meant that they also discarded potentially good genetic qualities.

The Berkshire became everyone's pig, widely used to improve other breeds and produce crosses for slaughter. It had already had its reputation damaged during the century by claimants who had no right to its name. A British breed society was formed in 1883/4 and by about 1890 the Berkshire had become a show pig, much too fat for the butchers and bacon-curers: it had lost a great deal of its former size during the second half of the century and the earlier practical, lengthy, broad and well-haired pig became fashionably short-bodied, smaller, short-snouted - pretty in the eyes of the fanciers but "as remarkable for its fat as the old Berkshire was for its proportion of lean." Prizes were being given to overfed fat young pigs as a sign of the early maturity that was considered so desirable. There was also the problem of its dark skin, disliked by pork butchers, though it was still primarily a baconer.

And so it began a slow decline in popularity, but not before it had been exported to many countries and set its indelible mark on many foreign breeds. Today it is a rare breed in its own country and has been through a long period of being considered too fat for modern tastes. What a shame that, back in 1890, the show-loving breeders had not heeded the butchers. What a shame, too, that they had all overlooked the Berkshire's perfectly lean cousin, the Tamworth.

It could have been a different story. An 1895 manuscript in the public library in Tamworth, Staffordshire, refers to an 1800 illustration of a **Tamworth** pig bred by John Bamford of Glascote Hall. This animal's external characteristics were "much the same in the shape of the head and general form as at present but the ears were more slouched and the colour white with black spots instead of the golden red that characterises the breed today." In fact that old picture shows a large pig with a light sandy rather than white background, with black spots. Clearly the Tamworth of the period did not necessarily have pricked ears or a plain red coat as it does today - if it was indeed a Tamworth.

The old Tamworth was usually a red-and-black pig, its colouring very like that in Low's illustration of the Berkshire, and in many other respects similar to the old Berkshire before its brush with the Asian pigs. The Tamworth did not go through the intensive improvement of the Berkshire: it retained its inherent leanness and hardiness. And while the Berkshires were bred away from their redness, the Tamworths were bred away from the black, though for a long time it was also known as the Grizzly or the Mahogany pig.

In 1799 the Tamworth was described as "spotted red and brown", of great size, with small ears, short legs, very broad sides, and only worth rearing if there was abundant food, else it would not thrive. Early in the 19th century it was being extensively bred in several midland counties as a woodland herd pig but it waited a long time to come into its own in the 1870s, when there was a demand for a bacon pig, and for a decade from 1877 it was given the "improving" treatment.

Not that it had much effect. James Long quotes a 19th century breeder who described the Tamworth as "a large, coarse, leggy pig, with a straight and thinly-set coat, and a dark chestnut-coloured skin, more or less spotted with black", with a long, tapering, wedge-shaped face and a tail "never curled". It had two major faults in the eyes of this breeder: it could jump over or through or dig under any fence ever invented, and it was "too prolific by half" - a fault because "his stock increased too fast, and that the longer he fed them, the further they ran into debt." Yet it was claimed to be an excellent breed!

It remained lean, very long snouted and a very dark red: older animals were almost black. In 1857 W.C.L. Martin, describing the way in which the Berkshire had spread all over England, said that Staffordshire could boast a strain from the progeny of "the Tamworth boar"; and William Youatt (1847) said "Berkshires" had been reared in various parts of England and that "some of the very best have come from Staffordshire, from the progeny of the celebrated Tamworth boar." It seems, then, that at this stage the Tamworth and the Berkshire were still similar and closely linked.

By 1860, however, the Tamworth or Staffordshire pig was going out of favour locally because of its "want of aptitude to fatten". On the other hand, many practical pigmen delighted in a Tamworth/Berkshire cross, which was said to produce the most profitable bacon pigs in the country, the Berkshire lending its Asian heritage of a better tendency to feed and earlier maturity. The cross litters tended to produce, not a mix of the two, but some wholly Berkshire in colour and some wholly Tamworth, and any second generation from the cross was hopelessly disparate, with a completely random collection of sizes, conformations and colours.

Still, in 1876 the Tamworth was alloted its own breed class at the Birmingham Show (it had been represented there since the first show in 1848) and in the 1880s Tamworths and Berkshires far outnumbered the white pigs at the show. At the 1883 Royal, held at York, the red Tamworths were mocked by northerners as "wild" pigs. They did well at subsequent shows, especially at Windsor in 1889, after which the breed began to spread all over England and south Wales - and eventually overseas, where its colour was appreciated in warmer climates and in cold. In 1882 Tamworths had been exported to the United States for the first time, and six years later they went to Canada as baconers - they proved particularly popular in Canada for their hardiness in cold weather but were never very numerous in the USA. Canadian Tamworths returned to England in the 1930s for a change of blood lines and to improve litter averages.

By the 1890s the colour of the Tamworth had softened; the skin was flesh coloured, with no black (the black spots had been eliminated in theory by 1880) and the hair was golden-red or clear sandy, though some claimed the latter indicated a white cross and that only the old deep red proved purity. (In the 20th century it was indeed crossed with Large White to keep its skin pale, whereas in Canada it often had black skin areas, either from the original red-and-black colouring or perhaps from crossing with the Berkshire.) That redness has been a point of much speculation by writers who have sought many a romantic ancestor for the breed - and for the Duroc in America, which is of a similar colour. The main sources considered have been Barbados, India or Ireland for the Tamworth, and for the Duroc from West Africa (Guinea), Spain and Portugal. Consider the theories:

(1) That in about 1812 Sir Robert Peel (at the time Secretary for the English Crown to Ireland) brought home some Irish pigs, probably descended from the **Irish Grazier**, to his Fazeley estate at Tamworth, Staffordshire, and that he kept the type pure until his death in 1850, by which time it was called the Tamworth. Sir Robert's great great granddaughter, Mrs Ann Petch, who has carried on the family tradition of top quality pig breeding, says that it had always been understood within the family that Sir Robert used a West Indies boar to form the Tamworth - he certainly had business in that part of the world.

(2) That Sir Francis Lawley, then of Middleton Hall, Tamworth, some three miles from Fazeley, imported from India a jungle pig, which was the foundation boar responsible for fixing the Tamworth's golden or chestnut colour. In 1814 this boar was presented to a farmer at nearby Glascote and became much in demand as a sire. (At the time it was all the rage for English in India to send young jungle pigs home as gifts to their friends. However, jungle pigs - the wild species *Sus scrofa cristatus* - are similar in colour to the fuscous European Wild Boar.)

(3) That in about 1750 a red, or red spotted with black, pig was imported from Barbados; it was used for breeding at Axford, near the Wiltshire town of Marlborough (a long way from Tamworth) and gave rise to a type called the Axford which persisted for many decades. By the 1930s, it is said, its name had been corrupted to "Oxford" but it still existed in crosses with the Berkshire. (The local Wiltshire pigs of the late 18th century were long in body, rising in rump, light in colour, with pointed ears of medium size.)

The Duroc by comparison is said to have originated from a combination of the Jersey Red (initially from Spain) and the finer red or sandy Duroc of Saratoga County, New York, said to have come from an *English* importation in about 1820 of a red boar and sow.

There was also in America the red or sandy Guinea hog, presumed to have been transported there from West Africa on slave ships. The American writer Coburn (1909) said he had been unable to find any domestic red hog in any country where the slave trade did not exist but that it *was* found in almost every country "where the captured Guinea negro slaves were landed". He also referred to a red or sandy Portuguese hog known in several eastern states before the Civil War. There had apparently been red and sandy pigs in the old eastern colonies right from the earliest days anyway, of unspecified origin.

The Guinea pig was described by Youatt as large in size, square in form, with short smooth shiny bristles, and it was known *in England* in 1767, if not earlier. The domestic and feral pigs of West Africa are descended from Portuguese pigs; the modern Alentejana of Portugal, for example, is a red breed, as is Spain's Extremadura Red, both being of the Iberian type which, some say, has Chinese blood. In the late 17th century, John Evelyn in England had a Portuguese pig said to have Chinese origins.

Christopher Columbus brought eight pigs with him in 1493 when he crossed the Atlantic from Portugal. They soon became feral and, with various others dropped off here and there by various navigators and explorers from Portugal and Spain, they rapidly populated the Spanish Indies, spreading in due course to mainland America.

Taking all those random ideas together, the Barbados-born Axford was probably of Portuguese descent but there seems to be no absolute proof that the Tamworth's colour came from an exotic source.

Colour changes apart, the Tamworth resolutely kept its long head and long straight snout with only the faintest dish to the face, its fairly long neck that gave it a racy look, and a straight back that was long in comparison with that of the Berkshire. It *looked* like bacon - indeed it had been acknowledged as a producer of top quality lean bacon in the 1830s - and it also had good enough hams. Sir Oswald Mosley had a herd of Tamworths early in the 1920s, when the breed was probably at the peak of its popularity as a baconer, though by the 1930s the numbers were dropping.

It was (and remains) an essentially active pig, capable of looking after itself and "fit to jump a five-barred gate" in search of acorns. Lean, hardy, vigorous and prolific, it was a practical farmer's pig, even if it did take a while to fatten, though early in the 19th century the farmers of Warwickshire had considered that the Tamworth could "grow into a sovereign quicker than any other pig". It was always a favourite at the Birmingham show, where on one occasion the Mayor was somewhat surprised when a party of foreigners he was escorting showed their disapproval of the magnificent improved Berkshires and whites but were full of admiration for the Tamworth - because of its legs. They valued its potential for walking itself several miles to market, as pigs still did until recent years in parts of Italy, for example, and in America and Australia. But perhaps it was that very ability and inclination to wander that prevented the energetic Tamworth from putting on weight as fast as its more docile and lazy improved relatives.

The Tamworth continued to be long-snouted and it was also prolific: 10-15 in a litter was common and the mother, who could breed very early, reared them well to produce fine-grained streaky bacon in properly long, deep carcasses, and splendid hams. It was improved by careful selection rather than by heavy outcrossing over the years. Yet it never became as widespread in its own country as some other breeds, though it was much appreciated overseas. One problem in the United Kingdom was that, early in the 20th century, it lost that valuable prolificacy and some of its hardiness, possibly from inbreeding. By 1943 the NPBA herdbook contained only 26 boars and 84 sows of the breed, and today it is very much a rare breed in its homeland.

That mystery "Axford" pig has been given some other imaginary roles. Its name is so similar to "Oxford" that there is bound to be confusion. The county of Oxfordshire lies immediately to the north of Berkshire, and is separated from Staffordshire by Warwickshire, home of the old-fashioned white or spotted farmyard type of pig. The pigs of Oxfordshire were sometimes described as a variety of the Warwickshire, mixed with small porky types of the Berkshire kind.

There was a good dairy industry in Oxfordshire, and where there were dairy farms there were always pigs to be fattened on whey and other byproducts. The old type of so-called **Oxford Dairy** pig was like the neighbouring Berkshire - lop ears, colour and all - but in 1837 the Marquis of Blandford (later Duke of Marlborough) imported two Neapolitan boars, which were used with Berkshire sows (some of them already with Chinese blood) by different breeders to create two different lines of jet-black pigs. The lines came under the same owner (Druce of Eynsham) who then used improved Essex boars on them and created the **Improved Oxford** - black, of fair size, with a fair quantity of hair, very prolific, good mothers and good sucklers. Druce also used black Suffolk boars; in fact, he would use any good black breed to increase the lean meat. The progeny, raised on dairyfarm byproducts, went in some quantity as pork for Oxford University.

Youatt describes the Oxfordshire pig as black-and-white spotted, found in considerable numbers in Oxfordshire, Northamptonshire and Leicestershire. It was very hardy, reasonably prolific and a great favourite with agricultural labourers and cottagers "to consume the garden and house waste during the summer, and then to be fattened in the autumn on the corn gleaned in the harvest fields." This popular animal was often known as the "plum pudding" pig because of its spottiness, and the background was often more sandy than white. Some claimed that the sandiness originated from a Tamworth/Neapolitan cross, or a Tamworth crossed with black-spotted pigs that had Neapolitan blood, or perhaps with the famous improver Robert Bakewell's so-called White Berkshire. Sanders Spencer, in 1905, said that at the end of the 19th century there had been attempts to classify the type as a county breed and also to establish classes for it as such at the county's shows, but that most of the prize winners had actually been spotted crosses, either a Tamworth/Berkshire first cross or selected coloured offspring from a Large White and a spotted pig of some kind. It was noticeable that the Tamworth/ Berkshire cross was strikingly similar in colour to the old spotted Berkshire: some writers described the original Berkshire as the "black and white and sand spotted pig of the midlands", and in the 1850s Youatt said that "cross breeds of the Berkshire strain" around Henley-on-Thames, in Oxfordshire, were known as the "New Oxford" breed and that they were sandy, black and white.

The spotted pigs were found all over the midlands, whether as "genuine" spotted Oxfords or as Tamworth/Berkshire crosses, and were further crossed to either Berkshire or Tamworth, in the former case becoming blacker and in the latter rustier.

The career of the pig that came to be called the **Oxford Sandy-and-Black** has been as patchy as its coat colour ever since. It seems to be very closely linked with the old Berkshires and Tamworths, regardless of whether it diverged from them as a breed in its own right or was the result of crosses between them or between either of them with other breeds. (Or was it even an Axford/Berkshire cross?)

The Oxford Sandy-and-Black, or OSB, has at least twice reached a crisis point when numbers were so low that extinction seemed inevitable. Unfortunately for the integrity of the breed, it did not have a breed society active enough to fix its colour and form more precisely; it never had a herdbook, nor were most of its breeders licensing their boars during the period in which licensing regulations were in force. In the 1960s it seemed that the only true OSBs were two or three sows, and one young boar which subsequently died. The last licensed boar had been registered back in 1947 and the Rare Breeds Survival Trust, when considering which breeds it should seek to help in the 1970s, decided that the OSB could not be recognised.

There was the added problem of the "war of

the ears". The 1950s OSB carried its ears horizontally, or lower, in a semi-lop style like that of many other pigs, for example in Sussex and Hampshire. The false OSB from the Tamworth/ Berkshire cross in later years naturally had prick ears like both its parents, and many assumed this to be a correct characteristic of the breed - so much so that when efforts were being made to revive it, some breeders deliberately discarded all but prick-eared offspring.

There was also a problem about the unfixed colour. The background "sandy" varied through sandy beige, light apricot, rich orange and deep rust; the degree of black spotting ranged from a little to almost total cover, even within the same litter. Frequently there were animals with pale to white feet, tail switch and face, which looked suspiciously like Berkshire trademarks. However, colour is a deceptive badge for a breed unless ruthlessly controlled. It is *type* that matters - and even that can change, so that the only certainty is in recorded pedigrees. And those have been lacking.

Sanders Spencer remarked in 1921 that "an attempt was made some years since to resuscitate the Oxfordshire Spotted pig but it was not a continued success". A new breed society for the Oxford Sandy-and-Black was formed in 1985, believing firmly that the original type persists, especially in its characteristic ear carriage. The 1950s pigs also had a "white tapir stripe" which ran down over the forehead to the snout - seen in photographs (now at the Museum of English Rural Life) taken at Mr Kilby's Chestnuts Farm, Mollington, Banbury, and Mr F.R. Roberts's Chadstone Lodge, Castle Ashby, Northampton, and above all in the photographs taken by John L. Jones in 1959 at the farm of Norman Bosely at Sarsden Lodge, Oxford, in which the sows have snouts as long as a Tamworth's.

The new breed society, appreciating the problem of lack of pedigrees, is determined to weed out any sign of prick-eared pigs, or any that produce black-and-white or plain red offspring, which would betray outside blood. The foundation herdbook registered 15 males and 67 females as breeding stock in 28 herds, which is a dangerously small number if inbreeding is to be avoided. But at least the OSB now has an active and determined society and at last has some formal breed standards as well.

Oxfordshire borders the county of Gloucestershire and it is sometimes suggested that the pigs of the latter also contributed to the OSB. It is a fair assumption: the Berkshire, Tamworth, OSB and Gloucestershire pigs probably shared their origins anyway, diversifying to a greater or lesser extent in the 18th and 19th centuries, particularly with the Chinese and other crosses. It has also been suggested that the original Gloucester pigs came from Devon.

The old Gloucester was typical of the widespread Old English type - large, gaunt, long-legged, hardy and prolific, and dirty white in colour, with a pair of wattles dangling from its jaw. This general description was still applied in the mid 19th century by Richardson, Youatt and others but the Gloucester was apparently dying out by then. It was an ordinary farmer's pig and no one bothered to remark much upon it, or try to "improve" it, or turn it into a breed, and its territory had been relentlessly invaded by the Berkshire since the 1770s.

Today the pig associated with Gloucestershire is a white lop with a few black spots, not unlike the so-called Staffordshire sow belonging to William Pitt of Pendeford and illustrated in 1796, when it was described as white or spotted, large-bodied and lop-eared. The question that puzzles the GOS Pig Breeders Club today is: where and when did their **Gloucester Old Spots** get its characteristic spots?

In 1989 the Royal Agricultural Society of England arranged a major art exhibition in London and among the paintings were two said to be of Gloucester Old Spots in the 19th century. One, by an unknown artist c.1840, shows a white sow with a few random black spots and with ears forwards above the eyes (which are visible); her piglets are prick-eared. The other, by Stephen Jenner (1796-1881) shows what looks more like the old Oxford Dairy pig - light coloured with darker patches rather than spots, and with semi-lop ears.

But there is a mysterious gap in the literature and the link between the dirty white Old Gloucester and the later spotted pig seems to be missing - except for one physical feature recently reported by Richard H.L. Lutwyche. Charles Martell, a Gloucestershire cheese-maker, told him of the memories of an old man of the county who said that the way to recognise a true Gloucester Old Spots was to feel two lumps around the jowl. Lutwyche's suggestion is that these might be the remnants of the wattles of the old breed. However, the old pigs of Yorkshire were once wattled, too, and others.

The GOS had a more secretive past than most of the other breeds in this group, until just before the First World War. In 1913 the Board of Agriculture announced a boar licensing scheme, which meant that nonlicensed breeds would soon vanish. A breed society was rapidly formed for the GOS and a herdbook started with a nucleus of 300 selected females and the best boars that could be found among 2,000 pigs inspected in the West Country. The initial aim of this Gloucester Old Spots Breed Society seems to have been merely to rescue a "heritage" breed in danger of quietly fading.

Then it was discovered that the GOS actually had some very useful qualities. Its bacon was as good as that of the Large White, its hams were heavier, and it was exceptionally prolific, averaging 14-15 per litter and quite capable of rearing 16 unaided - one sow produced 23 in a single litter, and reared them all, with the help of a foster. From the pig keeper's point of view, the sows had the added bonus of being docile and ready grazers, rather than rooters. They were very hardy and weatherproof, too, not softened by Chinese blood.

And then began an amazing public relations exercise, promoting the GOS as a baconer unspoiled by overselection. Soon the GOS was being exported and over the years it has gone to Hungary, Italy, Sweden, Africa, the British Virgin Islands (to upgrade local Caribbean pigs), Australia, and to America, where it contributed to the experimental Minnesota No. 3 and to the improvement of the "Spotted" type of Poland China. (Like the Berkshire, incidentally, it crosses with white breeds to produce all-white litters.) It also won its "orchard pig" title: a certain Kent orchard owner claimed that the GOS's manure improved the colour of his apples.

Seven volumes later there were 7,000 entries in the herdbook. Any spotted pig would do, and that began an equally rapid descent: far too many had been kept on indiscriminately for breeding. By the end of the Great War, the GOS was fetching ridiculously high prices and continued to boom through the 1920s and into the 1930s, and then collapsed.

In 1949 only 34 boars were registered; in 1955 it was only 27; and only 13 in 1974, when the Rare Breeds Survival Trust stepped in to help. It has changed in some respects during the 20th century: it is now lighter in the bone, for example, and it has become much less spotty. In the 1920s and 1930s some animals were more black than white but today breeders prefer as much white as possible (to avoid arguments with butchers) and allow only one or two small spots as a mark of the breed.

The Blacks and Saddlebacks of the South of England

The first volume of the NPBA herdbook published in 1885 included a section for "the Blacks", all of which were bred in the southern part of the country.

Like the midlands, the southern counties seemed to favour coloured pigs, especially solid black, or black-and-white belted (a pattern which is in effect a more formal grouping of black spotting on white). These two major colour types are represented today by two lop-eared breed groups: the **Large Black** <Plate 2>and the **British Saddleback** <Plate 2>. Both are amalgamations of similarly coloured breeds from the western counties with others of different origins from the eastern. There is also the modern **British Lop** <PLate 3>, defiantly white but otherwise not unlike the Large Black.

Samuel Sidney, writing in the 1860s, stated: "Black pigs and their crosses occupy almost exclusively the counties of Berkshire, Hampshire, Wiltshire, Dorsetshire, Devonshire, and Somersetshire. Sussex has a black county breed, and in Essex a black-and-white pig has become all black. In the Western counties, the prejudice against a white pig is nearly as strong as against a black one in Yorkshire. In Devonshire, white pigs are supposed to be more subject to blistering from the sun when pasturing in the fields." He then dismissed all black or black-and-white pigs except the improved Berkshire and improved Essex, while briefly mentioning that "Hampshire has an ancient, coarse, and useful breed of black pigs. They are inferior to Berkshire, and not in the same refined class as Essex, therefore not worth taking from their native county."

The prejudice in favour of black was perhaps justified when the big black pigs of the south west found much favour in warmer climates overseas, where they are still often known as the **Cornwall** breed. The original Cornish pigs were large, rough types with flat sides, heavy shoulders and long legs; they were described in the 18th century as "wolf-shaped". They had long pendulous ears; they were robust and prolific, and seemed to grow quickly when young. It is possible that they were of French origin (for example, Craonnais or Normand) though there is no documentary proof of such imports, and their type was also common in Wales. The type divided at some point into an old Welsh breed, a white English lop and an all-black - a colour apparently not known in the UK before the arrival of the Neapolitan and the Siamese.

There is a whimsical tale that during the 18th century a "slow boat from China" docked at Plymouth and unloaded a few black Asian pigs which had managed to escape the on-voyage pork barrel, and that some local Cornish farmers simply took a liking to them and rounded them up. Even more apocryphally, it so happened that a sister ship simultaneously docked in London, where some East Anglian farmers eagerly acquired similar black pigs, and so, in due course, would emerge today's **Large Black**, a breed which eventually drew together these two separate strands in western and eastern England, both with similar Chinese origins.

In contrast to that tale, the Large Black herdbook for 1929 claimed firmly (as breed societies are wont to do): "Undoubtedly the Large Black is one of the oldest breeds of pig in this country, if not in the whole world." An editorial then proceeded to trace the breed's history in the vaguest of terms, remarking that "Eastern pigs" found their way "to our shores, and with our equable climate and good pasture a small nucleus, in the hands of skillful breeders, laid the foundation" of what would become the Large Black. Yet the editorial continued by saying that a prominent breeder had traced the breed back to "the Old English Hog of the sixteenth and seventeenth centuries, and then on to the year 1807, which may be taken as the date of the origin of the modern type of Large Black Pig. Of them Parkinson wrote in 1810: 'They are distinguished by their gigantic size, they are the largest of the kind I have ever seen ... their heads are large, with very long ears hanging down on each side of the face, so that they can scarcely see their way.'"

Without explaining the details, the editorial implied that somehow the typical large, long-bodied lop-ear of the old English type, which was usually dirty white and spotted, became a solid black pig with the help of "eastern" influence. Some have suggested that the Large Black's coppery skin reflects the influence of the all-black Neapolitan. The mention of a date of 1807 is not explained.

Charles Vancouver, reporting to the Board of Agriculture on the county of Devon (published 1808 but surveyed since the 1790s), said: "The native hog of this country grows to a large size, stands high upon its legs, lengthy, of a large and coarse bone, flat-sided, and in its store state seldom seen in anything like tolerable condition; but proper time being allowed, will commonly fat to six score* per quarter." It was even then being improved by crossing to "the Leicester boar" for shorter legs, better conformation and performance, and then to Chinese to reduce size and increase profitability so that, when 18 months old and "fattened to its frame", this three-way crossbred could weigh "from 16 to 20 score* per hog". Crosses between the native Devon pigs and either the Leicester or the Hampshire could double their weight in 12 weeks on steamed potatoes with pease-and-barley meal. The subsequent cross with the Chinese would fatten in two-thirds of the time, again nearly doubling its weight. Vancouver does not mention the colour of either the old native, the Chinese or the crosses.

Sidney, despite his derogatory dismissal of all black pigs except the improved Berkshire and Essex, admitted elsewhere (circa 1871): "Devonshire has an excellent breed of black pigs, which partake, for the most part, of the character of the improved Essex and Berkshire. The climate seems to require less hair than the northern and midland counties." Apparently the "original" Devon pigs were valued solely according to their length - length of body, length of ears, of nose, of tail and of hair ("the longer the better, without reference to quality or substance") - and were of no particular colour or character. Within the last forty years before Sidney made his comments, however, the pigs of Devon had been "improved perhaps more than any other stock, by judicious crosses and importations." These included the Essex (improved by Fisher Hobbs) and the Berkshire, and in some herds the result was black pigs with short faces, thick bodies, small bone, little hair, and prize-winning conformation. But in north Devon the original type remained: "They will jump a fence that would puzzle many horses and some hunters." On the whole, however, the pigs of Devon were by Sidney's time far above average, "the black pig being, perhaps, the only foreigner who has ever been cordially welcomed as a settler in that very exclusive county."

Sussex also had large, very long, black or partly black pigs with very little hair and large ears hanging over their eyes. They were slow to mature and for that reason were often crossed with Berkshire (or later Large White) for very good bacon. The Reverend Arthur Young, in his county report to the Board of Agriculture (published 1813, with surveys in the 1790s) said that the hogs of Sussex were all either descended from "the large Berkshire spotted breed" or from a cross between it and "a smaller black, or white breed."

Sanders Spencer, in the 1920s, remarked that in Sussex there was a local and distinct variety, of unclear origins, with a strong local reputation for hardiness, prolificacy and pork. He said that the colour was locally termed "black" but was in reality more of a blue or slate colour. It was a long-bodied pig with short legs, rather coarse bone and short of hair, and its pork "contained a large quantity of lean meat." However, "it does not carry itself well, nor can it make good its claim to much style," he said dismissively.

* "score": a locally variable unit of weight, usually 20 or 21 pounds.

Its colour, formation and character suggested to Spencer "a good deal of Neapolitan blood". Certainly an illustration published in R.W. Dickson's *Improved Live Stock and Cattle Management* (1822) of "Different Valuable Breeds" included a black Sussex (depicted with a white "English" and a very spotted Berkshire) whose form is strongly reminiscent of the Neapolitan: it had a long, tapering snout, more or less prick ears, "mischievous eyes", fine skin, long but fine hairs, a slightly wrinkled neck, clean jowl, a slight dip in the back, good hams, and a touch of white on one back foot - this sow is not of the big lop-eared Devon type at all.

The little hill village of Rudgwick in north west Sussex (my own village for ten years) had its own "breed" at one time, said to be very large, very hardy, very prolific and a good mother. Harris misspelled the type as "Rudywick" in quoting Sidney on Youatt, who had said the Rudgwick was one of England's oldest and largest breeds, producing lots of excellent meat but slow to fatten. Baxter, the Lewes publisher of a comprehensive tome on agriculture (third edition, 1834), said that these pigs weighed 80-110 stone (at 8 pounds to the stone*) and made an admirable cross with the "Woburn spotted boar, introduced by the late Duke of Bedford".

Youatt described the Sussex as black-and-white sheeted, interpreted as "black at one end and white at the other" rather than as belted, and thought that it might be a variety of Lord Western's Essex (which owed its improvement to the Neapolitan), though others claimed it to be of original stock, and Sidney (1860) said the Sussex was wholly black and had been instrumental in changing Lord Western's old sheeted Essex into a black pig; but Sidney did admit that people tended to confuse Sussex with Essex. At the beginning of the 19th century, Lord Sheffield, in Sussex, was not only trying to decide between "Mr Western's Essex" and "Mr Ashley's Leicestershire" but was also experimenting by crossing with "the best China, and also with the wild kind."

Thus the trail of the big black pigs continued across the southern counties, but probably from quite different origins. The long-bodied Sussex blacks were also present in Wiltshire (according to Youatt) and in east Kent. A 1911 agricultural report said that the "old English long black pig with drooping ears" was still common in Sussex and east Kent (where it was known as the Kentish Black) but that none of the old unmixed herds had been registered and the breed would therefore probably soon die out or merge with the Large Black breed. Photographs show a rather shorter type than the Large Black.

During the 1930s the Large Black breeders had to change their pigs to keep up with the Danes: the rather heavy jowl and shoulder became finer. At the time the favourite bacon pig was the Blue-and-White (Large White x Large Black). There was a prejudice among butchers about the "seedy cut" - little black specks when the belly is cut open, at the roots of the bristles - but Large Black breeders would maintain that there is no seedy cut if the pig is well bred, i.e. with a thin skin and fine silky hair, and that anyway there is hardly any hair on the belly. Later there was a prejudice against fat in the breed, and indeed it still has a higher proportion of fat to lean than, say, the Large White.

Looking back through the Large Black herdbooks over the years, its fall from favour shows up clearly. In 1924, when the Large Black's own herdbook had reached its 25th issue, there two large volumes for the breed and there were more than 2,000 members of the society. Thereafter the size of the herdbook began to shrink. Only 31 boars were registered in 1985, for example, and this splendid outdoor pig is now a rare breed.

There were also *small* black pigs in the south and south west. In Cornwall, there had been smaller and larger kinds of black in the 19th century but a bacon factory was established locally and the demand for small fat porkers dwindled in favour of the large baconers. The porkers had been similar to what became known as the **Small Black**, an improved type embracing the Black Essex and Black Suffolk, which effectively also embraced an improved type in Dorset.

The county of Dorset, in the heart of Thomas Hardy's Wessex, should have been pig country in that it was home to many dairy farms, and even boasts a parish called Toller Porcorum (between Dorchester and Yeovil). Yet in the mid 19th century Sidney said that it had no reputation as a pig-breeding county and that one of the greatest of its dairy farmers had said, "All I know is, that our breed of pigs is very bad." They were at the time mostly black-and-whites of the Berkshire type, though James Long said that Sussex's black pigs were "evidently of a similar type to what the Dorsets were before they were improved by the introduction of the Coate's strain."

John Coate of Hammoon (a few miles north west of Blandford Forum) became renowned for his **Improved Dorset** pigs. Coate said that in about the 1830s he had purchased "a boar and sow in Somersetshire, of a breed said to have been sent from Turkey. They resembled in some measure the wild boar, being short on the leg, with very long, wiry hair, black in colour, and

*"stone": a unit of weight varying locally and according to what was being weighed - The modern standard is 14 pounds to the stone, but for, say, wool the unit can equate with 24 pounds.

very inclined to fatten. I was led to believe it was a mixture between the wild boar and Neapolitan breeds. I crossed them with some Chinese I had, and by so doing, *both ways*, produced the animals I named, when first exhibited, the 'Dorset breed', although not properly; but they had, from their beauty, previously found their way into many farm-yards in the county. I had two distinct breeds to begin with which I kept pure a long time for crossing; but as both wore away, have used my own stock as far akin as possible, and have once or twice introduced fresh blood by getting a boar as much like my own as I could. I have tried crosses with other breeds, but not liking their offspring, got rid of them again... With all animals, the first or second cross is good; but if you ever get away from the pure breed, it requires years and great attention to regain it, as the cross often shows itself in colour or shape years after it has taken place, when you fancy you are quite safe."

In later years, Coate's son gave a slightly different version of the tale, saying that a very hairy wild-type sent from Turkey was put to a Chinese boar, and her gilts to a Neapolitan boar.

The so-called "Turkey" pig was probably that illustrated in Henderson's *The Practical Grazier* under the name of the Black Wire-haired, as a Chinese/Siamese cross. The Siamese, of course, was often called a Tonkey or Tunkey (from Tonquin) - which sounds a more likely origin than Turkey. The illustrated Black Wire-haired was slightly sway-backed, with short prick ears, a fairly short snout but an almost straight profile, and the general shape reminds one of a modified pot-bellied pig from Vietnam (there is the Tonquin link, after all) or, more whimsically, a small rhinoceros. Sidney, who was familiar with Coate's black pigs, said they clearly owed a great deal to Fisher Hobbs's improved Essex - "they carry the relationship plainly in their faces." But that Essex owed a lot to the Black Neapolitan, which had reputedly been a progenitor of the black wire-haired pig from "Turkey".*

The "Black Dorset", or Coate's Improved Dorset, was more of a slate colour than black. Long described it as having "a bluish tint that is not seen in any other variety" and it was closer to the Neapolitan than the eastern small blacks. Its almost hairless skin was smooth, fine and bluish or pink; its small upright ears were carried forwards; it was fine in bone, short-sided, easily fattened, early maturing and prolific. The long head was somewhat narrow between the ears (which is typical of many Italian pigs of the Iberian type), the snout of medium length and straight. The sows were gentle mothers and good sucklers.

Low made no mention of any Dorset pig in 1842, nor Youatt in 1847, though in 1844 there were Dorset pigs at the Royal Show. In 1883 the "Dorset" was listed as "rusty black".

Much later, Dorset produced a very different and good-looking pig which had only a short life as a breed. This was the **Dorset Gold Tip** <Plate 2>, originally from a Tamworth cross (probably with Berkshire, and with some GOS as well), and very handsome too. The basic colour was a light Tamworth red with black markings, and the bristles had characteristic golden tips which really brought the coat to life. It is interesting to note that the ears were semi-lop, and one wonders about the parentage. The early-maturing Dorset Gold Tip did well at the shows in the 1920s and 1930s but by the 1950s there was only one known breeder; in 1949 only two boars were registered, and in 1955 but one. It was included in an exhibition of all of Britain's pig breeds, carefully gleaned from various parts of the country for the Festival of Britain in 1951. With no breed society to support it, the glowing Gold Tip gradually faded away and was already extinct by the time the RBST undertook its breed surveys in the early 1970s.

Most Dorset pigs had been black-and-whites of the Berkshire type, but the "ancient" Dorset pig was said to have been blue - possibly the original Blue Boar of the inn signs. It might have been a loose description for black - like the slate colour of the Coate pig - but it might have linked with the Sussex pigs or with a breed which developed in due course in Somerset: a blue-and-white, often sheeted or belted. This was a long, deep pig looking broadly similar to the WessexSaddleback, with ears over its eyes and a dished face. There is a photograph of the breed in the 1909 edition of Youatt's *Complete Grazier*, which shows the Dowager-Duchess of Devonshire's sow, Compton Daily Bread. There were moves at one time to set up a herdbook for this well defined type, which was highly commended for growth and prolificacy, but it came to nothing. Pigs of similar colours and characteristics were said to have been found "in years gone by" in Cambridge and Essex.

That the Sussex was sometimes described as a saddleback suggests a connection with the neighbouring county of Hampshire, where lies the great New Forest. The Forest was once the huge protected hunting ground of kings and for several centuries it offered an ideal environment for large herds of domestic swine on pannage, foraging for acorns and beechmast under the trees. The New Forest was almost the only stretch of forest still under pannage on a large

*Incidentally, the English had a habit of referring to anything exotic as being "Turkey" - hence the name of a bird that originated from America and had nothing at all to do with the country of that name. A "Turkey merchant", for example, might deal in, say, spices - not Christmas poultry.

scale at the end of the 18th century.

Sidney was characteristically dismissive of Hampshire's pigs: "There are some very pretty things to be said about the herds of swine in the New Forest, but they have been said so often that they are scarcely worth repeating." As for the "county" animal, the Hampshire of his time was black, or black spotted with red like the old Berkshire; it was also about the size of the Berkshire, but coarser - less attention had been paid to its improvement, though some steps had been taken in that direction. Etchings from Loudon (1825) show a pig similar in type to the old Herefordshire, with lop ears falling forwards, a thick coarse coat with a ridge of dark bristles along the back, sturdy limbs, a snout of medium length (sharper than the contemporary Berkshire's, and the head longer) and a dangling tail. In the area of Andover and Basingstoke, the type was described as longer than the Berkshire in body and in neck, disposed to fatten to great weights, and usually white or spotted.

The New Forest pig of the mid 19th century was long in body and flat-sided, with a long head and sharp snout. It was usually dark spotted (sometimes wholly black) but plenty of white pigs roamed freely in the Forest as well.

The dark "Hampshire hog" (a term apparently also applied to men of the county) was a useful pig but suffered from the same deficiencies as the Berkshire before improvement: "a want of thickness through the shoulder" and a tendency to be a slow feeder. Although flatter in the sides and with a longer head and sharper snout, it was clearly just a local version of the old and widespread so-called Berkshire type. No doubt it was also closely related to the Sussex pigs, though it was higher on the leg and larger - closer perhaps to the large black pigs of the south west.

The Isle of Wight's pig was a better, deep-sided and black marked variety of the Hampshire. Gradually the county breed was improved by a combination of selection and probably the use of some improved Berkshires and Small Blacks, so that it became much more stylish, more compact and with a better coat. Similar combinations had been used to improve neighbouring Wiltshire's pigs, which had originally been long and white but had been extensively crossed during the 18th century with Chinese and Berkshire to form a darker pig, often spotted, and hardy and amenable. The Wiltshire and the Hampshire were sometimes described together as the "dark spotted domestic English breed", a term which could equally have applied to the old Berkshire and others.

The dark spotted forest pig in Hampshire might have been crossed with the neighbouring black Sussex to produce one of Britain's more famous pigs: the **Wessex Saddleback** <Plate 2>. There was a local black-and-white belted pig by the early 19th century, described by Youatt as long, able to grow fast to great weight and produce excellent bacon. It was, said Youatt, very similar to the Dorset pig and had been improved with the help of Berkshire, Chinese, Essex and White Suffolk, and in 1820 it had travelled across the Atlantic to the United States. Low's illustrations of 1840 included the belted "Old English Breed sow from the midland counties", well-haired, with a long dangling tail, good-sized ears (black on the outside, white inside) forward over the eyes like those of a Landrace, white face, white forelegs but black shoulders and nape, black back end and white hind socks and tassel. She's almost, but not quite, a saddleback.

In the 1930s the Pig Breeders Annual described the origin of the Wessex Saddleback as a cross of "two old English indigenous bacon pigs, the black breed of the New Forest and the Old English Sheeted breed, uninfluenced by the Chinese, brought together first in the Isle of Purbeck when the forest area ran through the Cranborne Chase."

A consignment of this sheeted "Hampshire" was exported to New York in 1825, followed by others shipped from Southampton over the next few years, to become the foundation of the breed now formally known as the **American Hampshire** <Plate 21>. F.D. Coburn, in *Swine in America* (1909), noted that "the breed known in England as Hampshire is, however, of a different type, being black." He did agree that the ancestors of the American Hampshire (known in its early days as the "Thin Rind" hog) were said to have been imported from Hampshire in England to Massachusetts, between 1820 and 1830, by a Boston ship owner called Mackay, though it was not clear whether the pigs were belted. It was not until 1904 that the Mackay or Thin-Rind became officially the American Hampshire "in deference to their supposed origin". There is the obvious implication that the pigs might have been shipped from a Hampshire port, not necessarily bred in the county. The "saddleback" pattern was by no means unusual in Britain: there are several illustrations of 18th century pigs tending towards it, perhaps with a white belt, or white with black rump and head, the colour spreading to various degrees.

In the Forest, free-ranging inevitably meant that different sorts of pig interbred. However, a family at Plaitford and one at Landford kept their sheeted pigs pure, and in 1917 W.J. Malden recognised the handfed herds as "being the last of the Old English bacon pigs left in existence" - they had been maintained pure for more than ninety years. It was these, and their local descendants, that became the foundation of the newly named Wessex breed. In 1918, worried about the type's future (many pigs of all native breeds had been slaughtered during the war to feed the masses), people interested in the old New Forest pigs met under Malden's chairmanship and founded a breed society. The breed had almost vanished during that war but was saved by a Wessex Saddleback pig society which "threw its net so wide so that no good pig should be missed" with the result that quite a few "misfits" were drawn into it as well and a considerable amount of weeding out by the new breed society was necessary. Bearing in mind all the time a baconer as standard, they looked for prolificacy and quick maturity, and made a particular point of rejecting pigs with heavy fore-ends and jowls.

From the start Lord Melchett was the patron of the Wessex Saddleback. Within 17 years of the formation of the breed society, its ardent members had spread the breed into Herefordshire, "western Wessex", Hertfordshire, Norfolk, Nottinghamshire, Yorkshire, Northumberland and all. Malden made a nice comment to Wessex breeders in advising them against straining too much after length: "A thick, meaty pig will win in the end; it will load-up with more lean. The Wessex is of medium size, full of quality, can make the best porker-baconer. Too much attention to length draws away from the forest character and tends to bring out such relics of a coarser breed as may remain. Elastic can be stretched but it is no stronger for it. The same applies to the pig."

The Pigs of Eastern England

While the Wessex was developing in Hampshire, another saddleback had been evolving in the eastern county of Essex and in due course it would be combined with the Wessex as the British Saddleback in the mid 1960s. At the same time a small black type was developed in the eastern counties, and this would eventually contribute to the western counties' large blacks. In both cases, the breeds of the east and those of the west came from quite different origins and were merged (not altogether willingly) on the basis of a shared colour or coat pattern - a somewhat arbitrary foundation for their marriages.

The old **Essex** pig, as elsewhere, was the coarse, strong, gaunt Old English type. By the early 19th century there was a parti-coloured local variety of the type which was said to be a restless beast and an enormous eater, capable of fattening if it was given endless amounts of feed and time.

An early improver was squire Western of Felix Hall. It was he who first imported the black Neapolitan pigs from Italy. He crossed his thoroughbred boar with the big Essex sows to create his **Neapolitan Essex** or **Essex Half-Black** (black at one end, white at the other), a refined animal with prick ears, thin skin, light bones, short hair and a broad, deep body with a straight topline. The illustrations of "Mr Western's half-blacks" in Arthur Young's *General View of the Agriculture of Essex* (1807) show its early development: the boar and sow are long and level in the body, with slender legs, long tapering muzzles, a little wrinkling of the skin under the neck, ears of a good size erect and quite hairy. However, they can hardly be described as half-blacks as they are almost entirely black, with tiny touches of white on the underside, snout tip, lower legs and tail tassel. In general appearance they are very similar to Earl Spencer's Neapolitan boar and sow in Low's illustrations published in 1845.

Western's breed did very well indeed in the show ring and soon became popular as it matured very early and fattened rapidly. Unfortunately, he inbred them to such an extent that the type deteriorated in size, muscle, constitution and fecundity, until finally it was "more ornamental than useful" by the time of his death in 1844.

Every other breeder in Essex had benefited from crossing the Neapolitan with the big, vigorous, hardy local sows. It sired an excellent hybrid but proved less profitable as a purebred in local circumstances. Then one of Western's tenants, Fisher Hobbes of Boxted Lodge, used his lordship's Neapolitan-Essex boars on his own "large, strong, hardy, black, and rather rough and coarse" Essex sows, and eventually established what would by 1840 become the famous **Improved Essex**. It was a small black pig (with perhaps a slight tinge of red at the tips of the ears) with small bones, early maturity and rapid growth to produce a heavy weight of the highest quality pork. To modern eyes, perhaps, Lord Western's original Neapolitans look better animals than Fisher Hobbes's very fat pigs but the Improved Essex was soon being used widely in many counties to improve other breeds. It also superseded the Neapolitans and Chinese as an improver in France, Germany and the United States.

Sidney, in 1830, had referred to the old Essex as

being "a parti-coloured animal; black, with white shoulders, nose and legs - in fact a sort of 'sheeted' pig, large, upright and coarse in bone." Sanders Spencer pointed out that there was still a "sheeted" black and white pig in Essex and Cambridgeshire - quick feeders, light-shouldered, prolific, and good mothers - but he knew of only a few specimens. The type was good for both pork and bacon, with a good length and well filled hams; the milky sows were docile and good mothers. This saddleback tended to have a wider white belt than the Wessex Saddleback and it also had white on its hind legs up to the ankle. For some reason, Spencer decided that it was a cross between the Berkshire and Large White.

During the 1920s, it was rumoured that the saddleback Essex had been given Italian blood - but not from the Neapolitan. This time it was said to be from the **Siena Belted** (*Cinta senese*) of Tuscany. Wessex breeders were quick to point out that the Siena was only used in the Essex (if at all), never in the Wessex Saddleback itself.

Both the **Wessex Saddleback** and the **Essex** (which simply used the county name, not adding "Saddleback" to it) became popular outdoor sows, and both found willing buyers overseas, especially the Wessex. By the 1940s the Wessex was the second most popular breed in the United Kingdom, though the Essex was never as common. By the 1960s, however, these two breeds of such different origins were dropping rapidly in number and it was decided to amalgamate them as one British Saddleback. It was a decision much resented by pure breeders on both sides and numbers continued to decline, especially of the Essex, for which the amalgamation was disastrous. There were attempts to breed the two old types separately but many disgruntled purists simply gave up their breeds or, especially in the case of the Essex, simply did not bother to register their herds. There is probably only one purebred Essex herd in the UK today, with four male lines and eleven female lines. The Wessex Saddleback has done better as a purebred: there are eight male lines and 24 female lines of the old type even now. There remain differences between the two: the Essex still has a finer skin and lighter coat, a finer bone structure and lighter jowl; it stands higher on the leg, is a little shorter in the body, and its tail is set lower, and it retains its distinctive four white legs and a wider saddle. The ears of the Wessex Saddleback tend to pitch forward more; its ham is broader and deeper to the hock, and it is deeper in the flank, stronger in bone and pasterns. Otherwise the two are broadly similar in qualities, and they are also on the verge of a comeback. As the public begin to bring pressure on producers to move away from intensive systems, the Saddleback sows are ready to return to the outdoor systems in which they perform so well.

Eastern England had other pigs than those of Essex. In Suffolk a Mr Crisp of Butley Abbey was, according to Sidney, "a sort of cosmopolitan breeder, a purchaser of the best pigs he can find of any colour. His most celebrated pigs are quite black." Mr Crisp stole the name of Suffolk for his blacks and also for his whites, regardless of their origins; the two, though of different colours, were similar in type but the black had more growth, while the white tended to develop curly or woolly coats. This **Black Suffolk** was quite a good little prick-eared pig, locally hardy, contented by nature, early maturing, very prolific (average 10-11 per litter but up to 15-16, and twice a year at that), small boned, with sweet juicy meat, but inclined to put on too much fat. It was a Small Black type worthy to be included under that name with the Black Essex.

The term **Small Black** came to include Coate's improved Dorsets and the small black Sussex pigs with the mischievous eyes as well as the improved Essex and Suffolk blacks, but there were differences. The former pair had a greater resemblance to the Neapolitan, with their ears pointing forwards, for example. For the sake of "purity", the eastern Small Black breeders rejected any hint of a red tinge on the skin (as denoting a cross, albeit perhaps very distant). The hair was also important: "If it is found in abundance, it generally indicates a cross with Berkshires of the purest blood, having plenty of fine hair, entirely free from that woolly appearance which is so often met with in white pigs." The head was short but not exaggeratedly so; the nose short, and slightly uptilted, the ears short and erect. The Small Blacks as a group did well for many years but gradually disappeared into the Large Black.

Crisp was a great salesman and his propaganda was so good that the Americans were convinced that his white **Suffolk** was England's leading breed. However good or bad it may have been, it was not a Suffolk pig but in reality a small white with its origins in Yorkshire. The old Suffolk local pig was indeed white, but nothing like Mr Crisp's short-headed, short-legged, fine-haired cylindrical pig. Like the old Essex, the old Suffolk had a long head, lots of coarse hair, flat sides and long legs, and was said to be a good baconer. There were a lot of characterless pigs in Suffolk, mostly crossed with the black Improved Essex, and there were also some very good whites of the Yorkshire-Cumberland type which had been brought into Suffolk and went thence to Prince Albert's farm, where they changed their name to Windsor.

The pigs of Norfolk were described as indescribable, "the result of the mixture of many breeds in a *hocus pocus* or *porcus* style." Like the neighbouring old Suffolk, the Norfolk tended to be flat-sided, with a coat of harsh strong hair, and it produced "lean, hard meat". It was eventually absorbed into what became the Large White. It had been a great breeder - too much so for some farmers. "If they would have three or four less, and better quality, it would pay better," said one wryly. According to Youatt, the only noted breeder in the county concentrated on the Improved Berkshire. However, the Earl of Leicester bred better pigs - he was the famous agriculturalist Thomas Coke of Holkham (1752-1842), who became the Earl of Leicester (of Holkham, rather than of Townshend) in 1837. One wonders whether "the Leicester boar" often used by other aristocratic pig breeders might have been a Holkham pig rather than from the county of Leicestershire.

Early in the 19th century, apparently, one W.K. Townsend of East Haven, Connecticut, imported from England (according to Towne and Wentworth) some **Norfolk Thin-Rind** pigs said to be black, spotted with white or even sporting a white belt, which were used in creating the **Improved Chester White** in Ohio. The name Thin-rind also crops up in the history of what later became known as the **American Hampshire** (a saddleback) but this may be pure coincidence - Norfolk is not mentioned in the latter connection.

The Cambridgeshire pigs were also of a coarse type. They had strong, round bones, slouch ears over the eyes, and coarse, curly hair. The thick skin was white with patches or spots of blue. They were bred for the local climate and were very hardy, prolific and capable of reaching a great size, giving a heavy weight of pork but taking a long time to do so. In due course the Fenland pig was crossed with Large (or Middle) White to improve its general qualities without losing prolificacy and robustness: it still produced enormous bacon carcasses but was earlier maturing. Its coarse meat was used for heavily salted, dried pork "bacon". No doubt it was closely related to the white curly-coated pigs of neighbouring Lincolnshire.

The Whites

"The colour is best," wrote Markham in 1638, "which is all in one place, as all white or all sandy ..." The pig keepers and butchers of the north and east of England agreed with him. From Birmingham and the Fens to Lancashire, Yorkshire and Cumberland, the local pigs were white, perhaps with a few spots. There was none of that fancy Berkshire for them, none of those blacks or black-and-reds, none of those piebald or sheeted pigs. Apart from the western fringes (Cheshire's mixtures and Staffordshire's spotteds and reds) the lack of colour north of Birmingham was marked. And while the larger livestock farmers and aristocrats of the south were playing about with their coloured breeds and filling them with Chinese blood, the smallholders and weavers of the north were quietly fashioning their white pigs into what would eventually become world-beaters.

In the 17th century the county of Leicestershire was renowned for its pigs, which were very well fed on the local beans grown in great quantity. The Melton Mowbray pork pies of the county are still famous today, and it was in Leicestershire that the nation's pigs were most thickly congregated in the early 18th century. This was also the county home of the famous 18th century livestock breeder and improver, Robert Bakewell of Dishley (1725-95), renowned for his Leicester sheep and Longhorn cattle. He also turned his hand to pigs, for a while, but with nothing like so much success.

There were a lot of pigs in the county, most of them being bred and fattened for London and for markets which supplied ships. Bakewell, however, apparently ignored the local whites . Some writers claim that his pig was dark or black, some white or light spotted; Spencer said it was based on a native mahogany-coloured pig which Bakewell improved and then crossed with a black boar to produce the typical sandy, black and white spotted pig of the old Berkshire type. He used his typical in-and-in breeding techniques, which local farmers (quite rightly, it seems) thought would be disastrous with pigs, however successfully they had been employed in other livestock.

There was a **White Leicester** which would have a considerable influence on the big pigs of Yorkshire and on many others. Some said it was the result of white Chinese on the mysterious Bakewell pig; others that it had nothing to do with Bakewell but was the native county breed crossed with Middle or Small Yorkshire; others that it was named for the Earl rather than the county; but its origins remain vague. An illustration of a prize-winning pair of White Leicesters at the 1855 Paris Exposition is reproduced by Harris in his *Book of the Pig* (New York, 1870) but he says he could ascertain "nothing satisfactory in regard to the origin of this breed". All he could say was that Mr J.W. Williams of Somerset had been the principal breeder of them since he first exhibited in 1852, and that they were "the great improvers of the gigantic Yorks". The engraving, subtitled "White Leicester Boar and Sow - Small Breed", shows a very short-legged and plump pair of pigs with short, prick ears and a right-angled dishing to the face. Writing in 1902, McConnell included the Leicester under the headings "Brown" (which also embraced Tamworth, Cheshire, Worcester and Warwickshire pigs and fits in with Spencer's mahogany) and "Black" (with Berkshire, Hampshire, Devon, Essex) but not under "White". Youatt described the old Leicester as a typical midlands pig - big, flat-sided and slow-feeding - and "of a light colour and spotted with brown or black".

The White Leicester was a fast grower and a more refined pig than the original Yorkshire, with a smaller head, lighter bone and finer hair. Williams's pigs were crossed with Cumberland-Yorkshire to form the Small White and Large White.

To the south of Leicestershire were the once famous white pigs of Northamptonshire. They were short in the leg, with enormous lop ears hanging down almost to the ground, and thus blinkered were very gentle. They grew to a great size, especially in the Naseby area.

To the east of Leicestershire the large, windswept county of Lincolnshire always bred its livestock big and well insulated, whether red cattle or long-woolled sheep, or pigs. The pigs, according to Long, were "enormous" and the county type was "remarkable for its quantity of bone and coarseness of flesh. It generally had plenty of hair, a long snout, and huge flopping ears. Its chief qualities were its hardihood and prolificacy." He refused to grant these pigs the status of a "breed", saying they were merely a local subvariety and lumping them together with the Norfolk and the pigs of distant Westmoreland. Yet Harris talked about the "old Yorkshire or Lincolnshire breed" being the same - and, according to him, a bad breed at that. In 1810 Parkinson described the "Lincolnshire White" pigs as "being superior to all others except the Berkshire" and said: "Their ears are neither long nor short, standing rather near together, pointing forwards, sharp at the extremities, rather flat and turn up a little at the ends." The true breed was most numerous then in the marshes near Louth, though being white, he said, it was naturally tender - in Parkinson's view, a black or sandy colour indicated hardiness.

There is a fine painting of a Lincolnshire pig dated 1821 (the signature is possibly T. Coulas). It has a flowing, gently wavy white coat with a few black spots and a black head with a straight muzzle and prick ears (matching Parkinson's description in that respect). The inscription gives its dimensions and notes that its legs were only about 4½ inches long. Its belly, though not sagging, almost touches the ground.

A breed society was formed for what was called the **Lincolnshire Curly Coat** Pig <Plate 3>and suddenly a type which had been known for at least a century became respectable. "The farmers in Lincolnshire have taken up the matter in their usual whole-hearted manner, as though they were determined to give this thick-fleshed and hardy local pig an opportunity to prove its value," stated the new edition of *Youatt's Complete Grazier* at the time. "It is claimed for it that it is a refined type of the coarse, strong-boned, coarse-haired pig common in years gone by in the Lincolnshire, Norfolk, and Cambridgeshire Fens. No record appears to be available as to the general system of improvement: it may possibly have been due to the infusion of Large White blood and the continued selection of the breeding pigs possessing the greatest amount of style and quality. In these respects there may be still some room for improvement before pigs of the breed will be able to compete on equal terms with some other older breeds for the purpose of improving the general breed of pigs in other districts or countries; but there is no denying the fact that for the county of Lincoln with its system of farming and the in-boarding of a considerable proportion of the horsemen, shepherds, and stockmen, the Lincolnshire White Curly-Coated is wonderfully well adapted."

These big, curly-haired pigs were proudly reared in many local cottage gardens for fat home-cured bacon in the first half of the 20th century. The breed's daily weight gain was unbeatable and it could reach up to 60 stone. It was a prodigious producer of fat and an excellent and hardy forager - a factor of considerable importance to those with limited means. It had a longish snout, well dished face, large ears flopping forward over the eyes, and that distinctive fleecy coat; it was large, with a broad back, heavily fleshed, and both fatter and coarser than the Large White, and hardy, prolific and early-maturing.

By the 1930s it was at the peak of its popularity, overseas as well as at home. Its fat was greatly appreciated in Europe's colder climates - it was exported to Russia, for example, and was highly regarded in Hungary. The first Lincolnshire pigs had been imported by Hungary in 1873. They were still being imported during the 1920s, and used as crosses with local breeds. In particular there was an attempt to cross it with another famous curly-coated breed, the **Mangalitsa** lard pig - the crosses were nicknamed **Lincolitsa** - and the initial results were favourable. In its early days, the Lincolnshire made such a good impression that it convinced the Hungarians that they needed to change over without delay to the mass breeding of meat-type pigs and that the Lincolnshire was the breed of the future, especially as it was so fertile. But later it fell out of favour. Dorner said: "These otherwise well shaped, rapidly developing, easy to fatten, quiet temperament animals have the great disadvantage of being highly susceptible not only to infectious diseases but also to heart and lung diseases, in other words, show a high rate mortality. It is interesting that its almost degenerated poor physique, and often annoying high susceptibility to diseases are complained of by Germans as well."

In 1949, 82 boars were registered in England; in 1955 only two. By the 1960s it was disappearing fast, and the last known of the breed were slaughtered in 1972 after having been used by Unilever for virology tests - an ignominious end.

Yet its genes live on in the Chester White of the United States, which also perpetuates the genes of other extinct English whites like the Cheshire and the Cumberland.

The pigs of Cumberland were described by James Long as "not so large as the Yorkshire nor so symmetrical; their backs were very much arched, their skin was largely spotted with black, their quality coarse, and, in almost every respect, they were identical with the large pigs of Westmoreland, which were equally ugly, provided with huge legs, bony flanks, and very little capacity for laying on flesh."

Sidney explained that the so-called Small Cumberland breed was not really small at all but of medium size, short in the legs, with fine "clean" ears of medium size standing a little forward, a short nose, an even coat of short, fine hair, a broad, straight back, well developed ribs, and good rump and hams. The county was famous for its ham, and also the sauce that accompanied it at Christmas.

There was also a Small Yorkshire, which Sidney classed with the Small Cumberland. It had a short head with small erect ears; its back was broad, its chest deep, the legs short and bone fine. Three or four of them could be kept "fresh and symmetrical" on feed which would barely keep "one lean and gaunt large Yorkshire" alive. But Sidney said that although originally the Cumberland had been the larger, the two by his time were continually interbred (to advantage). People called them Small Yorkshire or Small Cumberland at whim, or Yorks-Cumberland, or Cumberland-Yorkshire. Ultimately they were called Small Whites - or a host of other names when they became so famous that the aristocracy tried to claim them as their own.

By the 1940s, the **Cumberland** breed <Plate 3> was shorter and heavier in build than the Large White, with a heavier jowl, wider shoulder and back, wide head, a very short and very dished face, broad and rather short ears hanging over the eyes, and fine sparse hair. It fattened readily and was a docile pig. A breed society had been formed in 1917 but the last boar of this fatty pig was licensed in about 1955 and the last sow in 1960.

Culley (1794) said that the large white native pigs of Yorkshire and Lancashire, very common a few years earlier, had "very large ears hanging over their eyes". Parkinson (1810) said that the Yorkshire of the late 18th century resembled the Berkshire in that both were spotted or black mingled with white, and it is said that the Yorkshire pigs were crossed with Cantonese pigs from China during that period.

An engraving of 1809 featured a massive piebald pig called simply "The Yorkshire hog", which belonged to Colonel Thomas Charles Beaumont, MP, and was of an "improved" type bred by Benjamin Rowley of Doncaster. It measured 9ft 10in (300 cms) in length, 8ft (244 cms) in circumference, and was the height of a pony (12 ½ hands) at four years old, when it weighed 1,344 pounds - and could have been been even bigger if it had not been "raised up so often to exhibit its stature": the beast's public appearances earned £3,000 in three years. His ears fell over his eyes, his snout was of medium length, his profile fairly straight, his body white with a black patch on the rump and tail and a black mantle over the shoulders, back, chest (not legs), ears and back of head, with the face white. And he had a good, strong set of legs to support all that weight.

Morton's *Cyclopaedia* (1854) described the old **Yorkshire and Lincolnshire** pig as "one of the largest breeds in the kingdom, and probably one of the worst". It was extremely long-legged, it was weak in the loin, very long in the body and "yielding coarse, flabby flesh, of inferior marketing quality". Its colour was chiefly white, and it had that long, coarse coat of curly Lincolnshire hair. Mr A. Clarke of Long Sutton, Lincolnshire, said at the time that breeders in Yorkshire outdid those in Lincolnshire only in point of size and he claimed that the pigs recently exhibited by Yorkshiremen like Abbot, Taylor and Tuley were "a size too large for any useful purpose, and would exceed in weight that of a moderately grown Scotch Ox."

By then it seems that the Lincolnshire "breed" had been merged into the Yorkshire, though breeders in the former county claimed that theirs was the foundation of what became the **Large White** <Plate 4>. The old type of Yorkshire, according to Sidney, took a long time to reach full size and "could be fed up to 800 pounds, but whether with any profit, is doubtful." Those exhibited at the Royal Show were colossal and produced high quality bacon but ate a lot in order to do so; however, the type was very hardy and prolific. Attempts were made to improve its slowness by mixing in some Berkshire, Black Essex, Neapolitan and other blacks, which produced a race of black-and-white pigs of varying quality: those from the Berkshire cross were hardy and useful but still slow to fatten, and the others became far too delicate for the northern climate as they had very little hair to protect them. Then the prick-eared White Leicester was tried, early in the 19th century, and this was a step in the right direction.

By Sidney's time the old type of Yorkshire had been banished to the northern parts of the county; the rest, in the grain-growing areas, clearly owed much to the White Leicester. Youatt said that the Large White was crossed with white Chinese pigs around 1830, and Sidney was told in 1860 that the White Leicester cross had been further improved by putting the largest and best of the crossbred sows to small white boars bred by the Earl of Carlisle at Castle Howard or by Mr Wyley of Brandsby (whose small White Leicester breed came to be called the Yorkshire) and thereafter breeding selectively among the progeny to retain the size and constitution of the large Yorkshire but to add from the small whites their symmetry and tendency to fatten. This process, it seems, formed the basis of the improved Large Yorkshire, bred mainly in the Aire valley around Leeds, Keighley and Skipton, and by 1860 they were already much in demand, not only all over the United Kingdom but also in France, Germany and the United States, where they fetched high prices.

That fame probably began in about 1851 when a Keighley weaver, Joseph Tuley, mentioned somewhat disparagingly by Mr Clarke of Long Sutton (above), exhibited his own improved Large Yorkshires. These were a huge success in many quarters; for example, the breeder John Fisher (manager for Mr Wainman of Carrhead, Yorkshire) is said to have built himself a cottage out of his proceeds from selling just one litter from a Tuley sow called Matchless. She and the Tuley boar Sampson became the foundation of some of the best Yorkshire strains, and the name of Sampson figured prominently in the first NPBA handbook, published in the 1880s. Tuley-bred pigs found their way to many parts of the world and fetched as much as a thousand pounds for one sow. They were in demand in Scotland, Ireland, Australia, America, Prussia, Holland and Spain even in the mid-century.

In 1876, an article in *The Field* claimed proudly that the large white pigs of northern England and Scotland were "uncrossed with foreigners", the writer's theory being that colour in the breeds of the midlands and the south indicated foreign blood. The pigs of Yorkshire, Lancashire, Leicestershire and Lincolnshire, he claimed, were "descended pretty directly" from the old English flop-eared type.

Although the big whites were common in Lancashire, Cheshire, Derbyshire and Lincolnshire as much as Yorkshire by the 1880s, and although Lincolnshire breeders continued to lay claim that their county's breed was the true foundation of the Large White, the breed was known (and still is) as the **Yorkshire** in many overseas countries, though in truth the name was bestowed on any type of pig imported from that county, and no doubt on any white pig that remotely resembled it. More precisely, there was a difference between the early Yorkshires and later importations of Large White, though they are usually lumped together abroad.

Whether Yorkshire or Large White, it gradually absorbed other county whites from the northernmost in England down to those of Norfolk. The breed was recognised in 1868, and its first herdbook was published in 1884.

By the 1870s the large whites had big overhanging ears, big long heads, long bodies lacking proportionate width, and flat sides in comparison with the Berkshires and Suffolks. The back had become level and the shoulder full, but the hindquarters still dropped and the bone was considered too strong. The coat quality was variable but "never the curly profusion which adds such beauty to the small white sort", according the *The Field* (1874). It was also less prolific than the old type (which commonly produced and reared litters of 16-18) but the sows, with litters of 10-12, were good milky mothers. However, the young had an "unfinished, inelegant appearance" and contrasted strongly with the "admirable proportions" of the smaller breeds that so pleased the show ring judges. Though not early to mature, they improved as they grew: at 12-15 months old they began to show "really grand proportions" and could become good baconers, though their large sides of bacon were only in demand for markets such as the large industrial and mining centres.

With so many contributors to the breed, it is not surprising that it was so vigorous and capable of meeting so many different requirements. Nor was it surprising that the type changed considerably as time went by. For example, the ears of an outstanding, prize-winning boar of 1890, Borrowfield King, were definitely forwards, almost drooping over his snout, rather than "slightly upwards and inclined forward" as the standard later required. In 1898 the question of colour was noted in the breed standards, which stated: "White, free from black hairs, and as far as possible from blue spots on the skin." That was for the large breed; no blue spots were allowed in the middle and small types. The large continued to show a few pale blue skin spots for many years, though they were selected against (especially by foreigners, who thought they indicated impure breeding), and there developed a very small **Yorkshire Blue-and-White** or Bilsdale Blue, which registered 35 boars in 1949 and only 7 in 1955, after which it became extinct. For a long time it was common practice to breed blue-and-white bacon crosses from Large White boars on Large Black sows.

By the 1930s the Large White was an enormous success all over the world, especially in countries with important bacon industries, like Denmark, Sweden and Poland. Before the First World War Sanders Spencer, author of several pig books, was one of the major breeders of both Large White and Middle White, having founded his Holywell herd in 1863, and he sold to North and South America, Russia and New Zealand, but above all to Denmark, making a substantial contribution to the creation of the Danish bacon industry towards the end of the 19th century and thus equally contributing to the development of the Landraces which would in due course challenge the Large White for supremacy.

Since then, of course, the Large White or Yorkshire has spread worldwide in huge numbers. It has formed the basis of countless breeds - the national Yorkshires of North America, Belgium and the Netherlands, the Large Whites of France, Poland, Russia and Sweden, the Edelschwein of Germany and Switzerland, the national improved whites of Bulgaria, Estonia, Latvia, Lithuania, Hungary and the Ukraine, and many more. All over the world it is used as the basis of commercial crossbred sows and as the terminal sire of their progeny, and its influence in the global pig industry has been even greater than that of the Dutch black-and-white cows in the global cattle industry.

For many years, the term "Yorkshire" included large, medium and small white pigs. William E. Bear, editor of a new edition of *Youatt's Complete Grazier* (already re-written by William Fream in 1893) in the first decade of the 20th century, said that the Large, Middle and Small Whites were originally all called Yorkshires "mainly because large numbers of pigs, principally of a white colour, were kept in that extensive county by the farmers, and to a very considerable degree by the mechanics in the neighbourhood of the larger towns, at some of which agricultural shows have been held for a great number of years. Indeed, the town of Otley claims to have one of the oldest societies extant. It is only within the last forty years or so that any particular attention has been paid to the sub-divisions into which the white pigs are now generally separated, and it is only fair that it should be recorded that breeders of white pigs not resident in the boundaries of Yorkshire have contributed most largely to that fixity of points aimed at in the three sections of what used in olden times to be called the Yorkshire breed of pigs." By then the large Yorkshire was more commonly known as the Large White.

At the Birmingham show in the late 1860s, there had been uproar when a litter of whites was disqualified on the grounds that they could not all be of the same litter: there were discrepancies in dentition and character. In fact they *were* of one litter, bred by Messrs Howard of Bedford, but of a cross between the large Yorkshire of Mr Wainman of Carrhead (near Keighley) and the Lincolnshire of Mr. Duckering of Kirton Lindsey.

Wainman was a well known owner of the large Yorkshire, though most of his success could be put down to his expert steward, John Fisher. In the early 1850s Wainman acquired some of the large Tuley "Matchless" pigs and crossed them with small or "China" whites or possibly Cumberlands. From the cross came a sow named Miss Emily, who, according to an essay in *The Gentleman's Magazine* in 1868, became the "principal mould in which the middle breed were cast and quickened", though the middle type was first officially recognised at

Keighley show in 1851. The same herd produced Lord of the Wassail, the "first middle breed boar that ever took a Royal prize", whose coat was 8½ inches long - to the delight of Wainman who, a keen angler, used the boar's hairs to dress his fishing flies. Another of his boars, Carrhead Duke, had such a thick hide that it was no good for anything but blacksmith's aprons: it was made into two of them, and the rest became a partition wall for a Keighley taproom.

Then there was Arch Trespasser, who played three different roles at the Royal. At one year old he was exhibited as a small white; at two years as a middle white; and at three as a large. Wainman's small breed owed its origins to a Cumberland sow crossed with one of Mr Watson's boars. Some of the offspring developed into small whites and some into middle whites which "combined the size of the large breed with the thriftiness and quality of the small, but there was no keeping some of them within growth bounds." Wainwright sold well to France and Germany.

The whites were gradually developed into three distinct breeds, distinguished nominally by their size as Large, Middle and Small Whites, but also by the degree of Chinese blood in the type. The Large showed least traces, the Small the most, and it altered their conformation and, very visibly, the shape of the face. The Large White's face was only slightly dished but both the Middle White and the Small White developed "squashed", shortened and extremely dished profiles. A couple from Leeds used to show a prize-winning sow called Lady Kate and such was their devotion to the animal that the wife would travel with it in the railway truck to all the Yorkshire and Lancashire shows. This cheerful dame "delighted to sit by her sow, and to reckon up on her fingers its thirteen crosses from the Chinese".

In due course it seems that the more practical breeders of Yorkshire and Lancashire concentrated on the large and middle breeds. Though never as popular as the Large, the **Middle White** <Plate 3> (with its own herdbook from 1884) grew in numbers over the years. The number of pedigree breeders increased four-fold between 1920 and 1925, and by the 1930s it was first choice as a specialist London porker. It was widely exported, in particular to Japan, where a shrine was even erected to a favourite Middle White boar, and in a letter to *The Ark* in 1980 Mr Hills, by then aged 84, recalled that his stock had been exported not only to Japan but also to Malaysia, Austria, South America and Africa. It was a good breed, like a Large White on a smaller scale, with that shorter head and dished face full of character, thicker in the body than the large type and with more hair. It was about the size of a Berkshire but much lighter in the bone and smaller in the head than that breed. The sows were just as prolific as the large and the progeny earlier maturing. Like the other whites, it often had a few pale blue spots on the skin (the hair from which was white) and these often increased in number as an individual grew older.

The Middle White has always been a pleasure to its keepers but is now a rare breed. Its demise was precipitated in 1933, when pig production boards were set up to develop the UK's pig industry but concentrated on bacon, ignoring the porkers and advising that pork should in future come from immature baconers. The Middle White had been a producer of quality pork but by the time the war years were over there was no such market: consumers had become used to "pork" from the immature baconers instead, and would not afford the quality product from the true porker. Middle White breeders did develop their own local markets but it was a very limited trade and the breed was no longer controlled by pedigree. In 1949 there were 157 Middle White boars - and by 1974 there were only five. It is now looked after by the Rare Breeds Survival Trust, and has proved a popular pig for farm parks; and for a while an enterprising breeder was producing suckling pigs for Harrods of London, from Middle White/Large White crosses killed at 3-6 weeks old. It is an ideal cottager's pig - kind and gentle, docile and thrifty, growing very quickly in the first four or five months, after which the growth rate slows down and it begins to put on a lot of fat. It is a comfortable sort of pig to keep, well liked by those who do so. It is not a miniature Large White at all, but a distinct breed with its own special qualities.

The Middle White has at least managed to outlive the **Small White** <Plate 3>. The Small had the misfortune to become a fancier's pig, the favourite of substantial land owners and princes, and that is probably a major factor contributing to its extinction. There was more Chinese blood in the Small than in the other two whites; in fact, some said that it was pure Chinese at first, originating from shipboard pigs landed at Plymouth and Bristol in the 17th or 18th centuries. John Fisher, the steward of the well known Carrhead owner, Wainman, said that the Small was first bred in 1818 by Charles Mason and Robert Colling of Durham (of Shorthorn cattle fame) and that his own first acquaintance with the type was in 1824, with the small whites of the Earl of Carlisle and Major Bower. Both had acquired their stock from Wyley of Brandsby, who had some Mason and Colling pigs known as the "Chinese".

Those who bred Shorthorn cattle seemed to take a liking to these little, dish-faced pigs, and they became the plaything of the aristocrats. Whether known as Small Yorkshire or Small White at first, the breed's face became very short and very dished, the broad snout turned up, the jowl very full, with a short, thick neck, and a general fullness all over. It had to be pure white, with small, short, erect ears, a fine silky coat, and an overall appearance of being small, thick and compact in comparison with other breeds. It was considered to be a greatly refined breed and far more attention was paid to its show ring appeal than to any practical characteristics, though it was early fattened as a roaster or porker or for small bacon.

One of the problems of being adopted by the rich was that each owner wanted to give the pig his own name. Lord Radnor was one of its early breeders but, as Sidney put it: "When any of Lord Radnor's stock pass into other hands in England, the produce generally cease to be called Coleshill. They become Suffolks, Yorkshires, Middlesex, according to the fancy of the breeder." (And in France, they were known as *cochons de salon*, or drawing-room pigs.)

Prince Albert began to exhibit small whites at Smithfield in 1843 and called them Suffolks or Bedfordshires. Two years later the Prince's pigs failed to win because, although they were "magnificent specimens of fat and cleanliness", they were also "absolutely gasping for breath" like overfed pug dogs. By 1851 the Prince had developed and was showing his Windsor "breed" - basically the same small whites with very dished faces but not as extreme as the earlier type, with short prick ears and, in a painting by Friedrich Wilhelm Keyl in 1858, perfectly cylindrical in shape and very short in the leg.

That "Bedfordshire" tag could be misleading - it was not the same pig as the **Bedford** or **Woburn** which flopped so badly in America and was a white or sandy breed with occasional brown spots and big lop ears. The Prince's Bedfordshires were simply Small Whites, derived from a mixture of medium-sized Cumberlands and small Yorkshires, whereas according to Baxter the "Woburn spotted boar" had been introduced by the late Duke of Bedford (Baxter was writing in the 1830s). The county of Bedfordshire could never really boast its own pig, and one farmer of the period remarked that he had not known it had a breed until he saw the name marked over one of Prince Albert's pens at a Smithfield show. Another merely remarked that the breed in his county was "wretchedly bad", and had been ever since he had known it.

However, because of its apparent royal and ducal connections the Large Spotted Bedfordshire or Woburn found a ready market in the United States of America. It was white or sandy with a few brown spots and was said to owe its origins to Chinese crossed with local pigs. It was slow and sluggish by nature (which helped it to fatten). As sketched in Henderson, it was a prick-eared pig with a tapering snout and random splodges of colour on its balloon-shaped body.

The Cumberland type used by so many aristocrats in their Small White mixtures was the so-called Small Cumberland that Sidney had explained was really medium in size. Most of the numerous small whites had dashes of Cumberland, Yorkshire and Leicestershire in them and were "highly fed crossbred toys" with very little to distinguish between them except their many names. Lord Ducie's was one of the most popular and was used by the Earl of Radnor (before it lost size and type) to produce his well known **Coleshill** based on Small Yorkshire or Yorkshire and Cumberland. Other Yorkshire/Cumberland herds became the **Buckinghamshire**, the **Middlesex**, the **Suffolk** (not to be confused with the Black Suffolk), the **Manchester** and various others, all virtually indistinguishable from each other or from the **Bushey** or Yorkshire bred by a wealthy banker, Mr Marjoribanks. The **Solway**, named for Solway Hall in Cumberland, was a Durham version - a branch of the Mason/Colling stock - which did in fact improve the Small White in general, both in constitution and size, with a greater proportion of lean to fat, and finer and more profuse hair (which the fanciers loved). The Solway influenced Wainman's pigs - especially that famous boar shown successively as a small, a middle and a large white.

And just to confuse everybody further, the Small White or Small Yorkshire was sometimes referred to as a White Berkshire, a name also applied (tongue in cheek) to the pigs that old Bakewell had tried to improve in the 18th century.

In the early years of the 20th century the Small White breed was described as much smaller than the Middle White, with very short legs, very short head, heavy jowls, a thick carcass "rather deficient in lean meat", and a profuse covering of silky, wavy hair. It was simply not a practical pig for the new century, and the 1919 edition of *Encyclopaedia Britannica*, though describing it as a beautifully proportioned pig, said that it was almost extinct.

Lop-eared Whites

Although the large old English type, with its big lop ears and long body, could well have been developed into one of what is today known as the Landrace group, instead it went in countless directions to become several indigenous breeds of various shapes, sizes and colours, as already described. The **British Landrace** <Plate 7> is in fact of entirely foreign origin: it was first introduced to the United Kingdom in 1949 from Sweden, when four boars and eight gilts were imported, with further importations in 1953. These were then carefully bred for British conditions and were very highly priced - yet it took only three years from their first release to the public for the breed to become the second most numerous in the country. The British Landrace Pig Society was established in 1953, and in 1956 the breed's supporters set up their own testing station to ensure that their new pigs remained highly commercial and profitable. With the Danish dominance of the bacon trade, and in spite of mocking references to the new pig's "ewe neck" and great length, the Landrace was soon challenging the Large White. In due course the two breeds settled into an amicable relationship and now form the basis of most commercial crossbreds in the United Kingdom.

There was a much older lop-eared white pig in England's west country, where small family pigs were traditionally kept to recycle household waste. The system was an informal one; boars were often shared between families and none of the pigs were registered, nor were they kept on large-scale systems. These white lops defied the local prejudice in favour of black and disproved the theory that white pigs could not stand the sunshine of the warm south west. They were thoroughly hardy and thoroughly practical farmers' pigs on a local basis.

The breeders of the type were independent by nature, and remain so today. The breed is now known as the **British Lop** <Plate 3> and is a minor one, with its own breed society based in Cornwall. The society was first formed in 1918 in reaction to the new legislation which had also prompted Gloucester Old Spots breeders to register their pig.

The British Lop has sometimes changed its name - it was known for a while by the cumbersome title of the National Long White Lop-eared pig (1921) and is sometimes called the Devon Lop or Cornish White. The main centre of its development was near the Devon town of Tavistock, on the western edge of Dartmoor near the Cornish border.

It probably has much in common with the old white Celtic pigs found in Wales and Ireland (for example, the Large White Ulster) and can fairly be called an indigenous landrace. It also had much in common with the **Cumberland** of the 1940s when the latter was a dish-faced, lop-eared, round hammed pig. The Welsh connection was stressed for a while when the Lop and the Welsh pig societies amalgamated from 1926 to 1928, though with separate herdbooks.

The earlier pigs, heavy-framed and very hardy, were ideal for the region's small farms, making use of farm wastelands and requiring minimal housing, living on stubble, grassland and woodland. The type was refined with some Landrace blood and from the early 1950s breeders focussed on ensuring that it graded for bacon. It remained local, though it spread to some extent into Somerset and Dorset, and it is now found over most of the west of England and up into Warwickshire, with outposts in, for example, Scotland - the biggest herd of Lops in the British Isles today is claimed to be at Coldstream in Berwickshire.

In 1929 the White Lop-eared was "threatened with expulsion" at Smithfield show and disappeared for a while, until the newly named National Long White Lop-eared was rescheduled in 1934. By 1970, however, its numbers had fallen very low, with only one male bloodline and three distinct female lines. Its popularity increased during the 1980s and the number of breeders grew to 60, with 41 boars, by 1983.

The old name describes the type - long, white and lop-eared, the long thin ears inclined well over the face, and the fine skin and long silky hair are white. It is one of the country's biggest breeds and can be used as a porker or a cutter; its conformation is comparable to that of the other south west breed, the Large Black. It is a very economical feeder, early maturing, producing well streaked bacon, and an economical outdoor grazing pig - hardy and self-sufficient. The sows are docile and long-lived and make excellent mothers: one of them managed to produce 17 pigs for her 21st litter. The sows are often crossed with Large White, Landrace or Welsh boars for good pork and bacon pigs.

Wales

The old Welsh pigs are said to have been driven into the country in Viking times, accompanying the Celtic minorities who also took refuge in south west England and up the west coast into Cumberland and over to Ireland. The *Mabinogion* saga tells of mass pig movements in Wales during that unsettled period.

In general, the Welsh pigs were mostly yellowish-white, sometimes spotted with black. From various reports, it seems that they were of the same type and origins as the typical old English lop - large and gaunt, and mainly left alone by the improvers with their Chinese and Berkshire pigs. Writing during the 18th century, Lawrence said that Cornish and Welsh pigs were "wolf-shaped" and long-legged - and no doubt those long legs were necessary. There were also some of the more primitive brown type, similar to the native Scottish pigs, described in the 1872 *Montgomeryshire Collections* as resembling "an alligator mounted on stilts, having bristles instead of scales ... gaunt and with a remarkable extension of the snout."

Sidney described how the dairymen of Cheshire brought in large numbers of pigs from Wales and Shropshire and then crossed them with the "Manchester" (Yorkshire) boar, producing "a larger and coarser breed than the small Yorkshire". A farmer buying Welsh stores would keep them for 12 months and sell them at 300 pounds, "which will scarcely pay for four months more keep than the Yorkshire, Manchester, and Shropshire sold after eight months."

Sanders Spencer agreed that most Welsh, like most Cheshire pigs, were not profitable, and said that the harsh coats of these whites indicated that they were slow to fatten. "One would have thought," he said loftily, "that the Welsh farmers were most favourably situated for markets" and should therefore have taken energetic steps to improve their pigs.

At the beginning of the 20th century the main Welsh breeding centres were in the counties of Cardigan, Carmarthen, Pembroke, Denbigh and Montgomery. The 1907 edition of *Youatt's Complete Grazier* described the Welsh pigs as chiefly white and "very much of the razor-backed, coarse-haired, slow-maturing kind, unprofitable alike to the feeder and the consumer" but capable of great improvement. And improve they did.

In 1922 the Old Glamorgan Pig Society, established four years earlier, amalgamated with the Welsh Pig Society and this combination joined in 1926 with the Long White Lop-Eared Pig Society in south west England to become known as the National Long White Lop-Eared Pig Society. Nobody seemed to like the liaison much on either side and they separated again in 1928, when the Welsh Pig Society was reformed. Between the wars, the Welsh was essentially a cutter, especially for the midlands markets, but it changed type after the second war by a combination of selection, testing and constructive breeding.

The modern **Welsh** <Plate 3> has become one of the more successful whites in the country, though its success is quite recent. By 1946 it had become very similar to the Danish Landrace - large and long, with a slightly dished face of the Large White type but with the ears tending to meet at the tips, short of the straight nose. It was good for bacon or pork - and clearly a winning type.

In 1949 there were only 33 registered boars of the new Welsh breed, but by 1955 (after the introduction of Swedish Landrace blood from 1953) there were 528 and by 1973 there were 671 boars. At Smithfield in 1962 there was a fundamental revision of the schedule and a few years later it included Landrace and "allied Welsh". By 1981 the Welsh had become Britain's third-ranking breed.

Scotland

The pigs of north east Scotland in the 18th century were much as they had been for many centuries: they were black or red, with coats so woolly they were a marketable commodity. The animals ranged freely and were independent, active, and sometimes said to be so ferocious that they became active lamb-killers in the Shetlands. That unfortunate habit apart, they were of a type that would have been recognised as familiar in medieval southern Britain as well. In 1761 free-running pigs were a considerable nuisance in Sutherland and were still a problem in some parts even in the 1890s.

Scotland today has no breed it can call its own and has never been such an ardent fan of the pig as England or Ireland. Before the mid 19th century, Scottish farmers rarely bothered to fatten their pigs for market, although they usually fattened one at home for Christmas. The most important pig keepers were the distillers and breweries, and the corn mills and dairy farmers, all of which produced waste products that could be fed to pigs. Sometimes a specialist might set up on a commercial basis: by 1784, for example, one George Ross had built himself a good pig unit on his northerly farm in Cromarty and was sending his own cured pork down to London, and even exporting it to both the East and the West Indies (the latter trade largely cornered by the Americans). His system involved the distribution of young pigs among his tenants and buying them back when they were ready for slaughter. The pigs were said to be of the large

Hampshire type commonly reared by the distillers of the period.

By the mid 18th century there was a thriving salted pork industry centred on Aberdeen. The pigs by then were an improvement on the semi-wild dark browns, but only just. They were lop-eared and had lightened to a dun colour, and began to be mixed with the newly fashionable Chinese. But towards the end of the century their numbers had declined, partly because of various factors affecting their feed sources. The growing urban centres were demanding more and better meat than could be supplied by the old type of long, lanky, bristly pig and before the turn of the century, they were replaced by improved Berkshire and Chinese pigs which were properly fattened on bran, potatoes, milk and meal.

Unlike English cottagers, most Scots rarely ate pork, and pig rearing was largely for the export of cured pig meat to London and other markets. Those who did keep a pig, however, would often house the animal as if it was a pet, perhaps tethered by the leg at the door or even inside the kitchen.

Early in the 19th century, improved long-eared white sows became popular in south west Scotland to meet the cured pig meat markets. The farms of south east Scotland preferred to rear smaller breeds and fattened them on farm wastes (barn-floor sweepings and the like) which produced a good meat for curing, and certainly not too fat. Unlike the English, the Scots rejected fat of any kind - and fat pork in particular. During the century customs changed and farm workers, living in the main farmhouse, began to eat boiled pork. Soon cottars were keeping their own backyard pigs in the English style and they began to lose their prejudice against fat. The pig breeders of the north, who had traditionally driven their herds down to the lowland counties to fatten them for English markets, now fattened them increasingly for the home market as well.

Yet still Scotland did not create its own breeds but brought in the improved English ones or relied on assortments. H.D. Richardson, in *Domestic Pigs* (1852), described in great detail the "very peculiar breed of swine" in the Orkneys, the Hebrides and the Shetland Isles. It was very small (no bigger than a "good-sized Terrier dog") and grey or brindled with a coarse, bristly coat. It ranged with total and joyous freedom, scavenging what it could, including newborn lambs. It was never given any supplementary feeding until its owners decided to drive their swine home for fattening, which the pigs achieved with surprising rapidity and a great increase in size. The diminutive Orkney pig had long, strong bristles on the back and was of "much variety of colouring" - usually dark red or nearly black, but sometimes brown, tawny or dirty white; the "wool" under the long bristles was so coarse that it was spun into ropes used by cliff-hanging egg collectors. The pig had strong, sharply pointed and upright ears and a peculiarly strong snout from its "constant exercise" in rooting. The flesh was in good quantity in spite of the lack of feeding and produced good pork for shipping stores, with an average weight of 60-70 pounds, at a time when Orkney, in the early 19th century, was doing a good trade in barrelled pork. But the fashionable Berkshires and Neapolitan-improved breeds gradually overwhelmed the old dark breed as the century progressed and it was already rare by the 1840s.

It had done well to survive so long. In early times, Scandinavian domesticated pigs were never found any further north than the Wild Boar would range, which was not beyond the deciduous tree level ("no pannage, no pig," as Anthony Dent put it in *The Ark* in 1977). There had been trees in Orkney and Shetland before the Norse settlers deforested the islands.

The native pigs of Caithness in the early years of the 19th century were small, short-bodied, and usually reddish or grey, or sometimes black. In the Highlands and the Hebrides the extremely hardy pigs grazing the hills were also small and grey, with shaggy coats of long hair and bristles, producing very good meat in the autumn and fattening readily down in the lowland counties, where the most numerous type was light and white, long in the leg, narrow in the body, with erect bristles from nose to tail, and slow to fatten.

During that century all these old Scottish types were replaced by improved English breeds, and there was still no "Scottish" breed by the early 20th century, when there were anyway only 144,000 pigs in the country in 1901, compared with nearly 2 million in England and 240,000 in Wales.

Ireland

On the isle of Aran there lingered, just, at the beginning of this century, the so-called **Irish Greyhound** pig - lean, lanky and wild-looking. In 1903 Sir Harry Johnston published a photograph of a piglet which was a cross between this Irish type and an improved breed, and it seemed to show faint traces of pale markings like the stripes seen in the young of the Wild Boar. Certain primitive pigs, all over the world, will produce striped young.

The Greyhound was deliberately named. It was tall and bony, with a very long head and snout, and so long legged that it was apparently an adept high-jumper. Its back was slightly arched and, whippet-like, the body narrowed at the waist, while the hams were best described as skinny. The coat was harsh, with a crest of bristles along the neck and back; its heavy ears hung down and below the throat dangled a pair of wattles - a characteristic often seen in the old flop-eared pigs of Gloucestershire and Yorkshire in England, for example.

Richardson's engraving of the beast in the 1840s shows something which seems to be halfway beween the Wild Boar and the domesticated pig. His description runs thus:

"These are tall, long-legged, bony, heavy-eared, coarse haired animals; their throats furnished with pendulous wattles, and by no means possessing half so much the appearance of domestic swine as they do of the wild boar, the great original of the race. In Ireland, the old gaunt race of hogs has, for many years past, been gradually wearing away, and is now, perhaps, wholly confined to the western parts of the country, especially Galway. These swine are remarkably active, and will clear a five-barred gate as well as any hunter; on this account they should, if it is desirable to keep them, be kept in well-fenced inclosures."

A better pig by far was the **Irish Grazier**, a general term for pigs with thin coats of various colours (often white) and of various sizes and types. There was quite a refined and long-bodied meatier variety, with a strong muscular back and full hams, standing on squarely set legs and with erect ears, for example. They were improved with the help of the old spotted Berkshire and later the large white Yorkshire pigs. Many of the type went to the United States in the 1830s and it is said that some Irish Graziers (white with occasional sandy spots - though these might have been Woburns) were introduced into Warren County, Ohio, along with some Berkshires, both of which were crossed with the Warren County breed and in due course produced what is now called the Poland China. The Irish Grazier had vanished from Ohio by 1842 but in the meanwhile it had also contributed to the Curtis Victoria in Saratoga County, New York. It was in Connecticut, too, where it was known as the **Grass** pig. Two brothers mated a Grass sow to a boar of some recently imported Norfolk pigs and the result was an early-maturing, quick-finishing cross which the brothers took with them when they emigrated to northern Ohio. Here the animals were crossed with another Irish Grazier descendant from Massachusetts, and more Irish blood was introduced into the mixture from a "Large Grass" boar bred in Ohio. These and others were gradually developed into the Improved Chester White.

James Long confirmed that, in Ireland, "the pig occupies a high position with farmer and peasant alike, and contributes more to its owner's contentment and prosperity than almost anything to which he devotes attention; indeed the treatment of the pig by the Irish, as a race, contrasts very favourably with that to which it is subjected, not alone by the Orientals, but by many of our own agriculturists of high degree."

By 1901 there were 1.2 million pigs in Ireland; on average there were more pigs per acre of crop, fallow and grass in Ireland than in England or Wales, and three times as many as in Scotland. But in Ireland, and only in Ireland, the pig population was diminishing rather than increasing, though in 1902 Sir Walter Gilbey wrote in *Farm Stock of Old* that the best and finest bacon in England came from Ireland.

Excellent Irish bacon and ham had been known for a long period but in the 1880s the large curers began to complain about the "form and quality of the fat pigs sent to the fairs from many districts" - which is a shame, as in 1802 a "truly surprising" improvement had been noted in the pigs sent to Ballinasloe Fair in Galway. The old-fashioned Irish pig - that gaunt and long-legged ranger - would be left to its own devices, foraging as best it could, until its owner decided he had enough pigs to fatten. That process, declared *The Complete Grazier* in 1893, was not easy. There had been attempts in some areas to improve the system and the pigs, by introducing from England the "old-fashioned long-bodied Berkshire or spotted boar", which had been successful until the "improved" Berkshire was used. The latter's beneficial effects were less noticeable in the cross.

Later, some of the Irish bacon-curers brought in young Large White boars but they were usually from the type of English herd that concentrated on winning rosettes in the show ring rather than being bred by practical, commercial pork farmers, and they tended to be too heavily jowled and thick in the shoulder (the least valuable part of the carcass), while being too light in the far more productive middle and hind parts.

The curers therefore formed a pig improvement society of their own and, said *The Complete Grazier*, "much good will result from it providing its managers do not form too high an opinion of their own stock, and thus fail to look further afield for the boars intended for distribution in the various districts where pig-breeding is followed." They faced stiff competition from Canada, Denmark and elsewhere, and adopted some of those countries' ideas such as constantly bringing in the best Large White boars that money could buy. The practice had led to "as good bacon pigs" being found abroad as in England, and they were better than the average Irish pig. The Irish needed to catch up with the opposition.

In 1937 there were 570,000 pigs in Northern Ireland (out of a United Kingdom total of 4.452 million) and 930,000 in Eire. The tradition in Ireland had been for pigs to be killed and hung to cool on-farm, which apparently gave the meat a distinctive flavour. It was then sent to the factories for cutting and curing in a method that differed from the famous Wiltshire cure: the carcass was boned, the ham and shoulder removed for separate curing, the skin left on, and the cured meat rolled and tied with string. The Second World War reduced the production of local cures and they were replaced by the Wiltshire method, which meant a loss of identity for the Irish product.

There was only one true commercial Irish breed of pig - the **Ulster** <Plate 3> of Northern Ireland. It had a thin skin favoured by the bacon curers but all too easily bruised in handling and transport. It resembled a Large White, and was usually known as the Large White Ulster or the Ulster White, but was shorter, finer boned, earlier maturing, with a silkier and much less abundant coat than the Large White, and it had long ears falling forwards like blinkers over its eyes. Probably of similar origin to the British Lop, the Cumberland and the Welsh pigs, it was a bacon breed and a useful grazer. Its history was brief. A breed society was formed in 1908 and opened a herdbook but there were only 32 registered boars in 1949 and the last boar of the breed was licensed in 1956; thereafter the Ulster became extinct.

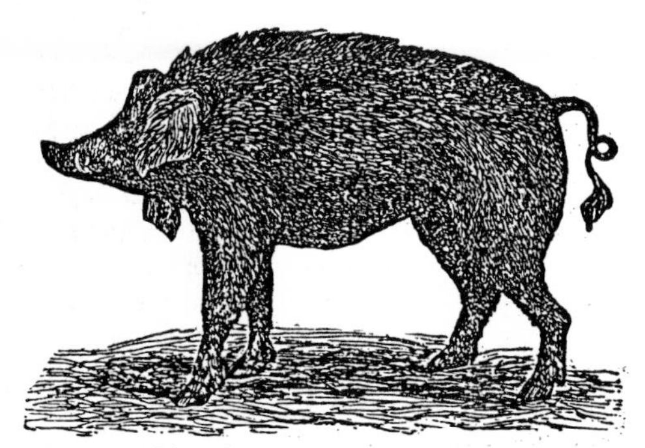

Fig. 13. Old Irish Greyhound pig [from Richardson, 1840s]

THE MODERN BRITISH BREEDS

Berkshire <Plate 2>

Now a rare breed in the United Kingdom, often crossed with the white breeds: the F1 progeny are all white and mature at a greater weight to give a carcass of quality. Docile sow has plenty of milk, high rearing percentage. Popular porker, also valuable as baconer in Large White cross or with Tamworth; early maturing, quick growing, good FCR, fine boned, plenty of lean meat in small quality joints. Carcass dresses completely white.

Originally large and lop-eared with red and black markings, improved in late 18th and early 19th centuries by Asian (before 1830) and then Neapolitan, to bring earlier maturity and other qualities. Now black with plenty of long, fine hair, and four white feet, white tail switch and white mark on face. Longer than it used to be, and lighter in shoulder, with dished face, medium length snout; ears fairly large and erect or slightly inclined forwards; legs short. Very hardy, in hot climates as well as cold. Widely exported since 18th century.

Origin of many breeds, including American and Canadian Berkshires, Kentucky Red Berkshire, Bayeux, German Berkshire, Dermantsi Pied, Murcian and others. Still bred pure in several countries. Herdbook 1884; American Berkshire Society 1875.

British Landrace <Plate 7>

Typical lop-eared white Landrace pig, long in body but not extreme. Originated from Swedish Landrace imported 1949 onwards; now second most popular breed in UK. Developed for quick growth, stamina, long lean carcass. Light fine head of medium length, straight snout; ears of medium size, drooping and slanting forwards; long slightly arched back, strong wide loins, full rounded hams, straight underline, legs of medium length. Soft skin slightly pink, hair white and fine. At least 14 teats. Good mothering, prolific and docile, widely used in crossbreeding, especially with Large White: crosses prolific, good growth rates and FCR. Breed society 1953.

British Lop <Plate 3>

Large white lop-eared pork or cutter pig, long and lean, similar in conformation to the Large Black, mainly in south west England. Practical and robust outdoor pig; economical grazer, docile and easy to manage. Originally from large Celtic lops of northern Europe, similar to old

Welsh and Cumberland pigs. Lop ears over eyes. Landrace blood 1950s. Now a rare breed.

Breed society/herdbook 1921. Also known as Cornish White, Devon Lop, Long White Lop-eared etc.

British Saddleback <Plate2>

Lop-eared black with white saddle; occasionally white socks on one or both hindlegs. White belt varies from almost non-existent to covering most of body. Excellent and favourite outdoor sow, good milkers, large litters, docile and hardy grazers. Also used in crossbreeding to Large White for very good blue-and-white bacon pigs (sometimes nearly all white). Very good FCR. Useful in hot climates. Originally from combining (1967) two distinct breeds of different ancestry, the Wessex Saddleback (in Hampshire) and the Essex (with white on hindlegs also) - hence variety in combined breed, and built-in hybrid vigour. Head of medium length, face very slightly dished, ears medium size carried forward; broad full hams, straight underline (at least 12 teats), strong boned legs, strong feet of good size; fine, silky, straight hair.

Froxfield Pygmy <Plate 22>

Variously coloured prick-eared miniature hybrid, bred for the laboratory at Froxfield, Hampshire, from Vietnamese pot-bellied ("I" type) and Yucatan hairless miniature. Currently coloured, often spotted, but will eventually be white; longer legged than Yucatan, good temperament, non-rooting. Also being sold to a few smallholders.

Gloucester Old Spots <Plate 2>

Large, hardy, lop-eared breed, now mainly white with one or two small circular black patches to identify it - used to be much more heavily spotted and was also sometimes black spotted with white. Traditional cottager's grazing pig. Docile, very good mothers, prolific, cheap to feed and able to convert rough feeds into lean meat, but will run to fat if incorrectly fed - quite good little porkers but must not be checked; also needs to be exercised to distribute the weight gain and avoid becoming overfat. Often crossed with Large White or Landrace - progeny all white. Now a rare breed. Has certain similarities with old Wessex Saddleback; possibly of common ancestry, with some old (unimproved) Berkshire blood, but no firm proof of link between present GOS and original wattled pigs of the county.

Meaty pig, with medium length head and snout, face slightly dished, ear dropping forward to the nose rather than at the sides; long level back, very broad loin, deep sides, large well filled hams, strong legs. At least 14 teats, and at least one clean, decisive spot of black colouring on the white coat. Herdbook 1914.

Large Black <Plate 2>

Black, lop-eared and as big as the Large White and originally deemed superior to it as a bacon pig. Similar in type to British Lop but whole black with a mealy hue. Excellent and hardy outdoor sow, exceedingly docile field grazer (ears hanging forward over the eyes). Early maturing, prolific, very good mothers with lots of milk, quick-growing litters; valuable cross with white boars for traditional blue-and-white baconer. Longer pig than of old; carcass still has higher proportion of fat to lean than Large White but has improved considerably in last 30 years; also much finer in jowl and shoulder now. Deep full hams, sound legs and feet.Well able to withstand hot climates and sunshine.

Originally bred as separate types, one in Cornwall and Devon, the other in Suffolk and Essex (from Small Black); combined as single breed, herdbook 1899. Now rare in UK; was widely exported in the past and known as Cornwall in many countries.

Large White <Plate 4>

Prick-eared, world's major white breed, with a long history. Often known overseas as Yorkshire; sometimes called Large English etc. Now in almost every pig keeping country in the world, and has been widespread for a century or more. Robust, adaptable, efficient and prolific, with excellent carcass and growth rates; universally used in crosses with Landrace. Boars strong and prepotent; sows very good mothers, large litters, heavy milkers, active and sound, long-lived.

Moderately long head, slightly dished face, snout broad and slightly turned up, wide between the eyes, light jowl, long erect ears slightly forwards and fringed with hair; long body, slightly arched back, well muscled; very good hams; good legs and feet; a large, strong, handsome pig, originally a rugged outdoor breed but very well adapted to intensive systems. Fine white skin without wrinkles or coloured spots, silky white hair. High quality bacon and pork.

Origins in Yorkshire and other nearby counties, with Chinese blood late 18th century; gradual divergence into large, middle and small white breeds. Large White recognised 1868, herdbook 1884. National types in many other countries as Yorkshires, Large Whites, Edelschwein and various Improved Whites.

Middle White <Plate 3>

Prick-eared white with short face much more dished than the Large White, and snub-nosed. Now a rare breed. Shorter in head and legs, fuller in the jowl, thicker and more compact in the body. Fairly large ears, fringed with fine hair and inclined forward and outward. Earlier maturing porker, grows well and ideal up to 130 pounds and can also make a cutter but not much good beyond 180 pounds. Well known as the "London porker" between the wars. Regarded with affection by those who keep it, friendly, quiet, and good mothers; consistent breeders; not much of a rootler; hardy and very economical, keeps in good condition and health on less than most other breeds. Usually as purebred but used to be crossed with Berkshire for fatter pigs long ago; now makes good cross with Large White to combine length and lean of the Large with very good pork texture of Middle. Widely exported in the past, and especially appreciated in Japan.

Sometimes said to have originated from Large White x Small White, but more likely simply selected on basis of size from the variable Yorkshires; recognised 1852, herdbook 1884.

Oxford Sandy-and-Black <Plate 2>

Sandy pig with black spots and semi-lop ears. Medium to large, general-purpose type. Slightly controversial breed which over the decades has apparently disappeared and re-appeared more than once. Ancestral links with old Berkshire, Tamworth and GOS. Never a major breed, recently revived as a rare breed with new breed society 1985 - 15 male and 72 female registered in first volume; 18 male and 114 female registered in 1990.

Medium sized semi-lop or lop ears carried horizontally or lower, somewhat similar to Welsh; prick ears indicates cross (usually Berkshire and Tamworth). Sandy red pig with random black blotches and often with pale feet, face blaze (described in old type as "tapir stripe" down forehead) and tail tassel. Proportion of black varies from a little to a great deal; colour of sand also varies, from pale beige to deep rust or rich orange. Back slightly arched, head moderately long with slightly dished face; legs strong boned and of medium length.

Gentle temperament, good mother, prolific and hardy. Good quality and flavour of meat, but can run to fat if overfed. Old type was poor doer, poor hams and long in leg. Produces commercial white hybrids when crossed with white breeds.

Tamworth <Plate 2>

Unmistakeable red prick-eared breed, now rare in the UK. Golden red and abundant coat of straight, fine hairs - shade varies from light ginger to dark red or chestnut. Slightly dished face, longer snout than most British breeds. Longer bodied than it used to be. Rather large and rigid ears, slightly inclined. Light jowl and neck, chest not too deep, light shoulders, strong legs with sprightly carriage; back long and deep, loin strong and broad, straight underline with at least 12 teats; well developed hams. Skin flesh coloured, occasionally with darkish spots, but carcass dresses white with no skin pigment. An energetic pig of character. Has always been lean, very little evidence of the old Chinese cross found in many other breeds, but Americans tried to breed away from bacon type, making shorter and thicker, which produced tendency to lay down more fat. Closely related to the old Berkshire; many theories about source of colour; originally bred in Staffordshire. Good cross with white breeds, also with Berkshire for good pork pigs.

Some strains nervous, some less prolific, though prolificacy used to be high throughout the breed. Tends to be slow feeder and slow to mature. Good grazers if they can be adequately confined; happy as woodland pig; long-lived. Does well in both cold and hot climates - very hardy, widely exported in the past, especially as bacon pig, and the English stock has been boosted in recent years with imports from Australia. First recognised 1850s; breed society and herdbook 1906.

"Iron Age" pigs <Plate 2> developed by crossing Tamworth with a zoo's Wild Boar, created originally in the Cotswolds to represent a primitive-looking pig in a television programme.

Welsh <Plate 3>

Popular and commercial lean white lop-eared breed of Landrace type (Swedish Landrace blood since 1953). Hardy in wide range of climates for outdoor systems; also adapts well to indoor. Apparently genetically distant from other white lops and a useful cross. Breed society and herdbook 1918, once known as Old Glamorgan.

Light, fine head, clean jowl and neck; landrace type lop ears forwards and tending to meet at tips short of the nose. Light shoulders, back long, strong and level; loin well muscled and firm, underline straight, full hams; legs of adequate length and good strong bone; white coat straight and fine, skin fine, blue spots undesirable. At least 12 teats. Prolific, with high carcass quality.

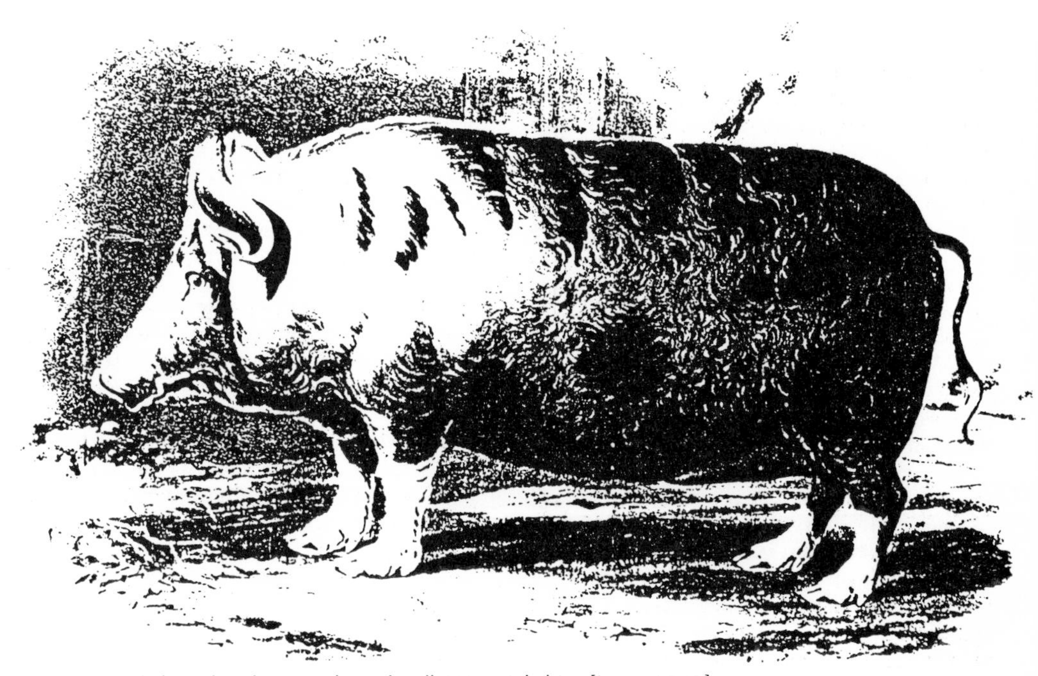

Fig. 14. Berkshire, bred at Mackstockmill, Warwickshire [Low, 1842]

SCANDINAVIA

Most of the land area of Norway, Sweden and Finland was too far north for the Wild Boar, or for the comfort of its domesticants. Yet Scandinavia has given the world the lop-eared and highly commercial white Landrace breeds which for many years have jostled Yorkshire's Large White for top place in pig populations worldwide. The **Danish Landrace** was the first to be systematically improved on a national scale and the Danes backed their skilled breeding with brilliant marketing. They were so successful that they imposed a ban on exports of their national breed, and the Swedes were quick to fill the vacuum with their own Landrace.

Denmark

"In Denmark," wrote journalist J.W. Murray, who chose to study Danish agriculture as part of his Winston Churchill Memorial Fellowship in 1973, "the farmer is important, and can feel that he is important. The country could not run without him."

When Murray wrote his book, there were far more pigs than people in Denmark (8 million to 5 million) and the country was the world's largest exporter of pig meat, half of which went to Britain. Indeed the national breed had been deliberately tailored to produce bacon for the British market.

This very small, flat and windswept country, where the climate allows pasturage for less than half the year, is a land of milk, butter and cheese, and of beef, pork and bacon, large proportions of which are exported - the Danes are a resourceful people and long ago learned that they had to export to survive. They have little in the way of mineral resources, and that is why their farmers are so vital to the national economy. Until the mid 19th century they exported grain but this trade was swept aside by the tidal wave of cheap corn that poured into Europe from the vast prairies of America when steamships changed the pace of Transatlantic shipping. For a while the Danes depended on their old trade of livestock exported on the hoof to Germany but returns were not sufficient until they decided, instead, to export the produce rather than the live animals: dairy produce and meat.

During the 19th century they began to succeed. Britain needed to feed its own rapidly growing industrial population and Denmark loaded the steamships with fresh produce for the voyage across the North Sea. But as they turned their wares westward, their valuable southern farmlands were ceded to Prussia and the large land owners began to lose their influence, while the farmers and smallholders began to increase theirs.

The second half of that century saw the emergence of the great movement that would radically change Danish agriculture and open the door to worldwide trade: co-operation. It began in the 1850s, initially in the form of credit institutions for the benefit of hard-pressed farmers. Then, in 1866, a pastor set up a retail distribution co-operative; his idea inspired others such as a co-operative dairy in 1882 and a bacon factory in 1887. There was no political factor involved - it was a practical scheme born of necessity in difficult circumstances.

Denmark came to rely heavily on its exports of bacon and butter to Britain, and faced potential disaster when, in 1937, Britain abandoned free trade. Salted meat had never been a Danish tradition; they had developed the bacon trade entirely to meet British demands during the 19th century and were sending 1,000 tons a year to that market in 1850, fifty times as much by 1900, and a huge peak of nearly 384,000 tons in 1932. Yet, at the turn of the century, James Long had claimed in his *Book of the Pig* that he had closely examined pigs in various parts of Europe, including the Scandinavian countries, and "in no case have we found anything in the shape of an improved race, or which deserves mention on account of its possession of any particular quality." He proudly proclaimed that Denmark, "which has long been sending us good bacon as the result of her enterprise", relied heavily on British breeds to do so.

The Danish pig was tailormade to produce bacon for the British plate, in a national breeding scheme that began in earnest at the turn of the century and proceeded with a high degree of skilled and co-ordinated breeding based on a relentless system of testing every aspect of the pig - conformation, carcass quality, fertility, viability and slaughter quality of the progeny, freedom from specific diseases and so on. Farmers were encouraged to use the best bred stock, the boars of which were subsidised by the bacon co-operatives. Thus improvements in the Danish pig spread rapidly and evenly through the national herd.

It was not only bacon that the co-operative

factories produced. There was a substantial export trade in canned ham and luncheon meat to the United Kingdom and the United States of America, also a wide range of byproducts such as lard, sausage skins, hogshair brushes, blood (for bakelite) and pancreas and pituitary glands for insulin and pharmaceutical hormones. With the formation of the Common Market, Denmark began to look much further afield and by the 1970s was exporting to 120 countries, with the emphasis on the uniformity of its produce and its prices. Denmark joined the Common Market itself in 1973.

In 1980, the country's pig population was 10 million. There was an outbreak of foot-and-mouth disease in 1982/3 which reduced numbers, but they had returned to the earlier level by 1986, in herds averaging 224 head. The number of herds dropped from 118,000 in 1970 to some 41,600 in 1986 when, as elsewhere in Europe, the herds were fewer but larger.

In the period 1972-1987, exports of live pigs had dropped from 117.7 thousand animals to only 17.6 thousand, and cured pig meat from 278.7 thousand tonnes to 142 thousand, but fresh, chilled and frozen pork had risen from 74,000 to 388,000 tonnes. Bacon remained the country's most valuable export of all agricultural produce and the UK was still its largest market for pigs and pig meat - though only just ahead of Japan.

Today there are 125 private "elite" pig breeding farms in Denmark, working with four purebred lines: **Danish Landrace**, **Danish Large White**, **Danish Duroc** and **Danish Hampshire**. There are about 7,000 purebred sows in these herds. The nucleus herds are still run by families, in the Danish tradition, and are visited regularly by breeding advisers from the association of Danish slaughterhouses. There are central testing stations for boar performance, and progeny testing is also carried out in individual breeding herds. Boars are measured ultrasonically for fat thickness; the nucleus herds are all put through the halothane test (0.4% of the Danish Landrace are sensitive); progeny test-groups are evaluated for carcass characteristics (the average proportion of lean is now more than 58% and expected to reach 61% in the near future). Very detailed records are kept on all the breeding families back to 1970 - which covers more than 340,000 animals - and individual pigs can be ranked on a national basis by an economic index. Fertility is an important factor and the BLUP method is used to calculate a family index for selection based on litter size, covering all the breeding pigs in the national programme. The main factors for selection in the breeding herd are daily liveweight gain, feed conversion efficiency and the percentage of lean meat in the carcass.

There are now 300 multiplier herds, with 25,000 sows, producing first generation parent females (Danish Landrace/Large White cross) for production herds. Artificial insemination is used extensively (60%) and crossbreeding is rife. The **Dan-Hybrid** <Plate 6> from the Danish Landrace/Danish Large White cross is the mother line for most of the 16 million slaughter pigs produced annually; sire lines include Danish Duroc (developed in Denmark as a lean type), Danish Large White, Danish Hampshire and Danish Hybrid boars. A **Dan-Line** hybrid boar has been created from Duroc/Hampshire crosses. More than 90% of the 900,000 sows in the Danish herd are now Dan-Hybrid, which boasts good fertility, good mothering abilities and a longer breeding life, and has been widely exported. The Dan-Hybrid can usefully be put to a Duroc boar for slaughter pigs with high growth rates, low feed conversion ratios and good carcass quality. Sadly, the famous Danish Landrace that was the basis of Denmark's magnificent rise as a bacon producer is no longer considered an economical breed in its own country except within a hybrid.

80% of the produce of slaughter pigs is exported, and live breeding pigs are exported to more than 40 countries worldwide.

Danish Large White

Now the most important breed in Denmark. White prick-eared all-rounder, mainly used for production of Dan-Hybrid gilts but also to produce terminal sires. Fast growth, low FCR, excellent carcass quality. Good sow fertility and mothering abilities. Very low incidence of stress susceptibility (less than 0.1%).

Danish Landrace <Plate 6>

Medium to large, strong and long-bodied white pig with fine hair, long snout, heavy lop ears over eyes, good legs. Very lean - no excess fat or wrinkles. Excellent fertility and mothering; world famous for carcass quality. Very low incidence of stress susceptibility. Dam breed in crossbreeding.

Danish Duroc

Red imported from North America 1977-79 as terminal sire in crossbreeding programme. Improved since importation, especially for meat content and intramuscular fat levels. Denmark now has Europe's largest population of pure-bred Duroc and is still expanding its herd. Performs very well as terminal sire with Dan-Hybrid females to give fast-growing slaughter pigs with low FCR. Halothane-free.

Danish Hampshire

Imported from USA and Canada at same time as Duroc, as terminal sire. Used mainly in production of crossbred terminal sires - popularly the Duroc/Hampshire F_1 which gives full benefit of heterosis on Dan-Hybrid sows. Hampshire gives lean carcasses and good meat quality, and is halothane free.

The History of the Danish Landrace

The medieval Danish pig, which survived even beyond the end of the 18th century, was of two types: a larger, long-bodied Jutland on the mainland and a smaller, short-backed, erect-eared Island type on Sealand with a high crest of bristles along its back. In 1804 Professor E.N. Viborg described the two basic national types of land pig and the description remained fundamentally the same in 1847. However, between about 1790 and 1820 there were recorded importations to the larger private estates on Sealand and Fyn islands of Chinese, Iberian and various English local or fancy breeds, especially around Copenhagen (a market for fresh pork). The big estates began to distribute breeding stock to smaller farms.

The old Sealand land pig came under foreign influence to a far greater extent than the Jutland type, and contemporary illustrations show the difference. A Sealand type pictured in 1844 was still much like the original land pig with its long legs and long, lean body; in contrast a Sealand sow of 1847 shows definite outside influence - she is black-and-white, effectively a saddleback with a wide white belt, and large ears beginning to fall forward, and a much deeper and fuller body altogether. Another, of 1844, has huge ears forward over the eyes and some random dark patches of colour.

A Jutland pig, in an illustration of unknown original date reproduced in 1883 <Plate 6>, is often offered as an example of the typical European land pig. It has long legs, a long lean body, slightly arched back, poor hams, a long, tapering snout, and horizontal ears growing forward, almost over the eyes. The Iberian type illustrated in Viborg (1804) is a black, short-legged boar with large, semi-erect ears, longish straight face and longish snout.

When pig breeding began to become important in the mid 19th century, with the loss of the grain trade and the development of dairying estates and their byproducts, breeding pigs were being brought in from Holstein and Schleswig in the 1840s to the dairy farms on the southern Danish islands. They were crossbreds, a combination of the local land pigs (still of the two original types) with English porkers such as Middle White and Berkshire. The crossbreds increased in numbers up to the mid 1860s as the basis of a live export trade in short, heavy pigs to Hamburg. At the same time the importation of pork-type breeding pigs from Britain was being developed. Germany stopped importing live Danish pigs from 1887, but even after the war of 1864 Denmark was beginning to look with interest towards the British market. British breeds were imported in larger numbers, especially the Berkshire for its rapid development and good health. The British porkers were favoured over the land pigs because they had been improved with Chinese and Neapolitan blood, and they strongly influenced the island pig populations on Sealand, Fyn, Lolland and Falster between 1840 and 1887. However, their numbers and influence were limited in north and central Jutland, where the original land pig remained largely untainted.

In 1865, a Scottish steamship line had opened up a regular crossing between Copenhagen and Leith, at the request of the Royal Danish Agricultural Society, to carry the produce of the newly built and privately owned bacon factories in Copenhagen and Aarhus. The demands of the British market encouraged the factories to import Large White breeding stock from the mid 1870s. Other private bacon exporters followed suit, bringing in mainly boars and distributing them to their upland pig producers. The main influx of Large Whites was in 1879-1896. Mr Magnus Kjoer, who became manager of a private enterprise bacon factory in west Jutland in 1880, had been trained in England and studied Irish bacon production (Ireland was Denmark's main competitor at the time); he realised the importance of changing not only production methods but also the type of pig to suit the British market - and radically, using a pig that was entirely different from the locals. The Large White was ideal for Danish bacon.

By 1879 the original Jutland land pig was still numerous, in contrast to the islands where so much crossing had already occurred - the original Sealand type had completely disappeared by the time of the 1871 census and the remaining so-called land pigs on the islands had been thoroughly crossed with the British porkers.

Kjoer became the main importer of Large Whites and, although only 200 breeding animals were imported from Britain between 1879 and 1896, their influence on bacon production was immense. Kjoer placed them in breeding farms, and salesmen then distributed the offspring all over the country. It was found that the first cross of a Large White boar on a land-type sow gave the best baconers but, with a shortage of breeding animals, crossbreds were widely used, with inferior results.

In 1896, a government livestock commissioner put forward a national pig-breeding plan in the face of increasing Canadian competition for the British market. For the sake of speed, his favoured scheme was the continuous distribution of purebred animals of both the Large White and the land pig so that commercial producers could breed first-generation crosses for export, and at the same time the land pig could be developed by selection from within the type. He proposed that it should be called the Danish Landrace.

In 1895, 7 Large White boars and 17 Large White sows were purchased as foundation stock for four new centres. By 1935, there were 252 breeding centres but only 11% of them kept Large Whites or Yorkshires. By 1962, the last Yorkshire breeding centre in Denmark had ceased to exist.

Now came the more arduous process of establishing the Danish Landrace. Its first 15 breeding centres were established in 1896 and by 1900 there were 91 of them. Government aid was available from 1898 to 1955, and by 1964 there were 249 Landrace centres.

The most difficult task had been to establish the Landrace foundation herds. Pedigrees were seldom available and Rasmus, who became the breed's most famous foundation sire and who was born in 1895, was of parents unknown. In the absence of paperwork, the only way to select the foundation stock was strictly by conformation, trying to keep as close to the original land type as possible. Although the British porkers had been so widely used for so many years, and in spite of intensive Large White crossing in the 1870s and 1880s, apparently the officials did succeed in establishing their typical foundation animals, though many had to be rejected as poor breeders.

It had been the tradition since the mid 19th century for certain farmers to keep Jutish land pigs for sale as pure bred as possible and they sold land-type weaners at rural pig markets. One important trademark of the old Jutland was its horizontal lop ears; it also had a straight profile untainted by any Asian dishing, and had a dense coat. With good maternal abilities, it was much better adapted to the Danish environment than the Large White.

The first Danish Landrace herdbook was produced in 1906, including first and second generation selected sires born between 1893 and 1904. There were 126 boars, 60% of them bred in Jutland, 21% on Fyn, 10% on Sealand and the rest on other islands. Progeny testing began in 1899, when it was shown that the Yorkshire took seven days longer to reach slaughter weight but its carcass had 3% more bacon for export.

With increasing competition for the British market, testing concentrated on carcass quality (previously growth rates and feed conversion were considered more important). Soon the Landrace became virtually the only breed in Denmark and it was greatly improved between 1927 and 1950 - it gained more length, better hams and a thicker belly but reduced its backfat. The rigorous breeding programme continued, still with very definite aims, and the breed consistently improved in its homeland. However, when it was bred in other countries the selection and management were often less strict and sometimes the breed developed faults such as weakness in the long back or the legs. After the Second World War, Denmark decided to restrict the export of its, by then, highly popular breed's pedigree stock, and left the field open for Sweden.

In the meantime the Danish Landrace had contributed to some highly successful Landraces in other countries - for example, the Swedish, Dutch, Norwegian, French, Swiss and South African. It has come to represent one extreme in the Landrace spectrum - that of the very lean and very long bacon type, which has managed to avoid the problem of stress susceptibility. In fact, long before the halothane gene was identified, the Danes had recognised a deterioration in muscle quality and in 1972 they altered the national programme to place the emphasis on quality rather than quantity of meat.

In deliberately selecting for length and bacon carcasses, the Danes found that their Landrace had become uneconomical. Its productivity was too low, and its carcass, bred for Wiltshire cure, became inappropriate in the European Community markets. They therefore imported the Large White once again and began to use their special skills in tailoring this breed to their needs, using it as a cross on the Landrace to produce the very successful Dan-Hybrid for intensive systems. Later they brought in the Duroc and Hampshire. In 1960, the Danish Landrace had been the country's only breed; today it produces only about a quarter of Danish bacon. But it was the blueprint and the genetic base for countries all over Europe to develop their own improved Celtic land pigs, albeit in many different directions. It is a leading example of deliberate breeding on a national scale aimed directly at a specific export market.

Meanwhile, on Fyn island today, there are still the remnants of the old Danish land pig on a rare-breed farm at Oregaard. Maybe one day someone will once again need these reddish animals with black markings, and wattles dangling from their throats.

Norway

Pig farming in Norway is often supplementary to other farm activities and the pig farms are small, averaging 15 sows each, not only because of natural conditions but also because of legislation which regulates production. In view of the country's strategic geographical position, the aim has long been self-sufficiency rather than export. The combination of these factors, and the costs involved, have restricted production to meet only the domestic market, in which consumption of pork is about 20kg per capita per annum. The average annual production is about 1.2 million pigs slaughtered at 100-105kg liveweight, with a mixed market for bacon and heavy pigs. Pork is the highest production factor in the meat sector, supplying 80,000 tonnes out of the national total of 195,000 tonnes (beef production is 75,000 tonnes, mutton 22,000 and poultry 18,000).

In 1988 there were 8,126 herds, 80% of which were of fattener-breeders; there were 4,271 sow herds with 20 or fewer sows each and only 30 with more than 70 sows, and there were 5,317 slaughter units with 50 or fewer slaughter pigs and 223 units with more than 500.

The country's only AI station is responsible for 75% of all sow inseminations. The national sow herd numbers about 60,000 animals, based on three breeds: the **Norwegian Landrace** <Plate 7> is the most common (65-70%), while the Norwegian Yorkshire and the Duroc have small purebred sow populations (500 and 50 respectively). Yorkshire sows in particular are used to produce hybrid market hogs from Landrace boars, and hybrid sows form 25-30% of the sow herd. The Yorkshire was first imported in the 19th century but the Duroc only arrived in 1984, from Denmark, to improve meat taste and to increase litter sizes. Under a control system covering 60% of all sows, current litter averages are 11.83 born (10.9 born alive) and 9.35 at 3 weeks old (weaning is at 5 weeks). Average age at first farrowing is 345 days; the average farrowing interval is 172 days. In commercial herds the average weight at 75 days is 25kg, and 100kg at 165 days, with an FCR of 2.8 and a carcass lean proportion of 59%.

Norsvin, the Norwegian pig breeders' association, was formed in 1958 as a non-profit farmers' co-operative embracing nearly all the country's pig production, and it began to base its breeding programme exclusively on economic criteria. By 1959, ultrasonic backfat measurements were being used on a large scale and organised AI was already part of the breeding programme; by 1977, they were producing frozen boar semen comparable in quality with fresh and in the following year the Norwegians established a boar data bank. Boars were station-tested and the best were reserved for AI. In 1982 they began to use computer tomography scanning in boar selection so that body composition could be ascertained without the need to slaughter.

Norsvin's breeding programme remains based strictly on economic factors, as a result of which the national breed has become perhaps rather plain in the hams and long in the leg. The most important traits are feed conversion efficiency, lean percentages, daily weight gains, carcass composition and quality, fertility and conformation. Within the breeding programme are privately owned elite herds, in which 83.6% (2,500 sows) were Norwegian Landrace in 1990, 15.1% (450 sows) Yorkshire and 1.3% (40 sows) Duroc. 40,000 pigs (including 5,000 boars) are tested on-farm annually to draw up an index for each animal. By 1989 it could be claimed that 75% of all pigs slaughtered in Norway had less than 14mm backfat at 100kg liveweight, and purebred averages for this measurement included 10.4mm and 10.2mm for Landrace and Yorkshire gilts, with 9.8mm and 9.7mm for the respective boars. In the elite herds, ultrasonic backfat measurements are as low as 8.8mm, with average daily weight gains of 978g at 2.04 feed units per kilogram of weight gain.

Norwegian Landrace <Plate 7>

By the 6th century AD, there were large herds of domesticated pigs in the woodlands of Norway and Sweden, all of them slate coloured, small and with plenty of bristles to protect them from the elements. Viking pigs gave rise to the modern Norwegian Landrace and long-legged, primitive domesticated pigs with striped, bristly coats and upright ears still foraged the huge forests in the 17th and 18th centuries. The Landrace evolved from local pigs which were crossed with **Large White** (and also **Middle White**) in the 1880s, and then with **Danish Landrace** in 1900. These early imports were carefully blended and selected for a Norwegian environment. The main breeding areas were in Hedmark and Oppland in the south east and in Trøndelag in the central region. Breeders in some areas liked black spots on their pigs and even now such spots are not unusual in the breed. More rarely, the spots have a yellowish edging.

Essentially, though, the Norwegian Landrace is a white pig of the Scandinavian bacon type - long and lean, with heavy, drooping ears. It is probably the most prolific of the Landraces, and the sows are good mothers. Daily weight gains are high, feed conversion efficiency is very good, and the carcasses are very lean and long. The problem of the halothane gene has been closely monitored in the breed and in 1989 no halothane-positive boars were found during station testing. The intensive use of AI has helped to control the potential problem: 98% of sows in elite herds are served by AI and only by boars selected to be sires of the next generation of boars, all of them screened for the halothane gene by means of test-matings in a deliberately maintained herd of 45 halothane-positive sows. None of the boars in AI service are halothane reactors.

The health status of the national herd is particularly high and tightly controlled; disease is almost unknown. This status, and the breed's good reputation, have helped Norway to achieve exports of its Landrace to many countries for quality pork production.

Icelandic

Compared with the Norwegian Landrace, the Icelandic pigs have larger heads, stronger legs, slower growth rates, similar or slightly lower reproduction rates and much higher fat levels in the carcass. Most of the pigs are white but some are black-and-white.

The importation of live pigs or of boar semen for breeding purposes is prohibited; the population, reared in isolation for several decades, has become inbred. There are only about 60 farms with pigs, and only six of these have more than 80 animals, accounting for some 40% of all Iceland's pigs. The national herd is about 3,00 0breeding sows and 300 boars. Most Icelanders greatly prefer sheep meat to pork.

The species was first brought to Iceland by Viking colonists and settlers from Ireland and the Scottish isles but became extinct during the 17th century. Pigs were introduced again early in the 20th century when Yorkshire and Berkshire stock came in from England along with Danish Landrace to form the basis of the present population.

Sweden

In Sweden, animal production is vital to farmers: it forms about 80% of their income. Cattle are considered to be the most important livestock but pig numbers are much higher. Most pig herds have fewer than a hundred animals each, though the number of small herds is decreasing. By the mid 1980s about 44% of the total number of pigs were in the hands of those who produced more than 500 slaughter animals, but these large producers represented less than 5% of all producers. In 1988, about two thirds of the pigs slaughtered were produced by some 4,000 specialist units; more than 2.5 million weaners are transferred each year from sow herds to grower herds and run considerable stress and disease risks.

In common with other Scandinavian countries, Sweden has had a national breeding policy to produce leaner carcasses and today all pigs are of the Landrace and Yorkshire types. In 1850 there were 560,000 pigs in the country; a century later there were 1.26 million and the figure has since more than doubled. Today, considerably more pork is eaten in Sweden than beef or other meat.

In 1880, agriculture employed three quarters of the 4.6 million population. A century later less than 4% (203,000) were directly employed in farming. The farms, as elsewhere, are becoming fewer and larger but a third are still only 2-10 ha and most are family enterprises, usually with no employees and often part of a co-operative group.

As in Norway, self-sufficiency in peace or war has been the aim in agricultural production, and the government helps northern farms with supplements for pork and milk. There tends to be a surplus to cover fluctuations such as the increasing demand for ham at Christmas. Retail price subsidies on pig meat were removed in 1980 and a decline in demand followed, but the trend has been reversed since 1986.

Recently, Sweden introduced new animal welfare regulations which have important implications for pig farmers and others. The regulations include, for example, a ban on dry sow stalls and they demand probably the most generous floor-space requirements in Europe for breeding sows and growing pigs. The whole industry is rethinking its approach and there is much more interest in deep-straw loose housing systems, with transponder-activated feeding stations, or outdoor systems where the climate is kinder. Early-weaning cages and flat decks are no longer allowed and the use of antibiotics in creep feed was banned in 1986, so that the weaning age (5-6 weeks) is high for a European country.

In a new Swedish scheme, top class hybrid sows are being leased to pig farmers shortly before farrowing. The farmer takes the litter through to weaning and then returns the sow to the pool for serving again in preparation for her next leasing term. Thus the farmer can specialise in farrowing and weaning, without having to incur extra capital costs.

Southern and central Sweden remain the most concentrated pig production regions, though the proportion in the extreme south has declined. The number of herds continues to fall while the size of remaining herds increases. The average herd size, however, remains comparatively low.

AI is much less used in Sweden than in Norway, especially for sows in the slaughter-producing generation. It is much more common in the breeding herds; most breeding sows are bought from specialised gilt producers and are usually Yorkshire/Landrace crosses.

Fewer than half the pigs now sent for slaughter are of that cross, however, and the long domination by the **Swedish Landrace** over the national pig industry is beginning to weaken. A premium is now paid for carcasses of Hampshire-sired three-breed crosses, which are marketed under the name **Pigghamn** and now account for about half the total slaughtered. The Duroc boar is beginning to make its mark, too, though only about 5% of slaughter pigs are currently sired by Durocs. The latest marketing name for the Duroc cross is the **New York Red**!

Swedish pigs suddenly became popular at the end of the Second World War, when Denmark restricted its exports of pedigree Danish Landrace and when the population of Germany's Large Whites had declined. Sweden emerged as a large-scale supplier of Landraces and Large Whites just as there was an increasing trend in most of Europe for lean meat and a decrease in the consumption of lard and fat meat. The change encouraged widespread exchanges of breeding stock between countries and a complicated network of crossbreeding and upgrading in which Sweden was able to play an important role.

The old Swedish breeds had become extinct by 1900, though recent attempts to recreate them superficially have used Wild Boar crosses (rather like the English experiment crossing Tamworth sows to Wild Boar for "Iron Age" pigs). However, the Swedish forests were once home to the same very primitive, coarsely bristled pigs that roamed Norway - erect-eared and long-legged dark brown animals of the same type as would have been seen in medieval times elsewhere in northern Europe's extensive woodlands.

Swedish Landrace <Plate 7>

White, with heavy drooping Landrace ears. High proportion of lean but not of extreme length like the Danish type. Emphasis on sound legs and feet, and on strength, with good liveweight gains, feed conversion efficiency, prolificacy and mothering. Fresh pork as well as bacon. Originated from imports, particularly of **Danish Landrace**. Breed society 1907, herdbook 1911. Exported to UK in 1950s as basis of **British Landrace**, and to USA to broaden genetic basis of **American Landrace**.

According to the *Guinness Book of Records*, a record price of 3,300 guineas was paid in 1955 for the Swedish Landrace gilt "Bluegate Ally 33rd", sold at Reading in Berkshire by Davidson Trust to Malvern Farms. This was the period during which Britain was forming its own Landrace, and some farmers belittled the Swedish pigs as "ewe-necked".

Finland

There are 1.4 million pigs in Finland, including 140,000 breeding sows and 5,400 boars. Pork is exported regularly. Canned goods, including luncheon meat and skinless sausages in brine, traditionally find a ready market in the Baltic countries and Russia, and are also exported to Scandinavian and other European countries, the United States, Japan and the Far East. On the domestic market, annual meat consumption is about 60kg per capita per annum, of which more than half is pork. There are about 10,000 farms producing slaughter pigs and they tend to be relatively small: only one in three can handle more than 300 pigs at a time. They are situated mostly in the west and south west of the country.

A third of the sows are artificially inseminated, which helps to maximise the national herd's genetic improvement. The purebred stock are either **Finnish Yorkshire** <Plate 4> or **Finnish Landrace**, in almost equal proportions, and commercial pork production is based partly on crossbreeding. Both breeds have excellent growth rates and slaughter characteristics, good feed conversion efficiency and fertility, good maternal ability, sound constitutions, vitality and stress resistance.

The overall objective of the national pig improvement scheme is to produce animals which meet changing market requirements and are also profitable for the producers. To meet those aims the scheme has long concentrated on FCE, improved growth rates, carcass and meat quality, constitution and health. Progeny and sib testing have been important since the late 1920s, and performance testing is carried out on farms and at central stations.

Of prime importance is the improvement of stress resistance in breeding stock, by a combination of halothane testing and test mating, intended to eliminate the halothane gene from the Finnish herd. The maintenance of Finland's well known good health status is also emphasised.

Finnish Landrace <Plate 6>

The white, lop-eared Finnish Landrace is unusual in Europe in that it derives essentially from Finland's own land pigs rather than relying heavily on imported Landraces. Thus it is set a little apart and is a useful source of heterosis in crossbreeding.

The two originators of the breed were the short-eared **East Finnish** and the lop **West Finnish** (with large, pendulous ears). These two thicker boned and rather coarse bristled unimproved types were brought together in the mid 19th century. A breed society for the combination was established in 1908 and it was not until the 1940s that some Swedish Landrace blood was introduced as well. The Finnish Landrace shows traces of its native origins in that some animals have blue spots. It is a popular improver for landraces in other countries.

THE NETHERLANDS

The total surface area of the Netherlands is more than 4 million ha, half of which is under cultivation. But only about 6% of the population work in agriculture. Dutch farming is, of necessity, intensively based and highly efficient, especially in livestock breeding. After all, it was this very small country which gave the world the black-and-white Friesian and Holstein cattle.

Much of Dutch produce is exported and this has been a considerable spur to efficiency, consistency and very good marketing. Livestock farming is worth some two-thirds of all agricultural production, in value, and pork is of particular importance in the intensive sector.

In 1935 there were about 1.4 million Dutch pigs. The total population increased from fewer than 3 million in 1960 to more than 12 million in 1985 (half of them fatteners, and about 1.5 million breeding sows) with the average herd size in the same period growing from 20 to 343, and the slaughter weight of pork rising from 435 to 1650 million kg. Meanwhile the 146,000 farms were reduced to 36,000. In 1985, about 19.5 million pigs were produced, 85% of which were slaughtered and the rest exported on the hoof. The home consumption of pork in that period rose from 23 to 40 kg per capita per annum.

Intensive pig farming took root during the 1950s and developed strongly in the 1970s when, as elsewhere, the number of units decreased but the average size of those units greatly increased. Such intensification demanded a different type of pig, by crossbreeding and selection, for higher production to meet higher input costs, and it also meant closer veterinary monitoring and legislation to ensure the welfare and health of the stock.

In parallel with this considerable growth in the industry, there has been a trend towards specialisation and the pig industry is now divided between top breeding farms, ordinary breeders, multiplication farms and fattening farms. AI stations offer top class boars throughout the country, and the national herd's genetic improvement is assisted by a carefully designed system which centrally tests boar performance and progeny. The National Pig Herdbook of the Netherlands checks pigs on the breeding farms and compares breeds and strains with those on its own research farm. The NPHB covers more than 12,000 breeding herds and has 50,000 sows available for breeding stock production on its breeding farms.

The most common female line is the highly prolific **Dutch Landrace**, widely used as a grandparent sow. Multipliers favour the **Dutch Yorkshire** dam line for production of parent stock, selected for good reproductive qualities, growth rates, feed conversion and meat production. The Yorkshire/Landrace parent gilt is prolific and scores highly for liveborn and weaned piglets.

The Dutch Yorkshire boar is by far the most popular commercial terminal sire, specially bred for high growth rates, good FCE and meat production with a high percentage of lean in the progeny. Crossbred and Duroc boars are also used. The Finnish Landrace is used on a small scale: 60 sows and 15 boars were imported from Finland in 1983 and then selected to fit the Dutch context, essentially as a dam line in cross with Dutch Landrace and Dutch Yorkshire for highly fertile F_1 multiplier sows. The Finnish breed's carcass is very long but well balanced and the breed is selected in the Netherlands for high prolificacy, strong constitution, high udder quality and reduced susceptibility to stress. There are only about 350 Finnish Landrace sows in the country.

The main structure of Herdbook pig production, however, is based on the Dutch Yorkshire sire line; Dutch Landrace nucleus sows are bred to dam line Dutch Yorkshire boars to produce F_1 crossbred multiplier sows, which are then crossed to sire line Dutch Yorkshire boars to produce F_2 slaughter pigs, so that the majority of slaughter pigs are crossbreds.

Recently a premium has been introduced for free-range pork production and, to offset costs, these strictly controlled units earn extra income by admitting paying visitors.

Dutch Landrace <Plate 7>

White, with large ears growing forwards horizontally. Long carcass, good musculature. High fertility, excellent mothering. Efficient. Originally from native pigs in the Netherlands, influenced by the German (Improved) Landrace (imported since 1902) and the Danish Landrace (imported 1929 onwards). Herdbook 1933, dating from 1913. In the 1940s and 1950s the Dutch Landrace was of the Danish type, bred more for length than stockiness. The Dutch population has been closed since then and was subsequently developed for a meatier type with heavier hams and a broader back, so that it became much closer to the German type but had nothing like the extreme muscling of the Belgian.

Improved by selection for specific dam line function (fertility and constitution important) - selection for better growth rates, feed consumption and slaughter characteristics. As dam, selection is for strong legs and feet, strong connection of shoulder/back/loin, sufficient length and depth of carcass, and width and depth of ham. In the past there has been a high level of stress susceptibility in the breed, with adverse effects on performance and slaughter characteristics; however, halothane testing and selection have lowered the problem permanently to less than 1%. About 40,000 Dutch Landrace sows in the herd, mostly served by Dutch Yorkshire to produce F_1 multiplier sows. Top 10-15% are used for pure breeding, all by AI on nucleus sows by station-tested purebred boars.

Dutch Yorkshire <Plate 4>

White, with erect ears. First Yorkshires imported from England at the beginning of the present century. Separated (1983-87) into dam and sire lines. Dam line boosted with British Large White (1988-90) and then closed and strongly selected; large solid carcass, average to good muscling, high fertility, good slaughter characteristics and constitution (strong legs and claws). There are about 8,000 Dutch Yorkshire dam line sows. Sire line as terminal sire selected for large strong meat type, quite heavy muscling, strength and quality of legs and feet, good gait, good width and depth of back, loin and ham. An efficient breed.

BELGIUM

Belgium is the home of the *culard* or "rumpy" livestock: cattle and pigs often display an extreme form of double-muscling which offers high weights of very lean meat, but with certain drawbacks.

In 1846, a few years after the Dutch had recognised Belgium's independence from the kingdom of the Netherlands, there were 497,000 pigs in Belgium. By 1910 there were 1.5 million but two world wars took their toll in a landscape which became a major battleground and by 1941, there were only half a million pigs. Their population had trebled by 1960, and was double that by 1970, and had reached 5.5 million in 1976. By the late 1980s there were 6 million pigs (and only 3 million cattle) in an agricultural industry dominated by livestock production.

The trend in Belgium, as elsewhere, has been towards fewer and larger pig units and greater specialisation, especially between 1945 and 1960 in the sandy regions where farms had traditionally been very small. By 1960 the pigs were on 130,000 farms; by 1978 they were on only 50,000 holdings and the average number per farm had risen from 10 to 105. Family farms by the thousand had been converted into specialist, thoroughly up-to-date enterprises.

The post-war period saw a growing home market demanding high quality fresh meat, which spurred Belgian breeders to improve their pigs. Fresh pork required much leaner pigs than the fattier type used for cured and processed pig meat. In 1950, in response to these pressures, a very special and localised village breed came to the industry's notice and soon became prominent in Belgium. It was a unique type for its unprecedented meatiness: it was solid muscle, especially in the hams, and with hardly a trace of fat. Indeed it had almost become extinct for that very reason - fat had been much in demand, especially during the war. It was, of course, the **Piétrain**, and its distinctive breadth and stockiness and its spotted coat made an impression overseas as well. It is now known all over the world for its double-muscled rump, a characteristic it shares with Belgian Blue cattle.

Belgium also produced its own **Belgian Landrace** and, again, it was much more muscular than other European Landraces. It is now often crossed with the Piétrain to produce rearing pigs, and both breeds have been widely exported.

Both the Belgian breeds became notorious for poor prolificacy and, more seriously, for high susceptibility to stress, until the breeders began to take these faults seriously. By the mid 1980s a hybrid breeding programme emphasised the two breeds' best qualities and masked their faults, and a third of the market share was taken by the hybrids. Now the combination of the two extreme breeds gives slaughter pigs that can kill out at an average 83%, with a lean content of 62%, though it has proved difficult to exploit that double-muscling without *ad lib* feeding. However, the Belgians are content with their stock and will no doubt continue to concentrate on larger, heavier lean carcasses with slaughter weights of at least 100 kg.

A more recent development is the **BN**, a Landrace line selected for negative stress susceptibility, the trait which is linked with extreme musculature which, in turn, is linked with the halothane gene and results in carcass problems such as pale, watery, soft fat, not to mention sudden death from stress.

The Large White is also used in Belgium, where it is being selected for prolificacy (the aim is for 20 per sow per year), growth rates (900g) and higher proportions of lean (56%). This big white prick-eared pig is basically the same as any other Large White - a strong, longish type, with a strong bone structure. The Belgians had long admired the prolificacy and maternal qualities of the Large White but noted that the British type had been selected more for absence of fat than positively for meat content, carcass distribution and dressing percentage.

The national breeding system is organised around provincial breeding associations within a national federation, with testing stations investigating the best strains of each breed. In 1987 the registrations for pure breeds gave top place to the Belgian Landrace (12,989) and Piétrain (6,573), with 261 Large White registrations and 926 of other breeds including, for example, the Duroc. The typical Belgian piggery today is intensive and highly automated, with correspondingly low staffing levels. Weaning tends to be early, at 3 weeks of age, and the Landrace in particular has been bred with intensive rearing in mind.

Belgian Landrace <Plate 7>

White, heavy drooping ears. Very muscular (selected for double-muscling). Quality fresh pork. Shorter than, say, Dutch Landrace but higher proportion of meat in lean cuts. Reasonably prolific but not necessarily good or milky mothers.

In its early years this Landrace was developed from local Celtic type pigs crossed with English breeds. It was established as a breed in 1930, when it was a short, fat and poorly muscled land pig. From 1930 until 1945 it was graded up to German (Improved) Landrace and after the war to Dutch Landrace which included a recent infusion of Danish Landrace. Thereafter the Belgians concentrated on selection for strength, fertility and improved growth rates and feed conversion efficiency. No doubt some Piétrain blood entered the type at some stage.

Sometimes known as the **Poppel** in France (where it is one of the four major commercial breeds), the Belgian Landrace is opposite in extreme to the Danish type. It is noticeably less long in the body and much more muscular, especially in the hams. It is large, with a long head and broad face, a snout of medium length, quite a slender medium-length neck, forward-growing ears hanging over the eyes, and a light but solid bone structure. It stands 80-85cm tall and is 160-170cm long, with typical weights of 340-400kg (boars) and 250-300kg (sows). The long body has a very wide back and those globular *culard* hams. It is a uniformly white pig.

BN

This variety of the Belgian Landrace is similar in appearance to the original but with less exaggerated hams and a stronger skeleton. It has at least 14 teats (the Landrace might have only 12) as it has been selected above all for better prolificacy without losing the high proportion of lean meat. It was bred in response to stress problems in the Landrace relating to the halothane gene, and screening tests for the gene were complemented with blood-typing in meaty boar lines. The ideal is a growth rate of 850g, a carcass with 58% lean and a production index of 19 per sow per year.

Piétrain <Plate 8>

Greyish white with black spots. Almost erect ears directed forwards. Solid and balanced medium-sized pig but double-muscled - bulging hams, extremely high proportion of lean meat for fresh pork (meat quality affected by PSE unless heterozygous for the halothane gene); backfat 7.8mm, dressing 75.9%, proportion lean 61.4% (French data). Early maturing unless otherwise selected. Height 75-85cm, length 150-160cm, weights 260-300kg (boars), 230-260kg (sows). Stocky, broad back, shorter legs than some; short neck, relatively light head; very muscular shoulders; large, deep, cylindrical chest. Boars precocious; sows docile, good milkers, usually good mothers (French averages 10.2

born alive, 8.3 weaned) though birth weights can be low and growth rates not necessarily fast. The black spots are large and irregular, often encircled by a bluish ring of white hairs on pigmented skin; red hairs are often present and the spots themselves are sometimes rusty red.

This is a romantic tale. In Brabant, there is a village called Piétrain, and it was near this little community that the breed was first noticed in about 1920 - but only locally. It was not until 1950 that it became more widely known for its quite exceptional and unique carcass qualities. There are various theories about its origin.

Some have suggested that the Piétrain has a mixture of Normand, Large White and Berkshire in its history; others that it owes its ancestry to a combination of the Bayeux (itself originating from Berkshire x Normand) with either Berkshire or even Tamworth, crossed with local Belgian pigs. It is interesting to note in passing that there were some large, strong, muscular types with semi-erect ears in France during the 19th century: originally the coat of this Périgord variety of the Limousin was grey-black but it developed into a black-and-white pied after certain crosses.

It is likely that a genetic mutation gave rise to the halothane gene and hence to the muscular hypertrophy that gives the Piétrain its exceptional conformation, and that this trait was subsequently selected for by its local breeders, whatever the original ancestry of their pig. For some two or three decades a few farmers continued to breed it, virtually unnoticed beyond the immediate environs of its village, and because of its extreme leanness it almost died out at a time when people craved fat during the war. All that changed in the 1950s, and by 1955 it was being imported by breeders in northern France. A herdbook was formed in 1958 but there were problems with the purebred and it was usually employed as a terminal sire. It was exported to Germany in 1960, and there it became even stockier - both Piétrain and Belgian Landrace were used to compensate for the poor carcass shape of Germany's specialist maternal breeds.

In due course a substantial prejudice built up against the Piétrain for its alarming tendency to "drop dead" under stress. This susceptibility is directly linked with the halothane gene that is expressed in the breed's muscling and the problem has been to avoid its drawbacks while retaining the very important advantages - which include, in comparison with (say) the Large White: a higher carcass yield for a given liveweight, a leaner carcass with a larger eyemuscle and more carcass weight in the ham, and a much higher ratio of lean to bone. (See Genetics section.)

The Belgian breeders are aiming for a growth rate of 700g, a prolificacy of 16 piglets per sow per year and a carcass with a lean proportion of 65%. The extreme type of Piétrain boar can have problems in covering sows because of short legs and lack of pelvis length, as well as the stress factor, and AI has therefore become increasingly popular. In France, they are trying to improve the boar's ability for natural service and have also been selecting over several years for larger animals with better hardiness and vigour.

FRANCE

In times gone by, there were almost as many pig breeds in France as there are departments. By 1979 there were only four officially recognised breeds, and all of them were originally imported. Today, the majority of France's pigs are improved whites and new breeds are being created during hybridisation programmes which now use south east Asian as well as American and European breeds.

The most important commercial pigs are the Large White and the Landrace, which France has developed to suit its own needs, and also the Belgian Landrace and Piétrain. The red American Duroc is increasingly popular and, since 1979, the indigenous pigs of China have played their part in France as well. The country also has an interest in the breeds of Vietnam and the tropical creoles of the Caribbean.

The most ubiquitous are the Large White and the French Landrace, used together in the production of parent hybrid sows. The Belgian Landrace represents only 3% of the selection sows and the Piétrain about 6%, but both breeds are used mainly as terminal sires. The stress-sensitivity gene is deliberately maintained in the terminal sire breeds but eradicated in the parent sow lines.

Production in some parts of the country has increased rapidly in recent years - by 43% in Brittany, for example, between 1980 and 1990. It has been greatly accelerated by a higher level of co-operation between producer groups. The pig population is now about 12 million, which is more than sheep but nowhere near the 23 million cattle. The human population is some 56 million, of which about three quarters live in urban areas.

The selection programme for all breeds in France is based on central and on-farm testing, with blood-typing to eradicate stress susceptibility in the French Landrace, and litter recording schemes to identify top-performance sows for an experimental hyperprolific Large White line. The breeding stock are produced by independent breeders, co-operatives and breeding companies supplying a multiplication tier of 800 herds (61,000 sows) to provide commercial farms with parental sows and boars.

French Large White <Plate 4>

White. Erect ears, directed forwards. "Brick" shaped body with long trunk, straight topline and underside, deep, with regular breadth; good hams, strong legs; height 100-110cm, length 185-200cm, liveweights 280-350kg (sows)/400-500kg (boars). Strong, large, short head with concave profile, large snout.

The large white Yorkshire already had an international reputation at the end of the 19th century, when it was introduced into France; a French breed society was formed in 1923 and a herdbook three years later. Plenty of Yorkshire pigs had been imported during the 1880s but they were of the smaller, snub-nosed types with plenty of fat - probably Middle Whites. However, in 1885 Large Whites, brought in for their fecundity and milkiness, were certainly imported. It was not until about 1938 that the French began to select for less compact conformation and less fat.

After the Second World War the Large White ousted local French breeds and today it is widespread, representing more than 55% of the sows in selection herds, where its adaptability, excellent growth rates (boars 926g per day at 2.49 FCR), good breeding qualities, and lack of stress susceptibility are appreciated. It is a thoroughly hardy breed, able to adapt to a wide range of climates and management systems; the boars are good workers and the sows are prolific (10.4 born alive, 8.9 weaned, 20.6 raised per annum per sow). Carcass quality is good; the average backfat thickness is 11.4mm, with 54.1% lean; the meat is of a good and even colour, with good water retention and little evidence of PSE.

French Landrace

White. Lop ears with the points towards the snout. Fine head; fine but strong skeleton; long body; 14 teats. Height 90-95cm, length 165-180cm, liveweight 350-450kg (boars)/260-300kg (sows). Of intermediate type between the very long Danish baconer and the shorter German and Dutch Landraces. Quite heavily muscled, with well rounded hams and a muscular look.

The French Landrace originated from Danish Landrace first imported in the 1930s (it was originally known as "French swine of the Danish type") but more extensively from the Swedish Landrace after the Second World War. The herdbook was founded in 1952. It took some time to breed the Landrace selectively to suit French systems and markets, but by 1970 it formed 30% of the country's purebred stock. It was developed as a dam line and, after a programme to eradicate the stress-sensitivity gene, its numbers have now settled down to about 25% of selection sows. It is used with Large Whites to produce F_1 crossbred sows. It has the typical Landrace qualities of docility, good mothering abilities and milkiness, good prolificacy (10.2 born alive, 9.0 at weaning, 20.8 raised per sow per annum) and sexual precocity. By selection, stress susceptibility has been reduced from 12% in 1981 to 2.2% in 1988 and still decreasing. Growth rates and FCE are only slight inferior to those of the Large White. The carcass is the longest of all French breeds (103.6cm, with 53.1% lean).

The rare and extinct breeds of France are of interest in their variety and the French are well aware of the importance of conserving the genetic reservoir offered by the old rustics that survive. They also make practical use of them in creating composite types for special circumstances, as shall be described. But many local breeds have already been lost during the present century, leaving only four in France and the mixed pigs of Corsica.

In 1887 there were at least 22 breeds, and there were still 19 before the Second World War. By 1956 they were down to 8 breeds, and 15 years later nearly all had disappeared. The **West French White** (a regrouping of the ancient **Normand** and **Craonnais** and others), survived with 70,000 sows. By 1970 the beautiful **Bayeux** had been reduced to 300 sows and the central, southern and Pyrenean breeds were all extinct, or very rare. The hardy little **Corsicans** had become endangered. In 1982 ITP (Institut technique de porc) and INRA (Institut national de la recherche agronomique) set up a plan to safeguard the remaining breeds by establishing genealogies, breeding young males to replace over-used boars, depositing semen stocks at INRA, registering basic performance data and creating new herds outside the traditional rearing regions. The first task was to prepare an inventory and this revealed that in 1984 there were only 200 **Normand** sows, 80 **Gascony**, 70 **Limousin** and 70 **Basque Black Pied** or **Bigourdain**. These few hundred breeding animals, all that remained of France's old breeds, were dispersed in 200 farms in three departments.

In general, the French pigs of the 19th century were coarse in bone but produced meat of high quality and were more prolific than the English breeds. James Long, in his *Book of the Pig*, described the French breeds under several groups, each including many varieties and local synonyms. (The Appendix lists synonyms and also the names of extinct breeds.) The first four were all lop-eared whites, which he divided into the "Common pig", the Normand, the Augeronne, and the Craonnais. The fifth group was the greyish-white Lorraine and the remaining groups were all of coloured pigs with semi-lop ears, including the grey-black or pied Périgordine, the saddlebacked Bressane and the black Corsicans. Long described the groups broadly in the following terms:

Normand: Coarse, thick-skinned and coarse-coated, with deficient hams, flat sides and thin collars, but good lean flesh. Very prolific, reached considerable weights (despite being "good walkers" - a useful quality for being driven to distant markets without losing finish).

Augeronne group: Similar to the Normand but many farmers in the Auge valley had taken greater steps to improve their pigs. Shorter heads and snouts and large flop ears. Still long-legged and coarse in bone but with broad, straight back, broad loin and "exceedingly good hams". Good fatteners, able to reach 650 pounds liveweight at 14-16 months, usually on buttermilk and skim-milk in the dairying regions that raised the pigs for Paris markets. Abundant but short and silky white hair over pink skin.

Craonnais: The most famous French pigs, centred in Mayenne. Large, upstanding animals, carrying their heads less close to the ground than most French pigs. Ears smaller but still hanging. Body unusually long and well formed, with wide-set shoulders, thick collar and broad loin, on short muscular legs. Better bred - finer skin and "hair of nice quality". Could reach 400-550 pounds at 15-18 months old (considered to be young for the period) and deemed to have the best flesh of all French pigs. Prolificacy relatively low. Valuable improver on other local pigs but unfortunately the name was used too liberally and bestowed on the unworthy as well as the good.

Lorraine group: Largely found in Moselle and Meurthe, also Alsace and Ardennes. Medium size - larger than Normand but not so well formed. Coarse-boned, large-eared and long-headed; body longer and narrower than Normand's and the sides flat. Greyish-white, often with black spots or patches. Meat of excellent quality and fat was "much esteemed" . Tended to grow slowly, perhaps because usually underfed in first month of life.

Périgord: Extensively bred in many departments, with many local names, including Limousin and Gascony. Strong, muscular limbs had become shorter in recent years; coarse animal, but highly esteemed locally and "entirely rustic", gentle in disposition and "fairly precocious in growth". Originally grey-black; had been crossed with Black Bourbonnaise to produce black-and-white pied pig, which breeders preferred: they were actively selecting for "a saddle, or black band, across the middle of the body."

Bressane group (including Black Bourbonnaise and Pied Charolais): Sows "most prolific and capital mothers" but no special quality to distinguish from other French races except colour: almost black, with white saddle or band across middle of body.

Corsican: "The only black pig claiming to be a distinct variety that is bred in France" and "practically the race of the Pyrenees". Ears erect, head large and long, body fairly well formed, hams lacking thickness, but flesh highly praised. The young "fatted with ease". Fine skin blackish brown, covered sparsely with fine black hair.

Those old French groups display nicely the two main types of European pig: the big, lop-eared, late maturing Celtics of northern latitudes, usually yellowish white, and the more compact coloured Iberians of the Mediterranean with their long snouts, medium sized semi-erect ears and concave profiles. The survivors of the latter type today include the **Corsican**, the black **Gascony**, the black pied **Basque** of the forests and the **Limousin** of central France, while the remaining Celtics were all combined into the **West French White** (1955) of which only the **Normand** still exists.

West French White (*Blanc de l'Ouest*) <Plate 8>

White, lop-eared, Celtic type. Large and deep, with sound skeleton but poor hams. Known for quality of meat. Tips of ears almost meeting at the tip of the snout. Not prolific (8.5 born alive, 7 weaned) but newborn piglets average 1.9kg at birth. Typically reared on pasture in small numbers.

The West French White was formed in 1955 as a group embracing the **Boulonnais** (found mostly near mining districts of Pas de Calais), the **Breton**, the **Craonnais**, the **Flemish** (which some say was crossed with the Piétrain to create the Belgian Landrace) and the **Normand**. It was thriving locally and expanding rapidly in the 1950s but by the mid 1960s it was losing ground to the Large White and Landrace; in particular, it was largely absorbed into the German Landrace.

Ultimately the West French White, known in France as the PBO (*porc blanc de l'ouest*), combined the **Normand** of La Manche with the large, dish-faced **Craonnais**, which had been France's most famous breed in the 19th century, though some said it had a mediocre carcass and was too fat. The fusion of the two under one name (though in practice the different types persisted, more or less) proved to be good for neither: it created an indeterminate type which did not adapt well to intensive systems and produced a carcass which lacked conformation and regularity. The individuality of the original breeds was further undermined by infusions of French and German Landrace from 1968 in an attempt to improve prolificacy. By 1974 there were only 4 boars and 48 sows.

It had been a good outdoor pig: free-range sows were on pasture most of the year and were peacable animals. The meat was of a good colour and quality, but there was not enough of it in the prime cuts.

Normand <Plate 8>

White, lop-eared, Celtic type. Large. Broad flat forehead, concave profile, large ears forwards over the eyes. Long, regular body, broad straight back, deep chest; long, strong, well muscled limbs; broad rump but mediocre hams. Good meat quality, especially for processing. Not prolific (8.5 born alive, 6 weaned) but good birth weight of 2kg and reach 7.2kg at 21 days. Adult boars to 450kg, sows 350kg. Smooth light pink skin with no black or grey spots; good coat of white hairs.

The Normand is a good outdoor pig with a long history. Its Celtic type was widespread towards the end of the Middle Ages - large pigs with lop ears and flat-ended snouts such as the Flemish, the Boulonnais, the Craonnais and the Normand itself. The Normand breed society was formed in 1937 and by 1953 there were 175,000 purebred Normands, forming nearly 20% of the national herd. The breed retained its identity for a while even after its fusion in 1958 with the Craonnais as the West French White: a few breeders refused to use Landrace in their herds and thereby saved the original breed. In 1983 the so-called pure Normand numbered only 15 boars and 199 breeding sows on 95 holdings. INRA therefore took steps to preserve semen from three boars for future use; it was a wise precaution at a time when many of the breeders were producing crossbreds rather than pure Normand.

It is a pasture breed and the sows shelter in little huts set up between the orchard apple trees. It is not a good traveller, and does not adapt to intensive systems.

The **Bayeux** was the result of crossing the Normand with the Berkshire. It was a meat type with shorter lop ears, a stockier body, and black-and-white markings which reminded an English writer in the 1940s of the Gloucester Old Spots. It disappeared during the 1960s through being crossed with the Piétrain.

Limousin <Plate 8>

Black-and-white, Iberian ears (small, slender, almost erect but pointing forwards); conical head, straight profile, long narrow snout - sometimes described as mole-headed. Medium sized. Thickset cylindrical body on slender legs. Rustic, vigorous, a good walker; slow-growing (takes 10-12 months to reach 100kg) and a good lard pig, also for sausage meat. Sows docile and prolific: only 10 teats but litters 9-10, good milkers.

This old breed of the west Massif Central originated on the borders of the Haute Vienne, the Corrèze and the Dordogne: it was also known as the **Saint Yrieix** pig and had been a recognised type since at least the 16th century. Its head is black; the rest of the body is white and irregularly speckled with round spots some 5-6cm in diameter; and the rump is covered with a neat black patch like a shield - another name for it is *cul-noir*. The pattern is also seen in German pasture pigs such as the Hanover-Brunswick and the Güstin. The hair is short and fine.

Traditionally, the undemanding Limousin was fed on potatoes, turnips, fodder beet or Jerusalem artichokes, and was finally fattened on sweet chestnuts, after which it was killed (in November and December) at weights of 180-200kg at 18 months old. It had a good reputation for its excellent fat - in the finished animal, nearly half the carcass was lard! The lard was highly prized in the countryside for cooking; it was white, firm and pure. The fat was the breed's undoing - only connoisseurs, it was said, could appreciate its tasty, firm, tender red meat.

In 1850 one Dr Escorne had described two ancient varieties, distinguished mainly by size: the smaller was plump and rounded, with upright ears (breeders complained that it rained inside them); the other variety was bigger in size and bone, its ears stronger and more horizontal, its hair more abundant and its body less bulky. This larger variety of the Limousin was the **Périgord**, which was crossed with the Craonnais and later the Large White to give the **Corrèze**. The Périgord had its own breed society from 1931.

In 1891 the idea of a herdbook for the Limousin was mooted but given up within three years, though the breed's first show took place at St Yrieix in 1895 with an entry of 186 animals. The first Limousin herdbook was finally published in 1935 in the face of infiltration by the Large White and Craonnais which were threatening the purity of the breed.

In 1953 there were 13,000 Limousin boars and sows but by 1970 there were only a few hundred and by 1983 just 8 boars and 68 sows, among 39 breeders mainly within 15km of Pompadour (Corrèze). All the sows were of proven descent but in no more than three distinct lines. It is now one of France's rare breeds and is carefully conserved.

Gascony <Plate 8>

Black, Iberian type. Rustic and vigorous, well able to stand hot weather, easily fed at pasture. Slow developer (100kg at 12 months). Very prolific (average litter 10), docile sows good mothers. Black skin; black hair, long and hard, thicker along dorsal line with whorls. Body cylindrical, back rounded, rump sloping with chubby buttocks, narrow chest; tail with thick tassel; limbs light but strong, good feet with black claws. Narrow upright ears carried horizontally, slightly inclined above the eyes; long slender head with pointed and mobile black snout. Good quality marbled meat and firm lard. Of medium size: about 75cm tall, 120cm long. Adults 200kg liveweight at 2 years old.

This useful and undemanding outdoor pig is claimed to possess an "Olympian calm". It is a vigorously rustic and self-sufficient breed ideally suited to the hot climate of south east France close to the Spanish border, where its black skin protects it from the sun. Its grazing includes herbs that give its meat a very special flavour and juiciness, though it is rather fat. It is slaughtered at 150kg but would reach 200kg at 2 years old.

It has a long history in the Pyrenean foothills. Its birthplace is in the Nebouzan and it probably represents the oldest type of pig known in France. It remained pure during most of the 19th century but developed some local varieties such as the **Tournayaise** (with very short ears and very pointed snout) and the **Bleu de Boulogne** of Boulogne sur Gesse (with semi-lop ears over a slightly retroussé snout, and with a shiny "blue" coat). This Boulogne region has since become the main breeding area for the Gascony.

From 1860 onwards it was crossed with **Lauragais** and Large White boars to produce the more precocious **Cazères** (white with a few blue spots) and from 1880 they were crossed with the Large White alone to produce the broadly similar **Miélan** (white, sometimes with small grey spots on the rump). Both of these breeds, and the **Piégut** variety of the Miélan, were better able to adapt to intensive systems than the Gascony but are now extinct.

The Gascony itself is very rare today, crossed

almost out of existence for the very maternal qualities which had been so valuable. In 1953 there were 10,000 in the breed; in 1970 there were several hundreds; in 1976 the population was estimated at 500 breeding animals and by 1981 the number had halved - and the only two boars were possibly not purebred anyway. The breed was disappearing fast, because breeders were still crossing with Large White. However, two years later it seems there were 15 boars and 82 sows among 39 producers, all within a 20km radius.

Basque Black Pied (*Pie noir du pays basque*) <Plate 8>

Black pied Iberian type, similar to Limousin. Docile but agile - used to wide-open spaces, heedless of wind or rain; undemanding feeder good for rough areas. Famous for tasty Bayonne ham (slaughtered at 1 year old at 120-140kg liveweight); also sausage meat. Cylindrical body, broad chest, slightly convex back, rounded belly and sides, good conformation, short loin, sloping *cul de Mulet* rump, hams developed but not thick; long, strong legs and sound feet. Of medium size (height 75cm, length 140cm). Broad muscular neck, long head, narrow face with straight profile, mobile snout; large fleshy ears half the length of the head, horizontal and inclined a little over the eyes. Black pied, with large well defined black patches; fine sparse hair.

This upland breed, originating to the west of the Pyrenees, slowly spread elsewhere and was known by various names such as **Bigourdain** (the most appropriate today), **Combrune**, or **Basco-Béarnaise**, or simply the black pig of Bagnères. There used to be at least two varieties: the **Béarnaise** was more slender in the body, with long legs and had more black than white in its colouring, but underwent numerous crosses with the Craonnais and Large White; the **Basque** was shorter in the leg, with a more compact body, and lacked the black patch in the middle of the back.

A good "runner", it is a thoroughly self-sufficient type on pasture and pannage in a challenging climate and, in typical Iberian style, a good lard producer, though traditionally slaughtered before the lard layer became too thick for the curers of dried Bayonne ham. The hams were heavy, firm and of a good colour.

It was very well adapted to its extensive environment, able to live on very little in unproductive and rough areas where it ranged widely. It has suffered from the disappearance of the native holm-oak woodlands.

In later years the prolificacy of the sows began to deteriorate, probably from a combination of inbreeding and lack of selection, though the mothers remained very milky and lost very few piglets. In 1953, the population was 1,200 but thirty years later it had dropped to 8 boars and 69 sows, on 32 holdings around Bagnères de Bigorre, mostly in herds of fewer than 3 sows (the largest had only 7); there were said to be about 500 "more or less" pure in 1981 but there had been quite a lot of crossing with the Gascony and many were of doubtful purity. Fortunately the Bigourdan breeders rarely used crosses but the genuine sows of the breed were of only three families.

Corsican <Plate 8>

The Corsican is a population rather than a breed or even a type - it is distinctive for its variety! The background is very mixed and the pigs live in an extensive system in which they are usually at liberty for many weeks, without supervision. They are often small and primitive in type, and typical colours now include black, black and white spots, grey, roan, fawn, white - and so on.

Their ancestors included the Iberian type of the western Mediterranean, especially those of Spain and Portugai with smaller ears and often with red coats like the Tamworth's, and the bigger lop-eared Celtic whites. There was also on Corsica and Sardinia a local subspecies of the Wild Boar, *Sus scrofa meridionalis*, usually with typically fuscous wild-type colouring grizzled by bristles tipped with cream or buff, and a facial saddle of white-tipped bristles, with a dense, smoke-grey underfur and dark to black ears, legs and tail. No doubt there was a degree of hybridisation between the wild and the ferals. Then the Large White was introduced, which was not at all well suited to the island but which added its genes to the pool so extensively that it is now quite difficult to find the relatively pure and largely Iberian island type. In 1978, INRA sought to conserve the pure, rustic Corsican.

The old medieval system of pannage - in which the pigs glean the forests in the autumn to fatten on acorns, beechmast and chestnuts - is still practised on Corsica and in south west Spain and Portugal. The Corsican pigs generally live as they please except at farrowing, when the young are confined to protect them from local foxes.

In 1983 there were 10,000 Corsican pigs but their numbers were decreasing. The old system is now under threat - partly, according to Julian Wiseman in *The Ark* (May 1988), because the traditional local products are being imitated and losing their reputation. It seems that large numbers of intensively reared pigs of ordinary commercial breeds are being raised for processing and packaging as "Corsican" pig meat without ever going near the woodlands or even being allowed to range on pasture. Somehow, they just don't taste the same.

New French Breeds

As the old breeds disappear, France is creating new ones and hybrids specifically for modern markets. In this respect, the nation's colonial history has been of considerable value: the French probably know more about the pigs of Vietnam, for example, than any other European country, and they have also made very good use of Chinese breeds.

The pig breeding companies, in co-operation with INRA and ITP, look for characteristics such as prolificacy and meat quality, either by developing within existing breeds or by creating something that meets their requirements. For example, there is a hyperprolific line of the French Large White, the **Hyper Large White**. The principal commercial cross in France is, as elsewhere, based on Large White and Landrace, with the "culard" races (Piétrain and Belgian Landrace) as terminal sires for better carcasses in the slaughter generation; there are also experiments with four-breed crossing using crossbred sires (for example, Piétrain/Hampshire or Belgian Landrace/Duroc) or crosses which use one of the sow parent breeds, such as Piétrain x Large White or Belgian Landrace x Large White, for three-breed crosses.

More exotic is the use of Chinese breeds for greater prolificacy. The **Tia Meslan** is a synthetic Sino-European line, bred by Pen ar Lan of Brittany, in which **Meishan**, **Jiaxing** and **Jinhua** boars (introduced to INRA in 1979) were crossed with Large White and Landrace sows in various combinations and proportions to combine the benefits of Asian and European breeds without also introducing the less desirable carcass and feed conversion traits of the Chinese pigs.

Pen ar Lan (in Maxent) derives its name from the Breton term *pen ar lan*, meaning "end of the heath". The company has produced several other commercial lines based on European and American breeds, such as:

Pen ar Lan 77: from Large White, Hampshire and Piétrain, line closed in 1973; 220 females in 1985 being bred pure; colour not important, and varied; intended as a male line for meat, semi-culard of the Belgian type, and to create terminal sire P76 (from crossing with Penshire P66); better muscularity and leanness than Large White; 430/290kg.

Penshire: from Hampshire, Large White and Duroc since 1977, line closed in 1984; 150 sows; colour varied and unimportant; bred as a stress resistant American-type male line to cross with P77 for terminal sire P76; weights as 77.

Laconie: one third each of Hampshire, Piétrain, Large White.

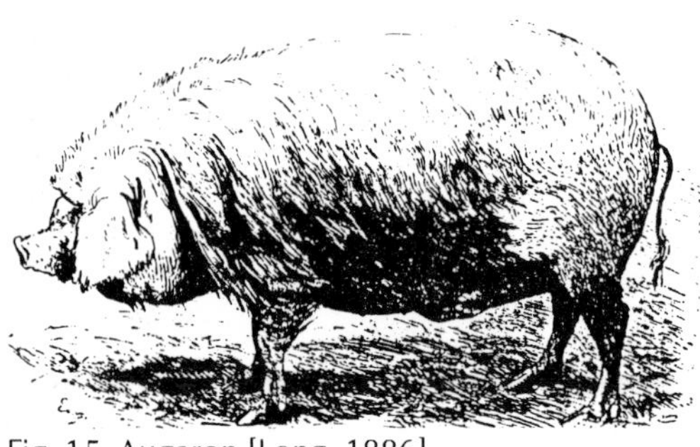

Fig. 15. Augeron [Long, 1886]

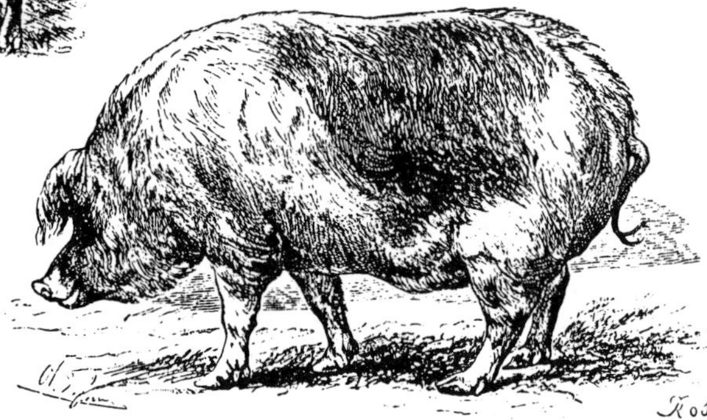

Fig. 16. Périgord [Long, 1886]

SPAIN AND PORTUGAL

The pigs of Spain and Portugal divide quite simply into the Iberian or Mediterranean lard types of the south - with long snouts, concave profiles, relatively compact conformation, medium-sized semi-erect ears, and black or reddish brown (sometimes pied) skin and bristles - and the Celtic type of the north with long lop ears, a leggier and longer body, flatter sides, late maturity, and often white or spotted or saddlebacked in colouring.

As elsewhere in Europe, most of the indigenous breeds on the Iberian peninsula are now very rare or extinct, having been swept aside by the Large White in particular - increasingly so as the two countries (especially Spain) cater for their tourist industries and set their sights on exports.

The Spanish pig industry has grown very rapidly and continues to do so. Production has increased by 680% in the last 30 years and vertical integration within the industry ensures that this increase is directly related to its markets. Producers in 1991 averaged some 17 pigs a year from each of the country's 1.9 million breeding sows. Spain's total pig population is second only to Germany's in Europe, but it comes fourth in terms of meat production, with a 1991 total of about 1.85 million tonnes, a lower rate per sow than in Denmark and the Netherlands. Spain is working hard to increase production levels and efficiency, and it is very much in the market for breeding stock.

Units integrated with large feed companies now account for about 80% of Spain's pigs, with some companies owning up to 40,000 sows. This can be a drawback as well as an advantage, in that it tends to mean that top growth rates and feed conversion ratios are not necessarily a priority. Another problem is the widespread use of the **Piétrain** as a terminal sire, with all the consequences of stress susceptibility and the effects on meat quality. But the Piétrain does meet the home market's demand for large hams and average carcass weights of 80-90kg. However, the trend is now away from the Piétrain.

Record-keeping and concern for animal welfare are perhaps less than whole-hearted, and slaughterhouse standards are low. The swine fever status of the national herd has long put a brake on exports, as has the high cost of concentrates, but Spain is so eager to take advantage of the export market that it is fully involved in sorting out these problems.

In this massive concentration on commercial pig production, most of the indigenous breeds are in decline. In 1965, only 25% of Spanish pigs were of imported white breeds (23% Large White, 2% Landrace) and local breeds accounted for most of the rest of the population. Today there are the remnants of perhaps two main groups of indigenous pigs - the Iberians of the south (**Extremadura Red**, **Andalusian Spotted** and **Black Iberian**) and the **Levant** type in the east. The Iberian group has the special advantage of producing exactly the right sort of marbled meat for Spain's dried ham.

Andalusia has a particularly rich inheritance of livestock types. Andalusian animals accompanied the great navigators and later settlers took them across the Atlantic to South America, where even now the Iberian stock are much in evidence. During the 1970s, the University of Cordoba began to take an interest in its native breeds, which had survived in large numbers in the first two or three decades of the present century but had begun to lose their identity with the introduction of intensive farming, when the demand for more productive imported breeds led to heavy crossing on the local livestock. It had reached a point at which some of the old breeds had become zoo animals and others were almost extinct.

In 1987, the Andalusian government recognised Cordoba's interest and a project was initiated to establish a census of each breed's remaining purebred stock and geographical distribution. Other aims were to learn more about them from those who still farmed them; to study the genetic status of each population, using scientific methods with genetic markers, blood-typing and biochemical polymorphism; and to discuss conservation plans for each breed. The Spanish government has now become involved as well and created a conservation farm for rare breeds at La Almoraima. Meanwhile a foundation (SERGA) to unify all Spanish rare breed conservation projects has been formed.

The two pig breeds identified for this conservation programme are cited by the university's Department of Genetics as "the IBERICO (black and red) and the MANCHADO DE JABUGO". That means, respectively, the **Black Iberian**, the **Extremadura Red** and the **Andalusian Spotted**.

Like the Spanish pigs, the old Portuguese breeds became widespread over the centuries and were taken not only to the Americas but also southwards and eastwards by navigators and traders. Portuguese pigs might well have been exported to England during the great breed improvement era of the late 18th and the 19th centuries. The 1934-5 edition of the *Pig Breed-*

er's Annual drew special attention to the "good properties of the old West of Europe wild boar of Portugal, which possesses most of the valuable features of our best modern breeds." This rather vague remark was accompanied by one of Professor Low's illustrations (published in 1840) of what was entitled "Wild Boar and Sow" of the Iberian type presented to the Earl of Leicester by HRH the Duke of Sussex. The original shows a blackish type with tawny red hairy ears and backline; the coat is rough but not long, except along the boar's back; the hairy ears fall forward; the snout is straight with a large flat disc and the sow's tail is curled, not straight. The whole conformation is that of a domesticant and suggests that this is not a wild pig at all but the **Alentejana** type, in spite of its rather wayward ears.

There was a particularly well known red Portuguese hog in North America before the Civil War. The breed's fame had spread across several eastern states since it had first been imported, destined for Daniel Webster's farm in Massachusetts. Webster had died before the pigs arrived and on landing they were sold to farms in New York and Vermont. They probably played their part in forming the Duroc - which today is being crossed with Spain's Iberian breeds.

Alentejana <Plate 9>

Once upon a time, Portugal had both Celtic and Iberian native pigs. The Celtic was represented most recently by the **Bisaro**, in the north of the country: it was black, white or pied. There was a black-and-white variety, the **Torrejano** of central Portugal, and also a local red pig with black spots, known as the **Freixianda**, in the Alvaiázere district of Coimbra. After the Second World War, however, the general transformation of European pig-keeping systems led to the Bisaro's downfall: it was increasingly crossed with the Large White and today it is represented by only one small group of animals and is virtually extinct.

The Iberian pig in southern Portugal is the **Alentejana**, named after its main breeding area. Sometimes it is described as the **Transtagana** or the Iberian or simply the Red Portuguese. Originally part of the general Iberian stock, it acquired some peculiarities over the centuries and was especially good at exploiting the groves of cork-oak and holm-oak for pannage. Acorns are not eaten by humans but the pig could convert these nuts into food for humans over a large part of the country.

Relatively speaking, it is still thriving. There were about 20,000 animals in a recent census, including 5,000 purebred boars and sows, mostly in the province of Baixo Alentejo. It is useful not only for exploiting the traditional extensive system but also as a gene pool of value to commercial pig-breeders.

It is quite a small pig, with slate-black skin and a few slender bristles in black, golden blond or russet red. The head is long and narrow with a slight angle between forehead and nose. The triangular ears are quite short and slender, directed forwards with the tips slightly outwards. The neck is of average length; the chest is described as "round", the back of medium length and breadth ("smoothly oblique"), the belly "somewhat sloping", and the tail has an abundant tuft of bristles at its tip. Like the rest of the pig, the legs are of medium length and are quite slender, with small, hard feet. Both boar and sow have at least 10 teats, and sows produce on average only 6 in a litter but rear them well if amply fed. Both sexes become sexually active at about 1 year old and the sows will breed for about 3 years, the boars for 2 years.

The breed's particular qualities include a high degree of rusticity and hardiness. It is an excellent walker and thus ideal for free-range pasturing. It also has a high aptitude for fattening and is in demand for its meat. It is very much a product of its environment, well adapted to exploit the oak woods and pastures. The Portuguese have recently appreciated that the dwindling of its numbers has led directly to the loss of the groves, especially of the holm-oaks, as the trees were grubbed out over large areas when the pigs were no longer there to give the woodland any economic significance.

Spanish Iberians

The "Ibérica" of Andalusia and Extremadura now includes black, red and spotted varieties - a mixture of colours which also characterises the region's cattle. The pigs are fortunate to have become the subjects of conservation efforts by the Instituto Nacional de Investigaciones Agrarias in Madrid, and its genetics department keeps a group of blacks at Oropesa, Toledo.

The breed as a whole numbers several thousands. The reds are greatly in the majority but are usually crossed with Duroc, so that only a small proportion are in fact purebred. The black herd at Oropesa numbers less than a hundred animals, and the spotted population had dropped to 7 males and 20 females in 1987, though they have since increased a little. However, the black and the spotted are on the verge of extinction.

The Iberians were originally lard pigs, though

the red has increasingly been selected as a meat type. The fat still serves a purpose in the production of special dried ham, a gourmet product for which lean breeds, even though well muscled and able to provide the large ham joints required, are no good: their lack of fat cover ruins the curing process and the meat simply dries out.

Apart from its meat quality and its adaptation to the local environment, the Iberian is too fat for modern tastes and the sows are not very prolific, nor are they milky nor particularly good mothers. The three Spanish breeds are as follows.

Extremadura Red (*Extremeña retinta* or *colorada*) <Plate 9>

This red pig of Extremadura and Andalusia, which is similar to the Alentejana, is the main Iberian variety in Spain. It is also known as the Red Iberian or the Andalusian Red, and is little different to the Black Iberian except in colour.

It originated as the **Oliventina** (now extinct) of Badajoz, also known as the **Raya**, which means "frontier" (it was on the Portuguese border). The Oliventina itself probably originated from the Alentejana of Portugal.

In recent years there has been much use of the American Duroc to improve the breed further, partly because of the similarity in colour. There is a theory that the Duroc originally owed that colour to Iberian pigs.

There was also at one time a whitish or golden **Andalusian Blond** (*Andaluza rubia* or *campiñesa*) in western Andalusia.

Black Iberian (*Negra iberica*) <Plate 9>

The Black Iberian, which is similar to the red just described except in colour, is also known as the Andalusian Black or Extremadura Black. There were two varieties, differentiated by their coats: the **Black Hairless** (*Negra lampiña*) and the **Black Hairy** (*Negra entrepelada*), which is now extinct.

The word *entrepelada* implies "between haircuts", while *lampiña* implies "clean-shaven", and the modern Black Iberian has no bristles on its unwrinkled, slate-black skin. Another name for it is the **Bald Guadiana** (*Pélon guadianés*) and its type can be seen in the equally hairless black **Pelón** pigs of Central America.

There used to be black or slate-grey wattled pigs of the Iberian type on the Balearic island of **Majorca**, but these have become extinct.

Andalusian Spotted (*Andaluza manchada; Manchada de Jabugo*) <Plate 9>

The third variety of the Iberian is an off-white pig speckled with black. It is now found in Huelva province and probably originated from crosses between the black and red Iberians, with perhaps some Large White blood in the late 19th century. In the 1940s this breed was one of Spain's two most important natives (the other being a Celtic type) and was described then as a large white pig with a straighter face and less pendulous ears than the Celtic; it was normally grown to a considerable size and carried a great deal of fat. A photograph of the period shows a balloon-like whitish pig with faint spots all over the body. In 1950 a spotted German pig was imported, possibly the Bentheim Black Pied, and there is perhaps some Berkshire influence as well.

It is now more often known as the **Jabugo Spotted** and was nearly extinct when it was rescued by the Cordoba University project. A recent paper by the University states that the present population is 30 females and 28 males and describes the breed in some detail.

It is about 90cm in height and easily reaches 100kg by one year of age; some adults attain 350kg. The conical head is rather small; the ears more or less horizontal and pointing somewhere between outwards and forwards. The back is arched, the ribs well sprung. The colouring is basically blond or yellowish-white with spots of various sizes spread all over the body - the general effect today is of more black than blond (except perhaps for the face and legs) with a mottled rather than patched or spotted look. Since the establishment of a herdbook in 1981, two lines have been identified: one is red with black spots and the other blond with black spots.

Spanish Celtic Types

There was once quite a famous hairless Celtic breed around Barcelona known as the **Vitoria**. In the 1940s, it was as popular as the Andalusian Spotted and was described as a large white breed with lop ears and a slightly dished face. (It was known as the *Chato de Vitoria*, the word *chato* meaning short-nosed.) Like the Andalusian, it became large and extremely fat. Its synonyms included Álava (its breeding area) and Basque-Navarre.

The so-called **Asturian** of northern Spain was similar to the Vitoria but was black; it originated from crossing Celtic and Iberian pigs but became extinct from being crossed with the Large

White.

The **Vich** or **Catalan** and the **Lermeña** of Burgos were local types similar to the Vitoria. The **Baztán** of Navarre was a local Celtic cross, either white, or white with a few blue spots; the **Galician** of the north west was a meat breed of the Celtic type and was white with small black or reddish spots on its head and rump - its synonyms included **Santiaguesa** and **Céltica**. All the Celtic breeds of Spain are now extinct.

Levant Group

The Levant type of eastern Spain was found from Castellón to Almería. It was the result of grading local pigs to the Large White, Berkshire and Vitoria. The only remnant of the group by 1987 was the short-nosed **Murcian**, a Berkshire cross, but there were only 4 males and 11 females.

Canary Black

The local pigs on the Canary Islands, which lie off the north west African coast, originated from a mixture of Spanish and African sows "improved" by English breeds, especially the Large Black and Berkshire. They are nearly extinct now.

ITALY

Depicted on a relief at the Forum in Rome is a surprisingly modern-looking pig. Its snout is of medium length, its back almost level, its ears pitched forward above the eyes. It is somewhat light in the hams and heavy in the shoulder, with a few wrinkles in the skin at the jowls and along the body.

A bronze Roman statuette of the 1st century AD looks rather like a playful Mangalitsa: her coat is curly, with something of a mane along the back; her body is plump, her legs very short, her small woolly ears erect, and her snout of modest length is slightly snubbed. On a Roman coin of c.80 AD there is a lop-eared, long-legged, almost hairless sow with well developed hams.

Roman writers described some very fat pigs of their time, when the principles of fattening were clearly well understood. Columella (3rd century AD) said that the ideal boar should have a pendulous belly and huge haunches, the sow likewise but longer in the body. He said that pigs kept in cold climates should have adequate hair, but those kept in towns could be hairless and white as they would spend some of their time in sties (some of which have since been excavated).

Such indigenous breeds as remain in Italy today tend to be late-maturing black, slate-grey or pied pasture pigs, and in most cases their ears are semi-lop, their snouts quite long and their facial profiles straight. In the warmer regions they are often hairless but dark-skinned, in contrast to Columella's naked townbred whites. However, although local breeds still accounted for nearly half the Italian pigs in the 1960s, today they are nearly all rare. By far the most numerous pig in the country now is the white, lop-eared **Italian Landrace**.

There are two theories about the origins of Italian pigs: that they belong to the same Iberian group as those in the south of Spain, Portugal and France, or that they are intermediates between European and IndoChinese pigs. Whatever is true, those hairless blacks of the warmer regions, especially the ones from the region around Naples, are of considerable importance in the history of the domesticated pig worldwide. At some stage - it is claimed in Roman times but possibly more likely in the 17th century - Italian merchants imported pigs from China to improve the indigenous stock's resistance to heat and sunshine. The breed that betrayed this Chinese influence in the slight dishing of its face was the **Neapolitan** <Plate 9>, which also developed other Chinese traits such as earlier maturity and a certain refinement in its thinner skin, quieter nature and an ability to convert food into fat and more delicate meat. It also inherited a sparse coat of fine hair, lighter bones and a general reduction in stature. The historical Neapolitan is described in more detail in the United Kingdom section.

There exists today around Naples a black, almost hairless breed known as the **Casertana** , with Siamese or IndoChinese blood, which is sometimes known as the Neapolitan - but it is close to extinction, which is a sad end for such an influential pig. There is, too, a black **Calabrian** which must have had a close relationship with the Neapolitan, but it is very local and rare today. It is ironic that the Italians have been using the Large White as the ideal pig for their famous Parma ham while the dark grey **Parmense** breed has become extinct within the last two decades.

In 1927, Mascheroni classified 21 races belonging to different Italian regions, with 8 subraces and varieties. Such diversity, he explained, came from a diversity of pig-keeping systems based on available feedstuffs - for example, wastes from cheese-making, or pasture, or pannage on acorns, or domestic waste, or vegetable waste. The most popular breeds of the time were the **Romana**, the **Casertana**, the **Siena Belted**, the **Maremmana** and **Macchiaiola**, the **Umbra**, the **Romagnola**, the **Pugliese**, the **Calabrian**, the **Sicilian** and the **Sardinian** - but only five of these survive today. Mascheroni listed many others, all long since vanished.

In 1949, more than half of the pigs in northern Italy were Yorkshires; 10.6% were still **Romagnola**, 6.9% **Modenese**, and 5.5% **Parmense**; old locals like **Garlasco**, **Cavour** and **Bergamasco** had practically disappeared. In central Italy in the same year, the Yorkshire represented 45.2% of all pigs, the **Siena Belted** 11.3%, the **Cappuccia** 6.4% and the **Perugina** 9.9%. In the south, where extensive agriculture was practised and the oakwoods remained for pannage, the Large White was only 29.7%, the **Casertana** 25.9%, and the **Pugliese** (including the **Calabrian**) 20.5%. In Sicily, the Large White represented a mere 4.4% and the **Sicilian** 81%; in Sardinia the local **Sarda** represented 90.7%, the rest being Large White.

By 1979, the few remaining pockets of local breeds had been thoroughly bastardised by continuous crossing and were threatened with extinction - breeds like the Siena Belted, with a documented history back to the 14th century, and the Casertana, which had contributed so much to the improvement of the English breeds in the 19th century. In the intervening years, as charted by Stefano Feroci, six old breeds had dropped to one tenth of their original populations or less (Friuli Black, Pugliese, Calabrian, Casertana Avellino, Casertana Caserta, Cappuccia) and the once top-place Romagnola had tumbled to no more than 200.

It seems that the Yorkshire or Large White has been the main culprit in the demise of Italy's local coloured pigs, as Stefano Feroci noted in his article *Salvare le razze italiane!* (in *Suinicoltura* VIII, 13-19, 1979). Until the 1870s, Italian pig-keeping had been based on the use of indigenous races. In 1873, Large Whites were first imported from England for their meat quality and especially for the production of Italy's traditional raw, dried ham. Crosses of Large White boars on local sows produced immediate improvements and the big white pigs soon spread right across the country. That was the beginning of the end for local breeds and over the next hundred years or so they would almost totally lose their individual identities, sacrificing their genetic heritage to the Large White and, later, to the Landrace.

Italy is unusual in the high slaughter weights it demands of finished pigs today, as every part of the carcass is processed except the loin, which is eaten as fresh pork. For example, flare fat becomes lard, collar fat is cubed for Mortadella, backfat is processed for lard and minced or cubed for sausages; fat belly is salted and seasoned for Felino salami; neck cuts are salted and seasoned, and hams are salted and seasoned for Parma and San Daniele ham. The ideal weight of a trimmed ham is 12-13kg, and of a Parma ham 9kg after seasoning, or at least 7kg after it has been seasoned for a year. That means the fresh, trimmed joint must weigh at least 10kg, and the cold carcass weight is 120-140kg. Fresh legs come from pigs weighing 160-170kg at 9-10 months of age.

The hams represent more than half the commercial value of the carcass. The traditional shape of the ham matters and so does the type and distribution of the fat. Parma ham needs a covering of white, firm, untainted fat of a good quality and with a high melting point. It is essential to have a layer of fat to help the salting process and preserve the characteristic sweetness and aroma of an Italian ham, and some breeds are simply too lean, lacking fat under the skin on the inner side of the leg. Without that layer of fat, or with a layer that separates from the meat, the ham tends to absorb too much salt. There are also processing problems if there is too much marbling in the meat, or too large an accumulation of intermuscular fat (pieces larger than a walnut at the centre, for example). These faults have increased with the use of Duroc boars on Large White and Landrace sows to obtain heavier pigs.

The meat itself must have certain qualities, too, for these uniformly pink raw hams. The unique flavour of the Parma ham is said to be due not only to the feeding of the pigs (partly on the whey residue from making Parma cheese) and the curing but also because the hams are matured in the good air of the Parmesan countryside, where the hillside climate is dry and airy. Even then, the locals claim that the most delicate and best flavoured hams must come from pigs fattened on those hillsides, not from salted hams sent in from, say, Lombardy, to dry in Parma.

It was only in the 1960s that the lean white invasion began to overwhelm the old breeds, yet some persisted on a local basis. Pig consultant Alexander Temple, in Monterchi, has seen the fairly safely established **Siena Belted** and also the rare **Casertana** and **Mora Romagnola** as well as two types from the **Madonie** in Sicily. There is now a rare breed farm in Portici and a tiny population of 12 Romagnola pigs under the watchful eye of an institute in Ravenna.

Italian Landrace

The white, lop-eared Italian Landrace came into the country much later than the Large White but has since become a firm favourite. The Large White/Landrace cross is the basis of the Italian pig industry, especially for its well known ham and salami products.

The Landrace originated from Scandinavian stock but has since been developed away from the extreme bacon type and selected more for meatiness. Like the Large White, it has been used to improve local pigs and is in demand for increasing litter numbers and for its maternal qualities, such as milk production and good mothering - traits which the Landrace boar imparts to his crossbred daughters.

The Breeds of Southern Italy

Casertana <Plate 9>

A synonym for the black or grey Casertana of Campania is Napolitana; another is *Pelatella* (plucked, bald). This is the almost hairless descendant of that influential Neapolitan of the late 18th and 19th centuries - but not for much longer. Its numbers are believed to be very low indeed (about 30).

The Casertana has slate-black, wrinkled skin and the faint look of a worried hippotamus with a wrinkled face. Its ears grow forwards on a conical head of medium length, with a slightly dished profile, and there are often two goatlike wattles (*tettole* or *barbiglioni*) hanging down behind the jaw. Its claws are somewhat splayed in typical Asian fashion: it is believed to have Siamese or IndoChinese blood.

Theories about its origins abound. In 1899 Professor Baldassarne made an elaborate case for a Casertana type in Roman times, drawing attention to all manner of images in terracotta, bronze, mosaic, bas-relief and so on at various sites. His researches led him to conclude that a "Roman" breed had lived in North Africa, Portugal, Spain, Italy and south west France, and that it was derived from crosses between Indian and European pigs - and that the Casertana was from this ancient union. Others prefer to describe it as an Iberian.

The Casertana is noted for its precocity, though not for its prolificacy. Sows can weigh 120-130kg at one year old, boars 150-160kg, and animals fattened for slaughter at that age might weigh 200kg. The average litter size is 6 (though sometimes as many as 9 or 10), born after a 100-day gestation, but the average sow is a good, milky mother.

In 1968 Matassino *et al* produced a very detailed statistical analysis of the Casertana (*Prod.Anim.* 7:173-247, Portici) in which they explained that the Casertana was also known as the Neapolitan because the Casertana pigs imported into England in several batches to improve local breeds happened to have been purchased in Naples, erroneously described as the principal breeding centre for the Casertana. By the end of the 19th century, the Casertana had a much wider distribution in Italy, no doubt because of its fame in England.

By the late 1950s, after years of fairly random breeding, standards were established for the Casertana, essentially that the skin was slate-black all over, without bristles, except perhaps for a little black hair on the head and neck; the mucosae pink and the hooves black. The conical head was rather long, with a straight profile; the ears were relatively short and grew with a forward slant; the neck was long and slender; the back slightly arched; the rump sloping; the thighs and buttocks long and muscular; the tail short and thin; the legs slender. The "two cutaneous appendages, more or less cylindrical" dangling under the jaw were vulgarly called *scioccaglie* (mumps).

Cavallino

This breed of north west Lucania, found to the south of the Casertana, may well be extinct by now. It was noted for its "frosted" appearance:

the black bristles were tipped with white. It was long-legged and a fast mover - its name means "pony". It was a pannage pig, given the freedom of the oakwoods to scavenge for acorns in the autumn and gleaning what it could in summer from stubble fields after the grain and legumes had been harvested. It grew slowly but the meat was of high quality for salami.

Calabrian <Plate 9>

This is another of the south Italian blacks, all probably related to each other, and sharing the problem of too much fat for modern tastes. David Kennett, technical manager of an experimental and demonstration farm in Calabria, has persuaded his regional Ente to preserve and promote indigenous breeds, especially the black Calabrian, though it is almost too late - perhaps a few hundred remain. Kennett eventually found some isolated remnants of the breed up in the mountains.

The Calabrian's former varieties included the **Cosentina** or **Oriolese**, the **Catanzarese**, the **Lagonegrese** (in south west Lucania) and the **Reggitana**. The group was spread throughout the province and the type is broadly similar to the Casertana: black, fairly long in the leg, with ears directed forwards.

Apulian (Pugliese)

There were several varieties in the ill-defined Apulian group and they were found in Lucania, Calabria and Molise as well as Apulia (Puglia). All have been extinct since 1980. They were unusual among southern Italy's pigs in that they were not black but white with black markings. The **Mascherina** (a synonym for the Apulian) was named for the masklike black markings on its head; the rest of the body was white except for another black patch on the rump. Varieties included: the white **Gargano**, with black markings on its hindquarters; the black **Murgese**; and the **Lucanian** or **Basilicata**.

The Apulian was a slow developer, reaching 80-90kg at one year old and possibly 130-140kg a year later if fattened. Sows would eventually reach 150kg, boars 170kg, at perhaps 3-4 years of age. Nor was this small pasture pig prolific, averaging 6 per litter, and it was often semi-wild, running free as a grazer and rootler. On such a system, however, it did produce good lean meat for salami.

Geographically suspended between the southern and the northern breeds of Italy was the black **Abruzzese**, with semi-lop ears, but it, too, is now extinct.

The Breeds of Northern Italy

Siena Belted (*Cinta senese*) <Plate 9>

This Tuscany pig is probably the best known of the older breeds, and dates back to the 14th century. Its pattern is similar to the saddlebacks of England and the Hampshire in America: there is a white "belt" around the fore part of the black body, including the shoulders and forelegs.

In 1980, Feroci put in motion a plan to rescue the Siena Belted from the danger of extinction and by March 1992 there were 92 animals on 8 farms (6 in Siena, the others in the provinces of Gorosseto and Firenze). It is a usefully rustic grazer and a forager in woodland and scrubland - an excellent outdoor type, and the sows quite happily give birth in winter.

It has a head of medium length with a straight profile; the smallish ears point forwards and slight downwards (it is a sign of impurity if they are large and hanging). The body is cylindrical, with robust limbs but poor hams. The black areas of the body have either shiny or smoky black skin with short, fine hair. The sows are quite prolific (average 7-8) and are good milkers; the average birthweight is 1.2kg, rising to 12-13kg at weaning (50-60 days old) and 40kg at 6 months, but only 70kg at one year old and 130-150kg at two years. It takes four years to complete its development at 170-200kg, but the meat is highly valued for processing.

In the 1950s, the Wessex Saddleback was imported from England (it was sometimes referred to as the Belted English) and became widespread in Umbria, often crossed with the Large White for grey-spotted commercial hybrids. With the shared colour pattern, it was also crossed with the Siena Belted to improve its hams.

The Cinta was crossed with the Large White to produce an F_1 hybrid known as the **Siena Grey** (*Grigia senese*) <Plate 9>, which was white with two large slate-grey patches (one on the head, one on the rump). These were bred as weaners, grown for export, especially at dairyfarm pig units in the Vale Padana. The Grey was an intermediate type between lard and meat - good for salami - and was both rustic and precocious.

The Siena Belted originated in the Montagnola uplands (up to 300m in altitude) in Tuscany and spread into Arezzo, Firenze, Pisa and the Maremma Grossetana, where it gradually replaced the small, black, semi-wild and primitive **Maremmana** that ran freely in the woods and scrublands. The Maremmana, also known as the *Macchiaiola* ("forest pig") or *Nera umbra* (Black

Umbrian), had prevailed from the late 19th century until about 1920: it was small, with black skin and quite a thick, shaggy coat; it had characteristic wattles from the throat and medium-sized, hanging ears. The long head had a straight profile and a good solid snout for deep rootling. Its skeletal structure was robust; the back was arched, the rump sloped; and it was a thoroughly rustic type, well used to adversity, and surviving in the autumn on acorns and roots in the oak and holm-oak woodlands. It was far from prolific and was only fattened with difficulty; it weighed perhaps 70-100kg at 12-14 months old, and 150kg at 16-18 months. However, it was extinct by 1949.

There had been nearly 195,000 pigs in Umbria in 1879; their numbers dropped by 1908 but thereafter grew until in 1952 there were 275,495 in the region. Apart from that little semi-wild forest pig, there was also the **Chianina** or **Casentino** of the upper Chiana and Tiber valleys. It was sometimes black but more often slate-grey, often almost hairless, and with a characteristic white "mask" - it was also known as the *Cappuccia d'Anghiari* (*cappuccio* = "hooded"). It had white socks as well. Its large head had a subconcave profile, and the modest ears grew forwards. It looked quite tall, standing on fine-boned long legs, with a long body, dipped back, sloping rump and poor hams. A good pasture pig, its prolificacy was quite good (8-10 in a litter) and the sow reared her young well. It was more precocious than the forest pig and quicker growing, weighing 110-120kg at one year old. But sows usually took three years to reach 150-160kg, and boars as long to reach 200kg. During the 1920s the Chianina was crossed with various breeds such as the English Large Black and the nearby Perugina and lost its reputation for being useful in semi-intensive systems, grazing in the woods with supplementary feeding in the piggery. It was still found as a diminishing population in Siena province in 1950 but had even then largely given way to the Siena Belted. It was widely crossed with Large White by the dairies that kept Chianina and Perugina sows for the production of hybrid rearing pigs and gradually became extinct as a pure breed.

The **Perugina** was a local type in the Tiber valley, rather than a definitive breed: it echoed the grey-and-white theme of the Siena Grey, being slate-grey with white areas on the belly. Its long body, sparsely bristled, was sway-backed with a narrow, sloping rump; its head was long with a straight profile and tapering snout, and its lop ears hung over the eyes.

Romagnola <Plate 9>

The English author H.R. Davidson, writing during the Second World War, described the Romagnola of Emilia as the only breed of any note in Italy, saying that it was not unlike the British Large Black. The Romagnola was important for more than half a century and even managed to resist the deliberate introduction of the English Middle White type in 1886, which was intended to replace it. One of two imported boars "accidentally" served a Romagnola gilt at pasture and the offspring were remarkable for their quick development and excellence as butcher's animals, so that the cross did indeed become widespread and commercial. Eventually the Romagnola did succumb to the 20th century white invasion and is now reduced to a protected handful of fewer than 50. In 1949 there had been more than 22,000 of them in Faenza.

It is sometimes known as the *Bologna* but more often called the *Mora Romagnola*, and indeed was officially named **Mora** in 1942. The word can mean "blackberry" or "mulberry" but also "Moor" with the implication of dark colouring. Another synonym is *Castagnona*, or "chestnut", in reference to its colouring, sometimes described as very dark brown with a coppery hue. The colour of the Mora is an important characteristic but variable and unusual: the remnants today tend to have light black or dark grey skin over much of the body, covered with bristles, but the skin of the underside (abdomen, inner surfaces of the limbs etc) is a rich, rosy colour. The young have hair of a fulvous colour in various shades (and sometimes with a faint trace of longitudinal striping), which becomes much darker as they grow and is almost black at the age of 50-70 days.

It has the typical long body and dipping back of the breeds of Emilia and Tuscany; its height averages 78cm (the sows are taller than the boars) and it is quite heavy-boned, with a long head, straight profile, and long, tapering snout which is almost covered by its long, forward-growing ears. The topline slopes upwards so that the rump is higher than the withers by several centimetres, and the back is dipped until the animal becomes more mature. It is not particularly muscular and the ribcage is quite narrow. The boars have a *linea Sparta* - a ridge of thicker, longer bristles along the back. The sows are quite prolific (10-12 born, 9-10 reared per litter) and good docile mothers. The pigs are useful grazers but, again, late developers; however, properly fed they can reach slaughter weights of 180-220kg in their second year, or later up to 250-300kg.

There were several varieties at one time. The most widespread was the **Forlivese**, with slate-coloured skin and black bristles tipped with white. The **Faentina** was a light red, the **Riminese** a dark red with a white star on the forehead. The hybrid offspring of a Romagnola crossed with a local inbred strain of the Large White (the **Bastianella** and **San Lazarro**) was knowns as the **Fumati** ("smoky") or Brinati, prized for its bulk, its high killing-out percentage and the firm, pinkish, tasty meat which was ideal for salami. But the Romagnola and its varieties began to disappear from the plains and their oakwoods as the Large White took over their area, though they survived for longer as purebreds in the hills and mountains.

Those inbred Large Whites, the **San Lazzaro** and the **Bastianella**, were originally formed soon after 1900, probably from the descendants of the 1886 English white imports which were presumed to be of the Middle White type. The two were about 62-68cm tall with long bodies, straight toplines, short legs, small prick ears, medium sized heads and medium length snouts - and very dished faces.

Another Emilia breed to be replaced by the Large White was the Black Emilian, or **Parmense** (actually a dark grey) or **Reggio**, which became extinct during the 1970s although it had once been the most widespread type in the province and had been recommended by Low as better than the Neapolitan - larger, with an even greater aptitude to fatten and able to produce equally delicate white pork. The **Borghigiana** or **Fidenza** was another Emilian casualty.

The black-and-white **Modenese** (probably now extinct) was developed in Emilia from 1873 onwards by putting Large White boars on local Iberian types; its predecessor, extinct in the 1870s, was the **Modena Red**.

Further north, the grey theme appeared again in the **Garlasco** of Lomellina in Pavia: it was grey with a white head but became extinct soon after 1949. Further north still were two more breeds which also died out: the black **Valtellina** lard pig of northern Lombardy and the **Friuli Black** or **San Daniele** in Venetia, which had been heavily crossed with the German Edelschwein between 1908 and 1940 and also with the Large White. It had become extinct by 1980.

Island Pigs

Sicilian

The **Madonie-Sicilian** is a small, late-maturing pig reaching only 100-120kg when fully grown. There are two ethnic types on Sicily, both of them grazers producing small litters (4-7): the black Madonie-Sicily, and on the inland estates the **Calascibetta** variety, a variable type whose colours range from black to white, with many examples of brindled crossbreds in between. Their meat is lean, tasty and ideal for salami. They probably originated from a mixture of local pigs with the part-Asian Casertana or Neapolitan, and also various English breeds including Large Black and Large White.

Sardinian

The Sardinian pigs, or *Sarda*, are even smaller than the Sicilian; adults weigh 70-80kg and stand 60cm tall at the withers. With their long bristles, they look very close to the Wild Boar, with which they frequently interbreed as they run in the woods. Their colours are very varied and include black, white, pied, speckled grey and "wolf" grey, and they have probably bred over the years with, originally, the French Craonnais, and subsequently the English Large White and Berkshire and the Italian Casertana.

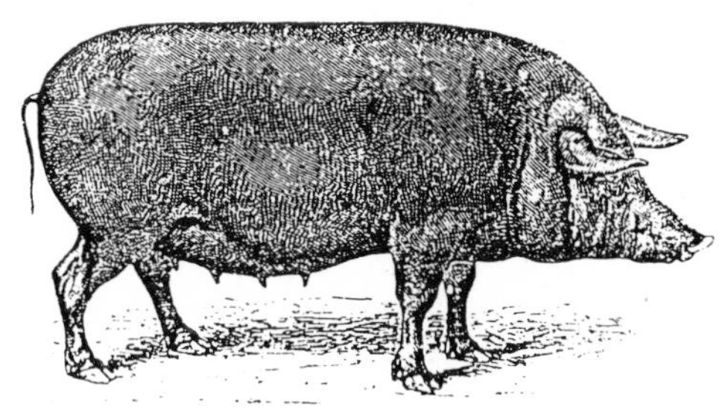

Fig. 17. Neapolitan sow [Long, 1886]

SWITZERLAND AND AUSTRIA

The two landlocked Alpine countries make the most of their upland and lowland meadows by grazing cattle, which are by far their most important livestock. But where a country has dairy cows, it also has pigs to use up surplus whey, skim-milk and other dairy byproducts. However, in common with other industrial nations, a large proportion of the pigs in these two countries are now fed on cereals and there has been a rapid change to fewer but larger pig units on an increasingly intensive scale, especially where land is scarce. Between 1967 and 1977, for example, Switzerland's pig population increased by a third to more than 2 million.

A few local types and crossbreds lingered a while but now the national herd is almost wholly of the typical European whites - prick-eared Yorkshire types (Edelschwein) and lop-eared improved Landrace. And, in a land of dairy cows, pork formed by far the largest sector of the Swiss meat market.

By 1985 there were 203,500 breeding sows and 8,800 boars, of which about 13% were registered in the herdbook. Of these, some 73% were Large White and 27% Landrace. The 1989 census recorded about 1 million altogether, of which there were 90,000 breeding sows and 3,330 boars. There are also a few Hampshires. Herdbook standards have been applied since 1976 and the Swiss have concentrated on good meat quality, using up-to-date techniques such as halothane testing, blood-grouping and the measurement of pH values. Breeders are divided into regional co-operatives or breeding units, all affiliated to three official breeders' associations (one for the Landrace, one for the Large White, and in the west the French-Swiss Smaller Livestock Breeders' Association). The nucleus breeding herd is about 6,000 sows and more than 3 million meat pigs are now produced annually.

Family farming is the mainstay of agriculture in Austria, where the consumption of pig meat is high (49kg per capita per annum) but apparently there are too many pigs in the country - or at least there is too much slurry. The pigs thrive on a diet based on maize and whey.

Güssing Forest Pig *(Güssinger Waldschwein)*

This semi-feral Austrian animal is not quite what it might seem. It is hunted in south Burgenland for its meat but is in fact a newcomer: it was deliberately bred from 1974 onwards from Wild Boar (*Sus scrofa*) crossed with an unusual mixture of domestic breeds from America (Duroc, Hampshire, Minnesota) and old-fashioned eastern Europeans like the Black Mangalitsa and black Yugoslavian pasture pigs. The females of this mixture were back-crossed to Wild Boar to produce a Forest pig which is three quarters Wild Boar and looks and behaves much like the wild type but grows faster and is more fertile. It is seen to be compatible with productive forestry, controlling weeds and pests and fertilising the forest soils without significantly damaging the trees. The pigs are given supplementary feeding and are selectively hunted in late summer to control the population and for their meat: they reach dressed carcass weights of 30kg at one year of age, or 60-70kg at 2 years.

Swiss Edelschwein (*Grand porc blanc, Schweizerische Edelschwein*)

The prick-eared white Edelschwein in Germany was originally based on 19th century importations of the Yorkshires from England - the Large White and the Middle White - and this is the Swiss version from the same origins, still sometimes known as the Swiss Yorkshire or the Swiss Large White. It is found mainly in the west of the country and is of the solid conformation and bone structure typical of the Large Whites. Its limbs and feet are strong and sound, well adapted for walking.

Swiss breeding targets include optimum distribution of meat in the prime cuts (without prejudicing quality), strong growth and the ability to make the most of feed, combined with high fecundity, good mothering, short farrowing intervals, regular litters, uniform piglet weights and a long productive life. Current test averages are: age at first farrowing, 353 days; 23.0 piglets born alive per sow per annum, 21.2 weaned; average 2.2 litters per annum; farrowing interval 164 days; daily weight gain of 889g from 25kg; FCR 2.58; carcass length 94.4cm; high meat quality (index of 3.6, where 4 is a top score); 53.6% better cuts. In most respects the Edelschwein outperforms the Landrace but has more intermuscular fat, though the backfat measurements hardly differ (12.0mm and 12.1mm respectively). Litter averages for crosses from the two whites are higher (22.3 weaned per sow per annum), while those of the Hampshire are much lower (17.8).

In 1986 the national herdbook registered about 25,000 out of the country's 200,000 sows and 9,000 boars (12% of the herd). Overall the ratio of Edelschwein to Landrace was 3:1.

Swiss Improved Landrace (*Porc amélioré du pays, Schweizerische Veredelte Landschwein*) <Plate 7>

The lop-eared white Swiss Landrace originated from Large Whites imported in the 1880s and German (Improved) Landrace imported between 1910 and 1953, crossed with native pigs. Switzerland's testing station was established in 1967, and ultrasonar testing was introduced in 1970. In the early 1980s Dutch Landrace and Danish Landrace were introduced to improve the Swiss breed, which is closer in type to the stockier German than the extreme Danish. It is found mainly in central and eastern parts of the country.

The standards for the Swiss Landrace specify a regular trunk, light head, harmoniously developed muscles in the shoulder and ham, a long carcass, well developed dorsal muscles, sound legs and feet. The aims in breeding are similar to those for the Swiss Edelschwein. Test averages are: 350 days at first farrowing; 22.4 born alive per sow per annum, 20.6 weaned, average 2.2 litters per annum; farrowing interval 166 days; daily weight gains of 863g from 25kg; FCR 2.67; meat quality 3.6; carcass length 98.0cm; 53.0% best cuts.

GERMANY

Pig-breeding has always been important in Germany. There was an enormous pig industry even in the 19th century in the northern lowlands, especially in Schleswig-Holstein, and a rapidly growing export trade that soon outstripped all except that of neighbouring Denmark. In the south, where the landscape was of foothills and uplands, the typical pigs were very similar to the French Lorraine type - of medium size, with long heads and large ears, long and narrow bodies with flat sides, coarse bones, slow growth rates, meat of good quality and plenty of fat; they were greyish-white pigs, often with black spots or patches.

In 1887, the talk of the Frankfurt exhibition was the change from the traditional late-maturing land pigs to the earlier maturing "improved Landrace", with the help of English pigs such as the Yorkshire and also the Berkshire (improved with Asian blood). Initially the term "German improved" applied to a meat-type pig whose progeny were repeatedly back-crossed to the Yorkshire large and middle whites until the breed resembled the Yorkshire. At the end of the 19th century these meat-types included the **Mecklenburg**, the **Meissen** and the **Westphalen** and these were typical early varieties of the improved German Landrace or "full-bred" pigs for the production of pork, as opposed to bacon or lard.

The term "Yorkshire" was applied in Germany and many other central and eastern European countries to a type described as of "much finer structure, much more pretentious" (Gaál and Gunst, 1977) than the English breed generally known as the Large White (which was only called a Yorkshire because it was originally imported from that county). The original "Yorkshire", which often included the curly-coated Lincolnshire pigs, proved much less successful in Europe than the true Large White, especially in peasant economies where the pigs either degenerated or perished under a system of management suited to a more robust and fatty type. But they did do well on large commercial farms. To confuse matters further, the name of Yorkshire was often applied to the genuine Large White and also the Middle White. However, James Long, who wrote extensively about the German pig industry of the early 1880s in his *Book of the Pig*, attended the German International Exhibition in 1883 and noted the German farmers' great progress with the British breeds. He even admitted that there were far more well bred Yorkshire pigs "of an exhibition type" in Germany than in England itself.

Lard was still a major German pig product in the 1930s and 1940s and the nation remained a high producer of pig meat, consuming it mainly as sausages or pickled pork (ham). The number of pigs in Germany exceeded considerably the total in all of the British Empire and Commonwealth countries combined (which in 1937 was 17 million) and before the Second World War there were nearly 29 million German pigs: it was the fourth largest national herd in the world.

The main breeds which were developed to meet the substantial German demand for sausage meat and pork were the *Veredeltes Landschwein* (**Improved Landrace**) and the *Edelschwein* (**German Large White**). The Landrace, which remains Germany's major breed today, was typical of lop-eared European landraces but much heavier in the bone with a thicker, heavier and shorter body than the Scandinavian type. The Edelschwein was very like the original English Large White but, again, of a broader, thicker build and more strongly boned. Both types, formally recognised in 1904, owed much to the whites imported from England in the late 19th century, crossed with local landpigs, and both became major influences in the development of commercial breeds all over north west and central Europe up to the Second World War.

By 1936 nearly all the other German breeds were so rare that most farmers had never seen any example of them. Yet in 1953 local breeds still represented 26% of Germany's herd, though by 1965 they had fallen to 5% in West Germany. The main breeds of the 1950s were Edelschwein, Improved Landrace, **Swabian-Hall**, **Angeln Saddleback**, **Güstin Pasture** and (for a while still) the English breeds, Berkshire and **Cornwall**.

The original German pigs, with a history stretching back many centuries and persisting through the 18th century, had been typical Europeans of the Celtic type, late-maturing, coarse in bone, flat-sided, with long legs, high backs and long heads. There were two types. The larger had hanging ears and a typical example was the **Bavarian Landrace**, a long-faced, two-coloured pig with the hind half red and the front (including the head) white. The second type was a smaller prick-eared pasture pig and there were two good examples. The **Güstin Pasture** (<Plate 10>) was long-faced and smooth-haired, white in the middle with black head and shoulders at one end and black rump and tail at the other; the **German Pasture**, also known as the **Hanover-Brunswick** or Hanover-Bismarck, was broadly similar but its copious coat was coarser, sticking up "in a way reminiscent of a rough-haired terrier", with a wide white belt from neck to ham.

The old breeds included several belted and pied pigs, often with long faces that suggested little or no Asian "improvement" - rather like England's Tamworth, a similarity remarked upon by an American, B. Dorner Jr, from Illinois, who saw red Tamworths in Hungary in 1919 and said that the type was "not a fine animal, similar to the German unbred (*unveredelt*) *Landschwein*."

After the Second World War the balance between the commercial German breeds began to alter strongly in favour of the Landrace which, by 1965, accounted for 92.7% of West Germany's herdbook entries, with only 1.6% for the Edelschwein; in East Germany the proportions were 63% and 29% respectively. The demand for well-muscled pigs persisted and the German Landrace remained much stockier and shorter-bodied than the extreme Scandinavian bacon type, with a very high proportion of lean (especially in the higher priced cuts) and a high dressing percentage because of its comparatively lower weight of offal.

In East Germany the agricultural system had changed after the war. The government confiscated the big private estates and also persuaded the peasantry to pool their land into collectives in which they would be shareholders. Then the collectives were divided into separate livestock and arable units.

In the west, by the 1980s a quarter of all the country's fattening pigs were concentrated in Lower Saxony. As in Scandinavia, there was a strong element of co-operation between farmers, in production as well as in marketing, among the many who were part-time or small farmers. In Bavaria the importance of small farms was even more marked in a hugely fertile area where farming and farmers remained politically influential and an important social factor in the villages. That situation is now changing rapidly throughout Germany: far fewer have any desire to enter farming of any kind today except on a part-time basis, so that the average age of farmers is steadily becoming older. The difference between north and south persists even now: Bavaria is still the home of village farmers who are perhaps more concerned about their local environment than the larger and more commercial pig farmers in the northern lowlands.

In 1989 there were about 25 million pigs in West Germany and some 39 million were being slaughtered annually - the country was the European Community's leading pig producer.

Half of all family farms had at least some pigs, averaging 17 sows and 38 fatteners on 400,000 farms. Home consumption of pig meat was very high at more than 60kg per capita per annum.

Nearly all of the German pig farmers, north or south, east or west, now rely heavily on the white German Landrace or its cross with the Edelschwein, but new breeds are beginning to make their mark as terminal sires and they are the same as in other European countries: the Belgian and American breeds. The Piétrain, for example, which has become more stocky in Germany, formed only 3.6% of the West German national herd in 1970, but 33.4% in 1988. The Belgian Landrace fell from 10% in 1980 to 4.8% in 1988, the year in which the American Duroc and Hampshire first appeared in the census figures. The red Duroc in particular is increasingly popular throughout Germany today, valued for its good marbled meat, its growth rates, fertility, hardiness and lack of susceptibility to stress. The belted Hampshire, a medium-sized American breed noted for its vitality, good growth rates, good carcass and meat quality, is used as a boar in crossbreeding. And Germany still finds a small place for the amazing **Mangalitsa** (described in detail in the Hungarian section), a small and very fat pig with plenty of long, frizzy hair, which used to be highly valued for its fat bacon. But the indigenous coloured breeds are gradually vanishing, though there are small populations of **Angeln Saddleback** and **Swabian-Hall**. Pure-breeding, though widespread, has decreased in recent years in favour of commercial crossbreds.

German Landrace (*Deutsche Landrasse*) <Plate 6>

White, lop-eared. Long head, slightly dished profile. Meaty and sturdy, shorter bodied than Scandinavian landraces. Boars 86cm tall, average 312kg (sows 80cm and 273kg).

At the end of the 19th century, various English breeds (mainly whites from Yorkshire) were crossed with large Celtic types of north lowland German landpigs, especially the **Marsh** pigs. A uniform type of German Landrace eventually emerged in the early 20th century and was recognised in 1904 as the *Deutsches Veredeltes Landschwein* or German Improved Landrace. It was also known as the German Long-eared or White Lop-eared (*Deutsches weiss Schlappohrschwein*). When public tastes began to change in the 1950s, breeders began to look for a less fatty and more meaty type with less length and imported Dutch Landrace pigs of Danish origin. (The Dutch Landrace had originated from imports of the German Improved Landrace in 1902.)

The German Landrace is a fertile breed (20.6 born alive per sow per annum, 19.0 reared - 1985 averages), with daily weight gains which improved from 749g in 1970 to 812g in 1985, and corresponding feed conversion figures of 2.91 down to 2.65, and the proportion of lean to fat improving from 1:0.58 to 1:0.36 over the same period.

The Landrace is the basis of crossbreeding schemes. Sire lines include the Piétrain for meat production and the best hams (though fattening is only average), the Belgian Landrace, and the Edelschwein for the best meat quality, excellent fattening and high fertility. The Edelschwein/Landrace cross also produces very fertile hybrid sows.

The **German Landrace "B"** <Plate 6>, which has a separate herdbook, began its development in 1970 at Pfalz, Rhineland, when the German breed was given better hams and a wider back with the help of imported Belgian Landrace and some Dutch Landrace. The boars are used in the production of lean pigs, but their growth rates seem to have been decreasing over the years.

Edelschwein <Plate 4>

White, prick-eared. Similar to Large White but stockier.

The Marsh landpig and the 19th century large Yorkshire white were also ancestral to the Edelschwein, with the help of the Middle White as well. *Edel* implies well bred, thoroughbred or noble and the type was first developed in northern Lower Saxony (Ammerland, near Oldenburg) but gradually spread into other areas until it was nationwide. It was recognised in 1904 as the *Deutsches weisses Edelschwein* (German White Thoroughbred). It is known for its excellent fertility and growth rates, and is used as a dam in crossbreeding programmes. Its growth rates are considerably higher than those of the German Landrace and its feed conversion rates are better, but its carcass has a higher proportion of fat and its numbers today are very small compared with the German Landrace.

Swabian-Hall (*Schwäbisch-Hällisches*) <Plate 10>

Saddleback, lop-eared. Strong, big build; long-lived, early maturing, very fertile; young grow quickly on sow's ample milk (average daily gains 850-900g); meat quality excellent, especially in cross with Piétrain.

The "German Saddleback" is not a breed but a general term to include the Swabian-Hall and the Angeln Saddleback, though they are of different origins. At the end of the 18th century there was a black-and-white landpig in the Württemberg region known as the *Hällische*. During the 19th century it was crossed with various types, including a "Chinese Masked", in a fairly haphazard way but after about the 1850s the crossbreeding became more organised, with Berkshire and other English breeds like the Essex. A herdbook and breed standards were established in 1925 and two years later the Wessex Saddleback contributed further to the breed's improvement. The Swabian-Hall became immensely popular locally but it began to decline as public tastes changed and the breed was found to be too fat. Unfortunately the breed society faded away in 1969/70. A few enthusiasts persisted with their fertile breed and the demand for it was revived from about 1980. A new herdbook was founded in 1983 and a new breed society in 1986, since when its numbers have continued to increase.

It is a fertile breed and well built. It has hanging ears and is basically white (including its legs and tail switch) with a black head and neck and black rump, thighs and tail. The black areas are edged with blue-grey, which is the effect of white hairs over pigmented skin.

Angeln Saddleback (*Angler Sattelschwein* or *Angeln*) <Plate 10>

Saddleback; lop-eared; robust; big build, deep; good growth rates (800g/day); milky sows, very fertile and good mothers.

Originally a black-and-white pied and unrefined Schleswig landpig, the Angeln was taken in hand in 1926 by a group of nine farmers who set up a herdbook two years later and worked to improve the breed with the help of the Wessex Saddleback and probably, later, Swabian-Hall. It had been recognised as a breed in 1937 and was popular as a fatty pig which formed 15% of the national pig population during the war. After the war, however, it declined rapidly until its breeders took steps to reduce its fat levels by introducing Dutch and Danish Landrace blood and, later, some Piétrain. They also re-imported some of the original type from Hungary (to which it had been exported soon after the war) and from East Germany, where there was a gene bank for the breed. In 1986 there were only 50 but the numbers soon began to rise with the help of the working group formed to save it from extinction. Its proportion of lean to fat has greatly improved.

It is a belted pig - the white belt includes the forelegs, but the head and back half are black. In recent years, with a market prejudice against pigmentation, it has been selected for a larger area of white.

Bentheim Black Pied (*Schwarz-Weisses Bentheimer* or *Buntes Schwein*) <Plate 10>

Spotted; lop-eared. Medium-sized landpig type, sturdy build, coarse hair, hanging ears; robust and healthy; slaughter weight 90-100kg; halothane-negative.

The Bentheim of south Oldenburg traces its origins to the common old lop-eared European landpig. It was widely distributed in Lower Saxony after the last war and was crossed with the Angeln Saddleback for improvement but during the 1960s and 1970s it had become limited to the Bentheim area, where it was being crossed with the Piétrain and others. It is also known as the Piebald or Spotted German pig, or the Bentheim Landpig: its coat pattern, described as "tiger" but more like a leopard's, is light grey with irregular splodges of deep black. It is almost extinct.

Baldinger Spotted (*Baldinger Tigerschwein*) <Plate 10>

Spotted; lop-eared.

Like the Bentheim, this breed in Donaueschingen, Württemberg, is described as a tiger-marked pig - greyish-white with black patches - and is also nearly extinct. There is a hint of the Berkshire about it and it was indeed the product of Berkshires crossed with local landpigs in the second half of the 19th century. It is earlier maturing than some as a result.

German Red Pied (*Rotbuntes Schwein*) <Plate 10>

Red-and-white.

This breed emerged in Schleswig-Holstein in about 1900 from red Angeln Saddleback sports, probably with Tamworth blood. It has been described as red with a white belt but some examples claiming to be *Rotbunte* seem to be of mixed colours, including something quite similar to the old unimproved Berkshires - quite long-haired and sandy with vague patches of lightish black or possibly very dark red. A breed society was formed in 1954 but the breed is now generally considered to have been extinct for many years. However, the sandy-and-black or black-and-red colouring is simple enough to reproduce, deliberately or otherwise, and there are no doubt pigs which might claim to be the *Rotbunte* but with no pedigree to prove it.

German Cornwall <Plate 10>

During the 19th century, the original western type of the English Large Black was widely exported to Europe from the south west peninsula and came to be known in Europe as the Cornwall. It is a big, lop-eared breed with a high reputation in its own country as an excellent outdoor sow (see United Kingdom section). Although quite popular for a while in Germany, its numbers became low after the Second World War and it is now extinct here.

Göttingen Miniature <Plate 10>

In the early 1960s, at Göttingen University, pot-bellied and wrinkle-skinned little pigs from Vietnam were crossed with the Minnesota Miniature (No. 5) from the United States to produce miniature pigs for research laboratories. The aim was to combine the small size and high fertility of the Vietnamese with the docile temperament of the Minnesota (itself bred for the laboratory from American ferals). Initially the Göttingen hybrid was coloured but the laboratories demanded white stock and the University therefore split the breeding group, retaining the black, brown and piebald types but also developing a slightly lighter-weight white by introducing the German Landrace. The Göttinger is very small, with small erect ears, a short snout and a dished face.

The **Munich Miniature** <Plate 10>, or *Troll*, was developed for a similar purpose from the Hanford Miniature (another American product, in Washington state, from ferals in the late 1950s); it is white-skinned with red or black hair, or spotted, and is about 43cm tall.

Various new meat breeds and hybrids have been created in Germany in recent years, including the **Leicoma** (at Leipzig, Cottbus and Magdeburg) which was based on Dutch Landrace with local saddlebacks and the Estonian Bacon (1971-75), crossed in subsequent years with the Duroc and local Landrace, and named in 1986. The **Schwerfurt Meat** type (***Schwer**in and **Erfurt***) was developed over the same period from Belgian Landrace boars on Piétrain x Canadian Lacombe sows.

EASTERN EUROPE

There have always been plenty of pigs in eastern Europe and pig meat is still a major product in Hungary, Poland, Czechoslovakia, Yugoslavia and Bulgaria.

At the beginning of this century, pigs were generally kept in ones and twos by families who reared them for the household, and in such circumstances there was little in the way of pig improvement on a national scale. But as the concept of breed creation and breed improvement began to spread through Europe, riding on the backs of England's Berkshires and Yorkshires and later the improved Landraces, so too did pigs become farm livestock rather than backyard animals and their numbers began to increase enormously. The traditional outdoor pigs, developed gradually over many centuries to suit local environments and markets, were no longer wanted and began to decrease in numbers.

Well within living memory, however, there was a great swathe of land running from Poland and the Baltic countries in the north to the Balkans in the south (bordering the large part of the world where pig-keeping is not practised) where much more primitive local pigs did survive. As in the west, they were broadly of two types: a large, lop-eared Celtic and a smaller, prick-eared pig. It was the latter that persisted in the south. The old pigs of the Carpathian basin described by Gaál and Gunst (1977) were still identifiable in many different races in the 19th century, when many of them were crossed with each other in a haphazard manner until the original types were no longer discernible. It was out of this melting-pot that the famous lard pig of the area emerged: the **Mangalitsa**.

In Poland, the Baltics and Russia, meanwhile, the old primitive pigs were rapidly being "improved" out of existence in the determination to breed commercial white pigs, and in the republics of the former USSR countless new breeds were being created, most of them relying heavily on the Large White. It was in the other corner of eastern Europe - in Bulgaria and Romania - that the primitives lingered longest.

The medieval pigs of central and eastern Europe can be divided into two main groups: a primitive larger type (though much smaller than modern breeds) with a clear relationship with the local Wild Boar, and a smaller type showing greater signs of domestication, especially in the shortening of its skull's lacrimal bone. Some have suggested that the latter type was influenced by Asian pigs, which seems reasonable in view of the 7th century domination of the area from the Black Sea to the Adriatic by the Avars, who were of Asiatic origin; but others believe that such skull changes were simply signs of the more advanced phases of domestication and that the Avars probably did not bring their own pigs with them.

The history of those pigs has been studied closely in Hungary (a nation which takes a considerable interest in its livestock heritage) and much of the information which follows is described in S. Bökönyi's invaluable book, *History of Domestic Mammals in Central and Eastern Europe* (Budapest, 1974). Other authors referred to include B. Hankó (1938) and Gaál and Gunst (1977).

For a while, Hungary itself was occupied by the Turks (from 1526), who were Muslims, and it was not until they had been driven out that there was deliberate and selective pig-breeding. Attempts have been made to identify the old regional types in Hungary and neighbouring regions, and Hankó made the following suggestions.

To the east, refugee Slavs living in the valleys of the Carpathian ring kept a mountain or **Surány** pig, while there was a rougher mountain pig with a crest of bristles along its spine in the Transylvanian mountains further north. In the west of modern Hungary in the region of the Bakony-Vértes mountains was the **Bakony** (a type which persisted late into the 19th century until it was absorbed into the Mangalitsa), which was similar to the Croatian **Bagun**. To the south west, on the other side of lake Balaton, was the Croatian primitive grey prick-eared **Šiška** in the Zselic region and on either bank of the Drava river, while in the plains around Zagreb (in Croatia) was the ancient **Túrmezö** or Turmezei breed. In between these two groups were the lowland pigs: there was a small lard pig on the Great Hungarian Plain between the Danube and Tisza rivers, which was known as the **Ancient Lowland** or **Ancient Alföldi**; while to the east of the Tisza in its flood plains with the Körös and Berettyó rivers was the **Meadow** or pasture type, known since prehistoric times; and slightly to its north was the primitive red **Szalonta** pig, common in the 18th century and once famed as a meat breed.

Hungary

Hungary is fortunate in having perhaps the best combination of soil and climate in eastern Europe. Much of the soil is alluvial Danube plain, ideal for arable farming.

The European land reforms of the 19th century did not occur in Hungary until 1945, and before then it was a country of smallholdings, semi-feudal estates and many landless peasants. The first changes came in 1945, when the Peasant Party won the first postwar elections; the Communists took control two years later, and after the 1956 revolt all land was farmed collectively by co-operatives of those who became land-holders in 1945, or by the state farms which had taken over the old estates. In 1989, when John Beynon Brown visited the region, the system was a command economy with farming directed from the centre through the large state and co-operative farms but there was still a strong smallholder section.

The opportunity to change from large co-operative agricultural enterprises is being greeted with caution. Before the state took over land in the 1940s, the average farm was only 6ha, which can hardly be considered a viable holding. The majority of farmland will be "privately" farmed by the end of the century; but probably by small groups within the structure of big co-operatives, using existing facilities but owning their own livestock.

Perhaps the most famous state farm is the 4,000ha HKG state farm at Herceghalom. This is the home of the **Hungahyb**, a hybrid derived from a combination of the Hungarian White, the Dutch Landrace, the Hampshire and one of the culard-type Belgian breeds (Piétrain or Landrace). It is now well known as a commercial pig in several European countries. However, the most numerous breed in the country today is the **Hungarian White** itself.

Although pig numbers have fallen recently, they still hover around 8-9 million and the country is ambitious to increase its already good export levels of pig meat. Its traditional outlet was the USSR. It is the most progressive of the east European pig-producing countries and wants to increase its EC exports to more than 400,000 tonnes per annum. Some EC countries are investing in Hungary, setting up processing plants there or offering venture capital and expertise.

Hungary takes an interest in conserving some of its few remaining rare breeds, which are sometimes seen in "traditional" farms in the national parks. Of the old pigs, however, only the Mangalitsa remains today.

The Mangalitsa Story <Plate 11>

The story of the Mangalitsa is the story of Hungary's pigs and also of the rise and fall of the European land pig. By the 19th century, there were two main types of pig in the region: the lard pig and the so-called meat pig, the latter being lean and thin in contrast to the grossly fat lard pig. The meat pig's conformation arose partly from genetics and partly from management. The group included, according to Gaál and Gunst, "Avar, Balkan, Bulgarian prickly, mountain prickly, Kassa, Polish (small-eared, large-eared), Moldavian, Romanian prickly, meadow, szalontai (Ugra, Görbred, Šiška)." "Prickly", in this context, should presumably be interpreted as "prick-eared", a trait in most of these small primitive types of Bulgaria, Romania, Yugoslavia and Hungary, though it might mean "bristled".

Although known primarily as a Hungarian breed today, the Mangalitsa lard pig's roots were in fact to the south, in Serbia, where the **Šumadija** had been carefully developed from the prick-eared **Šiška** on the Topsicsér farm owned by the Serbian prince, Milos, in the 1830s. Hence the Šumadija was often known as the *Miloševa.*

Southern pigs had been crossed over many years with the old Carpathian Basin pigs and in due course a small lard pig evolved as the basic Mangalitsa. It was then developed into a slightly larger and more uniform type by the deliberate use of the Šumadija. By the end of the 19th century, the Hungarian Mangalitsa was quite a large lard pig covered with thick, soft, curly hair (looking like a sheep from a distance) described as "fair" in colour, and it had black or dark slate-coloured hooves. A Black Mangalitsa was created in a cross with the **Black Syrmian** to the south.

In 1911 there were more than 6 million pigs in Hungary but after the Great War there were fewer than 2 million. The Mangalitsa was already deteriorating in type: it was described as of medium size, which was the farmers' preference as they said that the larger old type did not fatten so well. They preferred a pig both deep and long in the body, short-legged, with a medium-length snout and a big belly - it seemed that the bigger the belly, the better the pig's ability to convert its feed.

The breed was an efficient converter of maize into lard (maize remained Hungary's second most important crop up to the Second World War) and it was also a good grazer, very well suited to extensive systems. In its dual roles as a prodigious lard producer and an outdoor pig, it began to fall out of favour as consumers began to demand lean meat and farmers began to intensify their management systems. Yet in the early decades of the present century it did very well indeed, greatly helped by a national association of Mangalitsa breeders formed in 1927, which introduced herdbook registration and improved co-operation among the breeders. Although the breed's population had declined so abruptly in wartime, the breed society so improved its quality that numbers began to rise again and in 1931 the equivalent of 105,408 bacon pigs and 43,713 quintals of lard were exported. In the following year the figures were, respectively, 116,903 and 34,827: the type was already beginning to edge away from excessive lard production.

During the 1930s pure and crossbred Mangalitsas were also popular in Poland, Czechoslovakia, Romania, Yugoslavia and Austria but, as the central European countries increasingly tended to export their pig produce to the United Kingdom and to their own industrial areas, the Mangalitsa was being crossed with British and German breeds. Photographs from the period show an almost spherical Mangalitsa and prove that 19th century engravings of various "improved" and very fat European breeds were not exaggerated. The Mangalitsa's back bacon, smoked and cured, was eaten with bread as the staple diet for country workers all year round, and its lard was used at home for cooking as well as being exported. The whole body was covered with a mat of dense, curly hair which was claimed to protect the pig in Hungary's hot, dry summers as well as its severe winters. The heavy ears were also woolled and tended to fall forwards above the eyes as if shading them from the sun; only the face was fairly clean of wool. It was late-maturing, reaching full development at about 15 months old. It gave an average of 60-80kg liveweight (though in some districts it grew to 100-110kg) and it was far from prolific with only 3-7 per litter.

Between the wars, lard pigs were no longer so dominant in Hungary, though lard and bacon were still the only pig products demanded by the home market. However, as early as 1873 a national conference of pig breeders had agreed that they should see to it that meat-type pigs were raised for export, as well as the Mangalitsa lard type. In fact the breeding of pork pigs had started in the first decade of the 19th century, in association with dairy farming, but had always remained secondary to the production of bacon pigs.

The Mangalitsa continued to be in demand for its lard and was important to the makers of Hungarian salami; it was not in direct competition with the English porkers introduced in the early 20th century. A pattern gradually evolved: the Mangalitsa was used in extensive systems, while the less hardy meat types were in intensive systems, especially where they accompanied dairying co-operatives. Meat packers were demanding baconers and young ham pigs, and the English breeds were promoted strongly, though they were far more susceptible to diseases such as swine fever and infectious abortion.

There was a swing back to the Mangalitsa in the late 1930s, especially in regions where the climate was considered too extreme for the English pigs. The country's general economic situation was in crisis and, as economic conditions worsened, intensive farming became an increasingly unattractive prospect. The Mangalitsa and what remained of the primitive breeds, all well suited to cheaper extensive systems, came into their own again. It was realised that the meat-type pigs were only marketable if fed a great deal of expensive protein, and that there was much competition in those markets internationally. The self-sufficient Mangalitsa, however, could be kept very cheaply outdoors, all year round if necessary, and was supreme in its own market. Further, during the Second World War the demand for lard, and hence its price, increased considerably, and lard-type pigs also had the benefit of remaining duty-free, which the meat-type pigs did not.

A partial solution was to crossbreed, with all the advantages of heterosis between the native and the imported English breeds, and this was already happening in the 1930s on a fairly haphazard basis on smaller pig farms. At local markets peasants began to seek and pay higher prices for pigs of mixed blood or, as Gaál and Gunst put it, "spotted, pale, mixed, *baris*, *zerna*, spotted-bellied and spotted-dug piglets and young boars". The larger enterprises realised that crossbreds finished more quickly and fattened well. Some of the big estates were keeping separate pure nucleus herds of Mangalitsa as well as English porkers so that they could fatten the crossbred F_1 generation.

Perhaps the Mangalitsa's fate was finally sealed in 1923 by the formation of a highly efficient national association of meat-type pig breeders. Beginning with 80 pigs registered in its herdbook, it increased the number to 1,505 by 1938 and doubled it to 3,339 by 1942. The association had precise breeding aims and stuck to them to improve a white Hungarian meat-type pig with the English porker's qualities of fertility, rapid growth and excellent feed conversion.

In 1935 the Mangalitsa formed more than 94% of the Hungarian national herd but during the 1940s its population crashed to a mere 600 purebred breeding animals. In 1979 a new society was formed to rescue the breed at a time when they could only get together 80 females and 7 males for the new herdbook.

Though now dismissed in its native land as "grossly fat", the Mangalitsa still exists. It remains a "woolly" pig with slate-grey skin, and there are several interesting colour varieties. The yellowish-white "fair", or blonde, is the most typical of the original type; it can also be black, red or dark tan. Others include a Black Bellied, which is blonde with a black underside, and the reverse-pattern Swallow Bellied, which is black with a blonde underside. Some have been selectively bred for colour so that different strains are evolving. The piglets even now betray the breed's primitive origins: they are usually born striped.

It is an adaptable and contented sort of pig, delighting in a good wallow in hot weather, and extremely hardy in summer and winter, showing great endurance at low temperatures. The meat itself is comparatively lean and of high quality for sausages, but the backfat remains very thick and forms early. It is a small to medium-sized pig (slaughter weight 150kg) standing on strong, straight legs, with a deep, broad chest and wide, slightly arched back. Its short, conical head has a broad forehead, and medium-sized ears tipping forwards. The long, thick, curly coat of fine woolly bristles has a yellowish underwool; on the head and legs the hair is short, dense and straight, and often almost black.

In the early 1990s the British importers Harris Associates, of Redhill in Surrey, helped to save the breed from extinction by importing good specimens to England, despite acknowledging that the cost of feeding them would be prohibitive on a commercial basis. Yet the Mangalitsa's genes live on in many European pigs, especially in the eastern countries where it became the basis of many a new breed.

The Story of the Hungarian Meat Pigs

In the 19th century, Hungarian pig farmers began to hear of the larger-bodied and quick-developing English pigs, with their excellent feed conversion and high fertility, and as meat prices were beginning to rise in the 1870s it made sense for the Hungarian breeders to look more closely at those English types. Prime ham was being brought into Budapest from Kassa and Prague for wealthier consumers, who also delighted in Prague's pork chops and German-type cold sausages. Consumption of these imported pig meat products increased as the century turned and living standards improved generally. The government decided to support the development of meat-type pigs, and smallholders as well as large estates and dairy co-operatives were eager to raise them. For example, in 1905 the dairy co-operatives in Bácska and Torontál counties imported 500 English porkers, and in 1911 the southern counties received a distribution of 2,870 meat-type English sows. In 1926 more than 6% of the national herd was of the meat type but by 1935 it had become more than 20%.

The early breeders looked first to the famous Berkshire and the Essex. The **Berkshire** became a particular favourite in Hungary and remained so even in the 1970s in southern Bács country, where a herd based on stock first imported in 1890 still continued. It had been established as a pure breed in Hungary in 1884 and was found to offer fertility, rapid growth and excellent feed conversion - typical qualities of the improved English breeds of the period. There were additional virtues in the Berkshire: this black porker proved adaptable to extensive management and was able to tolerate strong sunshine and dry, hot summers, which was not a characteristic of later white breeds. It also produced an excellent cross from the Mangalitsa (a cross which, in the 1930s, would reach 260 pounds at 10 months old) or a good fattening pig from a cross with the white Yorkshire. The Berkshire/Mangalitsa cross became the basis of several breeds in neighbouring countries.

The **Essex**, introduced in 1870, played a lesser role and was often mixed with other belted pigs, especially from Germany. A type described as the Old Gloucester, said to be large-bodied, rough-coated, unpretentious and an excellent mother, was imported to a limited extent and also the red Tamworth, described one of the best grazing pigs.

Another English import of some importance was the Large Black, known as the **Cornwall**, which did very well in poor conditions. It did not develop quickly but kept its ability to "grow for a very long time and becomes a very fat animal". Of excellent fertility and mothering qualities, it was tough and hardy enough, not too sensitive to the weather ("due to its rough skin and thick fur"), though it was not very tolerant of intensive sunshine. It was a popular backyard pig among factory workers in the Budapest suburbs; it also produced a vigorous cross with the Mangalitsa and even during the 1970s remained locally popular in the Danube/Tisza interfluence. In 1945 a venerable specimen had the dubious honour of being killed and stuffed for the Magzan Mezögazdásagi museum in Budapest. A photograph taken just before slaughter shows a rather flat-sided but neatly proportioned old sow with enormous lop ears, a very dished and broad-snouted face, and a fairly sparse coat of long black hair.

The imported black or black-and-white breeds had many advantages, especially in extensive systems. The breeders and rearers liked them, but Bela Dorner de Enese (president of Hungary's pork breeders' association in the 1930s) made the following observation: "Strangely enough, the black English porker breeds are not willingly purchased by the Hungarian meat trade because of the darker skin and the black hair roots left behind in the skin and brawn. This is the reason why the white-haired and pale pink skinned foreign pork breeds are preferred in Hungary, although under Hungarian weather conditions the rearing of cold and heat tolerant, hardy black coated English pig breeds more resistant to disease and less demanding is more profitable and involves less risk. This differs from the demand of western countries or even of big markets of the neighbouring countries where only the quality and not the colour is regarded and paid for."

As well as the coloured English breeds (and the Poland China from America), Dorner described a whole range of imported whites - Dutch, German and English. The latter included the old Yorkshire, the curly-coated Lincolnshire and the middle and large whites, and it was these English porkers that were the most important in evolving the Hungarian white pig.

The Yorkshire and the Lincolnshire were from early importations and they did not prove sufficiently disease resistant. At the time the Hungarian breeders wanted to continue with the extensive systems for which their Mangalitsa was so well adapted. No doubt the old whites would have succeeded admirably if properly fed and housed, but as it was many of the animals died on the small farms to which the government had distributed them, especially the Yorkshire: up to 90% of the sows introduced in Transdanubia died.

The first Yorkshires were imported by sugarbeet factories in the north west. Large pig farms and estates soon followed their example and many large herds of the type were established between the 1870s and the 1920s. In spite of the breed's problems on smallholdings, it could and did thrive under more intensive management and proved to have an unparalleled feed conversion efficiency. It became the most widespread breed on manorial estates during the 1920s.

In less sophisticated conditions, other English whites did much better than the old Yorkshires and Lincolnshires, and filled a very obvious gap in the interwar pork market. There was a national move to import white (and black) English breeds through the NPBA in London between the wars.

The Great War had proved as catastrophic for porkers as it had for the Mangalitsa - or perhaps more so, as in such disastrous economic conditions people reverted to the native pig and the demand for abundant meals of bacon, sausage meat and fine pinkish ham remained high. After the second war, public tastes changed and people wanted smaller meals and more fine pork. "This change in demand," said Dorner in his report to the British pig breeders' association in 1934, "was intensively promoted and quickened by a modern 'fad', originating from the attitude of the young and less young ladies, desiring to slim."

The Middle White was widely used in Hungarian crossing programmes; for example, the Mangalitsa cross produced good fattening pigs. The Middle White was particularly favoured for its ham, and made a considerable contribution to the development of the white Hungarian breed. The Large White was ideal for bacon processing and quickly became more popular as tastes changed. Not all the Large Whites were imported direct from England: substantial numbers in 1923 came from Holland and Germany, for example - there had been some complaints that many imported Large Whites failed to acclimatise and were too long-nosed, too long-legged and too narrow for some Hungarian breeders, who decided to cross them with the Edelschwein.

Both the Edelschwein and the German (Improved) Landrace were added to the mixture that was forming the white Hungarian meat pig. A herdbook for the new Hungarian Yorkshire or **Hungarian White** was opened in 1923 and the breed was more fully developed after the Second World War.

Bulgaria

Bulgaria, a fertile and potentially valuable agricultural region, is Europe's most south eastern land and the pig's last stronghold. Beyond is Turkey, a largely Muslim country where pigs are not welcome, and from there eastwards and southwards there are no domesticated pigs of any note until China.

Writing to *The Ark* in May, 1978, Dr A.D. Richardson remarked that a few years earlier he had seen in a small Bulgarian village some pigs "about half the size of a Large White, black and covered with fur, which was curly. The fur was dark also. They seemed fairly well domesticated."

The primitive **Bulgarian Native** <Plate 11> type has prick ears, a straightish tail and a very hairy coat with a crest of bristles along the spine. It has long since been graded up to Large White, though there may be a handful remaining in the Botevgrad area. There is a primitive **East Balkan** in eastern Bulgaria which originated from crosses between Asian and European wild pigs; it is usually black (occasionally pied) and is prick-eared. Local pigs crossed with the Mangalitsa and the Šumadija produced the **Kula** in the north west, another lard pig which was black, red-brown or dirty white in colour.

Most Bulgarian pigs are now white. The national **Bulgarian White** was the result of grading up the native pig to Large White and Edelschwein, while the **Bulgarian Landrace** originated from Landraces imported from Sweden between 1957 and 1967. The new lean **Danube White**, also called the **Dunai White** (the river changes its name as it crosses into different countries), was developed from a combination of Bulgarian White, Large White, Landrace, Piétrain and Hampshire.

There is also an old mixture of Berkshire and native, with some Mangalitsa in it since 1940. This is the black-and-white **Dermantsi Pied** lard pig of Lukovit, in the north.

Dermantsi Pied <Plate 11>

The Mottled or Spotted Dermantsi was named after the Lovech village where it was created. It is a hilly region, in the foothills of the Balkans, with rather long cold winters and hot summers. The pig created for this setting was the result of crossbreeding primitive local pigs with Berkshires imported from England, and later with the Improved or "Noble" German Landrace, the Mangalitsa and the Cornwall or Large Black, also from England. The programme began in 1894. The colouring is sometimes like that of the Berkshire (black, with white points) or more often white with black spots - more black than white on the mottled body. The ears are of good size and almost erect. The cross to a Mangalitsa produces striped piglets, that to a Berkshire typical black with white points, and that to the Mirgorod (bred in the Ukraine) black-and-white mottled.

Romania

The grey, prick-eared **Romanian Native** pig of the Danube valley is typical of the east European primitives and can still be found here and there, its name sometimes charmingly mistranslated as the "Prickly" rather than the "Prick-eared". There is a mountain variety, the **Stocli**, and a marshland variety, the Marsh Stocli or **Băltăret**. Until recently there was also a **Transylvanian** local variety.

More developed Romanian pigs include the **Banat White** meat breed in the west, which originated from an early 20th century mixture of Middle White from England and Edelschwein from Germany crossed with the Mangalitsa, probably with some traces of other English breeds such as the Small White and Berkshire and also the German (Improved) Landrace. The **Bazna** of central Transylvania, known locally as the *porcul de Banat*, is a white-belted black porker developed from 1872 onwards from Berkshire and Mangalitsa. There is a **Dobrogea Black** (a minority of which are pied) developed between 1949 and 1967 from England's Cornwall or Large Black and the Russian Large White. The black **Strei** in Hunedoara, Transylvania, originated in 1877 from Large Black and Mangalitsa on local pigs in the Strei river valley.

The white breeds include a **Romanian Large White** and also the **Romanian Meat Pig** in the south (Bărăgon Steppe) which was bred from 1950 using Russian Large White on local Stocli sows, backcrossed to Large White.

The small republic of Moldavia, tucked into the south west corner of the Ukraine, looks culturally and historically towards Romania and its local pigs were no doubt of Romanian origin. The **Moldavian Black** was developed by crossing black local pigs with Berkshire and others from 1918 onwards but it is now extinct.

Yugoslavia

Many Yugoslavian breeds and local types owed a debt to the Mangalitsa, or to the Šumadija and Šiška. The **Šiška** of Croatia was another of the typical east European primitives - small, grey and prick-eared; the **Šumadija** lard pig of north Serbia was developed from it and contributed to the improvement of the Mangalitsa. The Croatian **Turopolje**, a black-spotted white lard pig around Zagreb, originated from the Šiška at the end of the 19th century, with Berkshire blood. The **Gurktal** of Slovenia is a similar type. Slovenia also bred the lop-eared, black-and-white saddleback known as the **Krškopolje** (now extinct), a local type crossed with German (Improved) Landrace and possibly Berkshire and Large Black.

The **Black Mangalitsa** (now extinct) of Syrmia was known as the *Lasasta* or "weasel": it was a swallow-bellied pig of blackish brown with a yellowish belly. Sows of this type were crossed with Berkshire and Poland China by Count Pfeiffer from 1860 onwards to create the **Black Slavonian** in east Slavonia, a meat and lard pig with semi-erect ears.

The Berkshire and Mangalitsa (and probably the Šumadija) were used also used in the development of the lop-eared, black-spotted **Resava** of Serbia. A similar mixture was the origins of the Serbian **Morava**, a lop-eared black meat-and-lard type later improved with the help of the Large Black. The spotted **Dzumalia** of Macedonia is similar to the Resava.

Ian Mason, writing in *The Ark* in November, 1981, remarked on some very hairy black **Macedonian** pigs he had seen twenty years earlier. Across the border, the **Albanian Native** is usually white, and its black-spotted variant is the **Shkodra**.

Whites include the now extinct whitish-yellow, curly-coated and short-eared **Bagun** of northern Croatia (cf **Bakony** in Hungary), which was obliterated by crossings with the Middle White. There is a **Slovenian White** and also the **Subotica White** of north Vojvodina, which is a curly-coated cross of Large White and Mangalitsa bred as a meat pig. The aim has been to use imported meat-type breeds (for leanness and economy) with local sows (for hardiness and meat quality).

Czechoslovakia

Czechoslovakia took gladly to the whites and to the breeding of numerous hybrids. By the early 1960s, 75% of its licensed boars were white - mostly of the Large White type. The older breeds include the black-and-white saddlebacked **Přeštice** (<Plate 11>), a meat-and-lard pig with horizontal ears lying forwards, which originated from local saddlebacks improved in 1957 with the Wessex Saddleback from England; it is a Bohemian pig, found in Plzeň. There used to be a **Rychnov** breed from an interesting mixture (since 1865) of Large White, Middle White and Poland China crossed with local sows but it became extinct in the early 1930s from being crossed with the Edelschwein.

Nitra's **Slovakian Black Pied** or Black Spotted lard pig was developed from 1952 onwards with a combination of Mangalitsa, Berkshire, Large Black (still being bred pure in the 1960s), Piétrain and no doubt other breeds, including the prick-eared **Czech Improved White** <Plate 12> of Bohemia and Moravia which originated in the late 19th century from English Large Whites and in due course German breeds (Edelschwein and Improved Landrace) with local pigs. This breed embraced the **Moravian Large Yorkshire** and was used between 1962 and 1979 to develop the horizontal-eared **Slovakian White** <Plate 12>(recognised in 1980 and sometimes faintly spotted), with two-thirds of the genetic material being contributed by a landrace.

A combination of the Czech Improved White, the Slovakian White and the Czech Landrace <Plate 12>produced the **Slovhyb-1**. The Belgian Landrace, Piétrain, Duroc and Hampshire are also bred in Czechoslovakia and other hybrids include the **Nitra Hybrid** (from Czech Improved White, Slovakian Black Pied, Czech Landrace, Hampshire, Slovakian White and Large White), the white semi-lop **Synthetic SL98** (Belgian Landrace and Duroc), the prick-eared blue-and-white **SL96** (Belgian Landrace and Hampshire) and the **Czech Meat** hybrid (originally half Landrace, quarter Duroc and quarter Hampshire, recognised in 1991). In addition there is a **Czech Miniature**, developed at the veterinary research institute in Brno from the Göttingen and Minnesota Miniatures with the Landrace.

Poland

Pigs are the traditional livestock of Poland. In 1991 there were some 22 million of them and they contributed about 29% of the value of all agricultural production. Of the 62.9kg per capita per annum meat consumption in Poland, 36.8kg (58.5%) was pig meat. The human population is about 38 million.

The 1990 figures revealed that about 71% of the pigs were on private farms - in sharp contrast to most of eastern Europe. There are more than 2.6 million private farms in the country and 1.6 million of them have pigs, with an average herd size of 8.5 head. The average number of sows on these farms is only 2, and 400,000 of the farms have but one pig.

Before the Second World War, many Polish farmers and their workers were relatively prosperous. After the war, there was a government policy of confiscating private land to create state farms (mainly in the fertile west and north - the majority of private farms today are in central Poland). Although the state farms cover only 20% of the cultivated land area, they benefit from 80% of investments in agriculture; yet their production levels, even now, are less than those of the private sector. But that private sector, over the years, has become a veritable galaxy of very small holdings, less than 5ha each.

One of Poland's most promising exports is pig meat, especially prime ham and pork. In the 1970s, the FAO noted that 90% of Poland's fattening pigs were produced on private farms, whereas in other east European countries the proportion was exactly the reverse (80-90% was produced by collective and state farms). It is much easier to spread the benefits of improved pig breeding to very big units than to countless very small ones, and the Poles are by nature an independent race of determined individuals. Yet Poland was the first of the east European countries after the war to change its breeding goals from fat production to meat pigs, ten years ahead of the rest.

Most of the commercial pigs are of course whites, and Poland also breeds Duroc and, more recently, Hampshire. There are also some interesting native breeds, past and present.

Polish Native <Plate 11>

Poland is one of the few European countries to have, even now, a healthy Wild Boar population in its forests, and some are tame enough to approach the smallholdings quite fearlessly. The two major components of the primitive Polish Native, now extinct, are said to have been domesticated from different subspecies of the wild pigs.

The **Small Polish Prick-eared** (*Mała polska ostrovoucha*) <Plate 11> is considered in Poland to have originated from *Sus scrofa mediterraneus*. It was a short pig, weighing up to 120kg, with an arched body, a deep, flat chest, and short, rounded, erect ears. It carried a bushy, heavy coat of pure black, white or red, or pied. The type persisted between the two world wars in south east Poland (the Pripet Marshes), where it was known as the *Poleska* or **Polesian** breed. After the war there were still a few of the type near the Bug river, where they were known as the **Nadbużańska** breed. The Polesian, or **Sarny**, bred with English pigs to give the **Krolevets** lard pig in the Ukraine.

The other type was the typical Celtic lop-eared pig that was the basis of so many national landraces. The Poles say that this *świnie zwisłouche* originated from *Sus scrofa ferus* and was brought into northern Poland by Dutch and German settlers from the 14th to the 18th century. After acclimatisation, it came to be called *Połska świnia zuławska*, or **Polish Marsh** swine. They were late-maturing pigs and much larger (up to 200kg) than the Polesian, with large lop ears, and probably of the type which contributed to the German Landrace. In 1978, when the pure form of the Polesian could still be found on the Ukrainian side of the border, local Polish village pigs were described in *The Ark* as showing almost no trace of the Chinese "improving" influence: like the original Celtic pigs, they were still tall, lean and slab-sided, with lop ears, and were usually white with black spots.

The **Large Polish Long-eared** breed (*Wielkapolska długoucha*) was an intermediate form between these two basic types, weighing from 100-150kg, and was found in central and northern Poland. Its fairly large ears were nearer erect than semi-lop, carried forward but well above the eyes. Its snout was long and tapering, with a straight facial profile. Its colours included black, red and pied.

Złotniki <Plate 11>

Some very primitive long-eared strains, whose piglets were often striped at birth, were still kept in several regions in the late 1940s and were saved from complete extinction by Professor Alexandrowicz, who bred them using modern husbandry methods. His new breed, recognised in 1962, was the **Złotniki Spotted**, based on the primitives with Large White - a combination that would also be used to form Poland's commercial white breeds.

The Złotniki, which is now rare, is named after a research station run by the College of Agriculture in Poznań, where the professor also developed a white meat pig. He bought the foundation stock between 1944 and 1950 from Poles who had been moved from Vilnius and were resettling in Olsztyn province: their livestock included a mixture of the local lop-eared primitives and some short-eared pigs, with a few pure whites as well which were mainly Large White.

The professor wanted a pig suited to Polish farming conditions, able to compete in productivity with the superior imported whites but excelling them in hardiness - hence the use of the primitive stock. The Swedish Landrace was included in the breeding programme, and the **Złotniki White** usually has dropping ears as a result. It is a large pig (about 82cm at the withers, 250-300kg) with a long straight snout, a medium-length body, fairly long but strong and heavy-boned legs, and often a sloping rump and pear-shaped hams. The meat quality is said to be excellent, and it is a good cross with white boars. A long, dense coat proves its hardiness; it is less refined than a Large White and later maturing. Litter sizes in 1990 averaged 10.39 born alive (9.76 at 21 days, weight 65.52kg); average backfat 16.8mm.

The **Złotniki Spotted** has small black patches and is a meat-and-lard type. In 1990 its litter averages had improved in the last ten years from 8.70 to 9.43 born alive, and from 7.80 to 8.59 at 21 days; the 21-day weight had increased from 46.10 to 49.69 and the daily gains from 473g to 533g. The backfat thickness remained at about 18.4mm.

Puławy <Plate 11>

This coloured, prick-eared breed was developed by Professor Zdzisław Zabielski on the Borowina research station. The farm was managed by the State Research Institute of Farming in Puławy, hence the breed's name. The foundation stock was a mixture of primitive local pigs and Berkshire. Berkshires had been imported from England at the turn of the century and were being bred on estates along the Wieprz river before the First World War. They had considerable local influence at the time. The indigenous primitives were by nature slow-growing, late-maturing and long in the leg; their meat tended to be dry and stringy. With the help of the Berkshire, they became very early maturing and fast-growing producers of fatty meat, and this was typical of the early Puławy: it had a small head, erect ears, short snout and dished Berkshire face, with short legs and the typical cylindrical, deep, broad, short body of a fat-meat pig. But its native inheritance gave it the ability to accumulate its fat around the muscles, so that the meat itself was not too fatty for processed products. However, its tendency to fatten too early had several drawbacks. For a start, it was sometimes difficult to reach high finishing weights. Secondly, it seems that the early-fattening tendency contributed to lower fertility and the Puławy sows were producing only 6-8 in a litter, though they mothered them well and gave ample milk.

The Puławy's fat was much in demand between the wars and immediately after the last war and, being such an easy breed to fatten and so well adapted to Polish farming methods, the breed became very popular. When the demand for fat decreased, the breed was changed to supply more meat by reducing the rate of maturity, lengthening the body and decreasing the fat content of the carcass. The agent of these changes was a combination of selective breeding and the use of the Large White.

Today the Puławy is a much trimmer pig. Its backfat in 1990 averaged 17.0mm; its daily gains had increased in ten years from 524g to 589g and its litter averages from 10.56 born alive to 11.17, and from 9.72 at 21 days (weight 59.69kg) to 10.32 (63.55kg) Its characteristic colouring is black-and-white pied, but with more black than white, and as the black pigmentation is only in the epidermis the carcass dresses white, though inadequate scraping leaves some black bristle roots. Some animals have smaller red patches as well as the black and white - something like the Berkshire in 18th century England.

Polish Large White <Plate 12>

This group includes all the country's large whites, regardless of source. In about 1880, white prick-eared German pigs (which had already been influenced by the Yorkshire or Large White of England) were brought into Poland. They had smaller heads than the Large White, and smaller, more upright ears; they tended to be big and too heavy in the fore part. They were improved in the 1920s with the help of Large Whites and became known as the **Pomeranian** (*Pomorska*) breed, which was graded to the "thoroughbred" German white Edelschwein during the Second World War. By 1956 the various prick-eared white pigs had become so similar that it was decided to call them all *Polska wielka biała* (Polish Large White) and a herdbook was formed combining the Pomeranian, the German prick-eared white and the English Large White. The English type had been selected for bacon (including quality and carcass length) and the German for the internal fresh meat market. There remain two different types within the breed today: a bacon and a general utility pig. Sows produce litters of 10-12 and the average 21-day weight in 1990 was 62.47kg. The backfat at 110kg liveweight averages 15.5mm.

Polish Landrace <Plate 12>

Poland imported lop-eared German pigs as the foundation of its own Landrace, and after the Second World War the Swedish Landrace played an increasingly important role in its development. Apparently the old lop-eared Polish Marsh was not involved. However, the first lop-ears were brought by Dutch immigrants into the regions of the lower Vistula and Warta rivers. During the Partitions, the territory was occupied by the Germans (Great Poland and Pomerania) and the Russians (some of south east Little Poland) and for a time there were two groups of lop-eared pigs. Before the First World War further imports were made, mainly from Westphalia; also during the Second World War.

The early type of Polish Landrace was less refined than the Large White. Its back was slightly arched, its rump gently sloping, its skin thick and folded, its growth rate less and it was later maturing. The modern type, however, has a straight back, long sides and well developed hams; its head is of medium size and its large lop ears reach forward in typical Landrace style.

The Poles developed different Landrace lines based on the Norwegian (line 21), the German (line 23) and also on the Welsh (line 24), but from January, 1992, these were all combined with the line 20 Polish Landrace and are all in the same herdbook.

Litter averages in 1990 were 10.35 born alive, 9.75 at 21 days (weight 60.48g); daily gain 576g.

RUSSIA AND THE REPUBLICS OF THE FORMER USSR

The huge area of what was formerly the USSR covers a diverse range of cultures, climate and terrain. It stretches from the Carpathian mountains of Europe to the Pacific coast of Asia, and from the Arctic Ocean to the borders of the old fertile crescent of the ancient world and the central Asian deserts - from almost polar to subtropical climates, from humid to arid, from temperatures as low as -68°C in north east Siberia to 50°C in the central Asian republics. The old Union covered an area of 22.4 million sq.km, stretching 10,000km from west to east, in both Europe and Asia.

The European republics, when under Soviet power, drastically reduced the populations of their indigenous pig breeds in the cause of "improvement", largely by grading up with imported Large Whites, Landraces and Berkshires. There have been deliberate attempts to create many new breeds suited to different environments, based on the indigenous pigs contributing their hardiness to the imported breeds' productivity. An unknown number of native pigs lost their identities in the process and a huge reservoir of regional genetic variation has vanished. Too late, steps were taken to preserve the remnants in the 1980s, in recognition of their potentially valuable traits such as hardiness, disease resistance, good constitutions, quality meat and any hidden assets which had not yet been appreciated.

Today there are more than thirty breeds over the area as a whole (including the Asian as well as the European regions) but very few indeed are of the old indigenous types, though most of them carry a small inheritance from the native pigs. The common east European theme of large intensive units has been carried to extremes and there are a few, almost town-sized, hybridisation centres capable of housing thousands of sows with the aim of providing first-generation crossbred gilts and boars to groups of collective farms. The centres have no land except for the housing, and all feed has to be bought in. In the Ukraine, for example, they offered pigs of 26 breeds, but 80% of those pigs' genetic material was Large White. The standard sire was the **Estonian Bacon**, which remains the typical pig in the European republics and is based on the Landrace.

Before the break-up of the USSR, about 80% of the 80 million pigs throughout the union belonged to the state. Many farm workers could keep a pig or two themselves in the traditional backyard manner, along with perhaps a cow and some poultry. At the beginning of 1991, 96% of collective farmers, 98% of pensioners' families and 78% of the families of other rural workers and employers had allotments, the average sizes of which (for each group respectively) were 0.29, 0.32 and 0.13ha. On those allotments could be found 22% of all Soviet cattle, 27% of all sheep and goats, 35% of all poultry and 22% (16.4 million) of all pigs - an increase in the latter species of 2.47 million since 1985. From these private allotments people were selling significant quantities of produce, including 260,000 tonnes of meat and fat. As the state agricultural section collapsed, the allotment holders profited considerably: they were not only almost self-sufficient but could also find a very ready urban market for their surpluses.

Although barely discernible now, the original indigenous types were much the same in the European republics as in countries to the west and there was the typical grouping seen also in Poland: the smaller European prick-eared and the larger Celtic lop-eared were the basic native pigs in the republics. Types described as "long-eared", incidentally, tend to be semi-lops, usually more prick than lop.

The formation of "breeds" began in the latter half of the 19th century and was practised on a grand scale in the 1930s, 1940s and 1950s. Typically, native pigs selected for, say, disease resistance, a strong constitution and general fitness and suitability for local conditions, were crossed with the improved and highly productive European breeds until a stable type was established through several generations of progeny selection. The term "strong constitution" is an essential one in the context: it embraces factors such as good health, well developed bone structure, strong legs and feet, a good coat and a smooth, elastic skin. It is also associated with high productivity, especially reproduction.

Soviet pigs were divided into three broad types - general purpose, meat (pork and bacon), and lard - and were developed according to market requirements. Fashions changed, of course. The extreme lard type was the breeders' favourite in the 1940s and 1950s but meat quality and better finishing performance are high on the agenda of any breeding programme. Maternal lines are usually from the general purpose group, selected for best prolificacy, while sire lines are from the meat group. The lard group is quietly disappearing.

In 1989 there were, officially, 32 pig breeds, breed groups and types. The terms "breed" and "breed group" are specific. During development, a population of animals becomes a breed group when certain levels of productivity and numbers of animals are achieved: there must be at least 3,000 breeding sows and 300 boars, with not less than 3 breeding lines and 6 families in the population. As numbers and lines increase, the breed group becomes a breed: the threshold is 5,000 sows, 500 boars, 6 lines (each of at least 2 branches) and 12 families. Thereafter, breed improvement is a continuous process of testing, selection and, where necessary, crossbreeding to bring in new blood or to develop new regional types.

There is a danger in this concentration on productivity. The greater the degree of "progressive" breeding, the further the distance from the important qualities of the native pigs - for example their adaptation to the climate, their low nutritional and housing demands, their general healthiness and hardiness, their resistance to stress and the quality of their meat. It is a danger that is beginning to be recognised in many European countries.

In 1980 there was a proposal for a book on the animal genetic resources of the USSR, as there was no comprehensive publication in English covering that most interesting subject. The book was at last published by the FAO in 1989 and forms the basis for much of the breed information which follows.

The republics have been divided geographically. The Baltic countries include Estonia, Latvia and Lithuania; the west includes Belorus and the Ukraine (Moldavia's pigs are included with Romania's); Transcaucasia, where Europe meets and mixes with Asia, includes Georgia, Armenia and Azerbaijan; Russia includes the whole of Siberia. Many of the central Asian areas are Muslim and therefore pigs are inappropriate, but Kazakhstan has a couple of interesting breeds which are described at the end of this section.

The Baltic States

The republics of Estonia and Latvia were annexed from Sweden during the reign of Tsar Peter I (1696-1725). In 1918 the Bolsheviks were forced to surrender Estonia, Latvia and Lithuania to Germany and Austria, and the three Baltic republics became independent until annexed by the Soviet Union in 1940. Through all the chopping and changing, each preserved its regional identity and each now has its own modern white breed of pig. Those of Latvia and Lithuania are classed as general purpose types, while Estonia has its well known bacon pig.

Estonian Bacon (*Estonskaya bekonnaya*) <Plate 12>

This white meat type pig, recognised in 1961, was developed from local long-eared sows, crossed with Large White (and some Middle White) and several improved Landraces - German, Finnish, Swedish, Welsh, and most influentially, Danish Landrace boars. It is quite a long-bodied breed, deep and wide in the chest, long and wide on the back and with full hams. The head is of medium size, the face straight or slightly dished, and its large Yorkshire-like ears tend to droop forwards, but not over the eyes. It is a white pig, occasionally with small coloured spots. It looks very like a landrace but claims a better daily weight gain and FCR, a longer carcass, less backfat, more weight in the bacon carcass and a higher protein quality index (the latter being the ratio of tryptophan to hydroxyproline—amino acids which are protein building blocks). It is widely used as a paternal line in crossbreeding systems, and also more locally as a maternal breed. There has recently been a little injection of Duroc as well.

Latvian White (*Latviískaya belaya*) <Plate 12>

Very similar in type, constitution and conformation to the Large White, the prick-eared Latvian white general purpose pig was developed by crossing Large White (and to some extent Edelschwein) on native pigs. Officially recognised in 1967, there were more than 500,000 of the breed by 1980 (about 96% of the total purebred Latvian herd) and it is used as a maternal breed in crossbreeding systems throughout the republic.

Lithuanian White (*Litovskaya belaya*) <Plate 12>

The use of German Landrace boars in this general purpose breed's development is shown by its lop ears. The Landrace was used with Edelschwein and Large White on native pigs; its type, constitution, conformation and productivity are similar to that of the Large White. The Lithuanian White was recognised in 1967, and by 1980 its population was more than a million. It has its faults (sometimes individuals have weak pasterns, depressions behind the shoulders, or insufficient hair) but the breed has been divided for improvement in meat quality, fattening performance and uniformity into five populations, one of which has been infused with Swedish Large White and another by Landrace. As well as being dominant in Lithuania, it has been used in crossbreeding schemes in Georgia, Kazakhstan, Turkmenia, Belorus, Moldavia and Russia.

Belorus

The native lop-eared and short-eared pigs of Belorus formed the basis of the republic's modern pigs in a breeding programme that dates back to the 19th century, when they were crossed with various improved English breeds. The indigenous pigs included, for example, the **Polesian**, a variety of the Small Polish Prick-eared pig found in the Pripet Marshes on the Ukraine border - both the Ukraine and Belorus share a frontier with Poland.

The English breeds imported in the 19th century included the Yorkshire, the Middle White, the red Tamworth and the Large Black, and the type that was developed in Belorus was a black-and-white pied pig. One of the breeding groups which never reached breed status was the **Slutsk Black Pied** in the west of the republic, created before 1919 but now extinct. The main breed is also pied. A **BKB-1** is being developed as a strain of the Russian Large White.

Belorus Black Pied (*Belorusskaya chernopestraya*) <Plate 13>

The 19th century crossbreeding of the assorted local and English breeds produced a large number of improved native pigs bursting with hybrid vigour. They were taller than the original locals, earlier maturing and with larger litters, and they retained their native ability to thrive despite poor feeding and management. During the 1920s this improved Belorus was further interbred with Large White, Middle White and Berkshire, and in due course was also influenced by Estonian Bacon and Swedish Landrace. The Belorus Black Pied was recognised as a breed group in 1957 and as a breed nine years later, but its numbers were never high: there were 102,000 by the early 1980s and it accounted for only 0.3% of the total population.

It is described as "black pied" and the proportions of black and white areas vary considerably. It has a light head with a straight face, and medium-sized ears growing forwards in a semi-lop style. The body is of good depth and width, the back straight and broad, and the hams are described as "moderately plump". Its resistance to disease and stress is good. It is also sometimes known as the **White-Russian Pied** or **Spotted**.

Ukraine

The Ukraine is the second largest of the republics, after Russia. It, too, has historical and geographical links with Poland, and it shares borders with Czechoslovakia, Romania and the Black Sea. Its most common native pigs were short-eared and spotted, and it was these that formed the basis of its improved breeds. It is the home of the **Mirgorod** and the **Ukrainian White Steppe**, two of the four most prominent breeds in the 1940s and still around today. They form the basis of the two main pig groups in the Ukraine.

Mirgorod <Plate 13>

This interesting, well-tried pasture pig - a lard type of various colours with small prick or semi-lop ears - is thoroughly adapted to the Ukrainian forest steppelands. Recognised as a breed in 1940, it was originally developed by crossing spotted, short-eared Ukrainian native sows with English breeds, especially the black Berkshire, the Large White and Middle White, and also to some extent the red Tamworth, and this mixture is revealed in its colouring. In tune with the times, it was intended as a lard breed and its rapid descent in numbers since then reflects the change in tastes away from fat. In 1960, there were 744,000 Mirgorods; by 1980 the total population was 186,000. In 1983 the average backfat thickness was 28mm, though in a champion boar for meat quality it was 37mm.

Like the Ukrainian White Steppe, the Mirgorod grows well even when fed on nothing but straw in a cold building. It is a solidly built pig, broad in the chest with a straight, wide back and strong legs. Its head is of medium size, the snout of good length and the face slightly dished. The small ears are usually erect, pitched forwards, but occasionally are slightly drooping. The unwrinkled skin is hard but elastic, with an even covering of dense bristles over the whole body. The predominant colour is black-and-white pied but some animals are black, or tan, or black-and-tan. It is fairly prolific, averaging 10.8 per litter in breeding centre tests in 1983.

Other breed groups of a similar type are now extinct. The black pied **Podolian** in the west was developed from locals crossed with Berkshire, Middle White and Large White. The **Dnieper**, in Cherkassy, was a black spotted lard pig derived from local short-eared natives crossed with Mirgorod, and then with Berkshire (1911) and Large White (1937-8). The **Krolevets** in northern Ukraine was black or black pied and originated from English breeds crossed with the local **Polesian** or Sarny of the Pripet Marshes.

The **Poltava** (named for a pig breeding research institute) is a meat hybrid developed since 1966 from Mirgorod with Russian Large White, Landrace, Piétrain and Welsh. It is now contributing to a new **Lipetsk** type in Russia, in formation from 1991, which is Poltava x (Poltava x Belorus commercial hybrid), as a variety of the new **Soviet Meat** breed. The latter is based on the Poltava with some Kharkov and Belorusa hybrid blood and includes varieties such as the **Central Russian** and **Steppe Meat** hybrids. The **Kharkov** meat hybrid is a cross of Russian Large White, Landrace and Welsh. There is also a **Dnepropetrovsk** hybrid from Russian Large White, Berkshire and Landrace.

Ukrainian White Steppe (*Ukrainskaya stepnaya belaya*) <Plate 12>

The development of this breed, recognised in 1932, was a new Soviet experience and it became a blueprint for many other breed creation schemes. It was also the first breed to be developed specifically for combining the hardiness and local adaptation of native pigs with the high productivity of imported improved breeds. The consolidation of this marriage of qualities was achieved by deliberate inbreeding, with rigid culling on the basis of a rugged constitution so that it was better suited than the Large White to the area's continental climate. It became the third most populous breed in the USSR and there were 812,000 in 1964, though by 1980 numbers had decreased to 636,300. Although bred for Ukrainian conditions, it also spread to neighbouring Moldavia and eastwards to parts of Azerbaijan, Armenia and Turkmenia.

The original cross was of Large White boars on the south's native spotted **Ukrainian** breed (now extinct) and it is similar to the Large White in conformation but more rugged and solid, denser in the bone, and deeper and wider in the body. Its large ears droop slightly, shading the eyes; the head is of medium size, the face slightly dished. It has strong legs and dense white bristles.

Ukrainian Spotted Steppe (*Ukrainskaya stepnaya ryabaya*) <Plate 13>

During the development of the Ukrainian White Steppe, selected spotted females were crossed with Berkshire and Mangalitsa boars. Thereafter the blueprint of close inbreeding was followed, with rigid culling for constitution and productivity, and the Ukrainian Spotted Steppe was recognised as a breed in 1961. Its numbers have never been high: at the time of its recognition there were 28,00 but they had dropped to 7,000 by 1980. It is better adapted to the hot southern climate than its white cousin, though it is similar in type, and evaluation figures seem to be identical. The coat is black-and-white spotted or black-and-tan, and some individuals are wholly black.

Transcaucasia

The Transcaucasian republics form a melting-pot where Asia and Europe meet, mix and argue, and where the two great religions of Christianity and Islam sometimes clash. Georgia (bordering Turkey) and Armenia (bordering Turkey and Iran) are mostly Christian but Azerbaijan looks towards neighbouring Iran and is a mainly Shi-ite country, not interested in breeding pigs.

There are two particularly interesting pig groups in this part of the world: the very primitive **Kakhetian**, and an Armenian type developed for forest and mountain zones. Local Georgian pigs contributed to two now extinct breeds, the **Imeretian** (with lop-eared Polish Landrace blood) and the **Kartolinian** (with Large White blood). In Russian territory just to the north of the Caucasus mountains there is a black pied **North Caucasus**.

Kakhetian <Plate 13>

This group of primitives in eastern Georgia remain fairly close to the Wild Boar in their cranial structure, and their piglets are striped at birth. They were once widespread in Georgia but now the main centres for the purebred type are in the regions of Akhmeta, Telavi, Kvareli, Gurjaani and Dusheti. Their numbers are dropping rapidly: there were 6,000 in 1969 and five years later there were 2,000 with only 1,200 in 1980 when there were just two pure breeding boars and 103 breeding sows. Steps are being taken to protect this rare breed and to add its qualities in constitution and disease resistance to the improved breeds. It is being crossed with the mangalitsa in the Georgian mountains.

The Kakhetian, a lard and meat type, is quite long and strong in the leg and short in the body but well built with a deep, wide chest and broad, straight back. As befits its extensive lifestyle, it has tough feet and a coat of long, hard bristles. The head is relatively small, with a straight profile and a fairly long snout. The upright ears tend to tip forwards.

Forest Mountain (*Lesogornaya porodnaya gruppa)* <Plate 13>

The native grey pigs of north and east Armenia were developed with the help of Large White and Mangalitsa to form a breed group which numbered 7,000 in 1964 and increased to twice that within five years but dropped down to 2,000 in 1974 and only 569 purebred in 1980, with 16 breeding boars and four boar lines. Bred specifically in the 1950s for Armenia's forest and mountain zones, it is well suited as a pasture pig but also adapts to confinement: the practice is to keep the young on pasture to 6-8 months of age and then fatten them for 60-80 days. More Large White is being introduced to improve the fattening performance.

A thoroughly hardy pig, it is sometimes white or occasionally black. The ears used to be of medium size and horizontal but have become increasingly large and more upright as the proportion of Large White blood has grown. The chest is deep and broad, the legs long and the feet strong for ranging, the body long with a good covering of bristles and an undercoat, and in winter the coat grows long. In comparison with the Large White and various meat breeds, Forest Mountain carcasses have a higher fat content (9.9%), a lower moisture content in the meat and a more intense meat colour.

North Caucasus <Plate 13>

Local Kuban pigs in Krasnodar, the territory bordering the eastern shores of the Sea of Azov and to the north west of the Caucasus mountains, provided the basis of the North Caucasus when they were crossed with Large White, Berkshire and Edelschwein at state and collective farms around Rostov. The breed was recognised in 1955 and there were 141,000 in 1964. By 1980 they had increased to 195,000, with the best at breeding centres in Gornya (Rostov) and Krasny Vodopad (Tashkent), and the Pobeda breeding farm and Donskoe training farm in the Rostov region, and the Alexseevski state breeding farm in the autonomous republic of Mari. The breed, selected for improved meat quality and fattening performance, was developed for use locally and also in parts of the Ukraine, Georgia, Armenia and some of the Asian republics.

It is a black pied pig with a dense coat of soft bristles and erect or semi-erect ears.The chest is deep and wide, the back and loin broad and of medium length; the hams are full and plump, the legs strong. Its broad head has a slightly dished face.

The **Don** type, recognised as a separate breed in 1978, is a highly productive meat pig developed by using Piétrain boars on North Caucasian sows. Development of the **Rostov** breed group of meat pigs began in 1973 as a combination of Russian Large White, Russian Short-eared White (from imported Edelschwein to Krasnodar since 1927), Piétrain and Welsh; the mixture is similar to that of the Ukraine's Poltava. There also used to be a *Pridonskaya* or **Don** breed group in Rostov (at Kamenski, near the Sea of Azov) from Large Black, Cornwall and long-eared whites crossed to local Large Whites, but it is now extinct.

RUSSIA

Most of Russia's breeds have developed from local pigs (usually lop-eared) with Large White, and most are now white. Their development tended to centre around Moscow, though over a wide radius. Several persist but several other breed groups in that general area became extinct - for example, the **Alabuzin** at Kalinin (white lard pig, occasionally spotted, originally from local lop with Large White and some Middle White and Berkshire in the late 19th century), the **Meshchovsk** at Kaluga (local with Large White), the **Kalikin** at Ryazan (grey pied lard pig from local lop with Large White and Berkshire), the **Ievlev** at Tula (lop-eared black spotted land pig, sometimes black, white, or white-spotted, from local pigs to Large White, Large Black and various black or black spotted breeds), the **Dobrinka** at Lipetsk (bred from 1932 from Large White on local), and the **Rossosh** at Voronezh (black pied lard pig bred in 1940s from a mixture of local with Large White, Berkshire and Mirgorod).

There are also more generally distributed whites and hybrids based mainly on the Large White and grouped below under **Russian Large White** for simplicity, as it was by far the most numerous breed in the old USSR, accounting for 86.5% of all pigs of recognised breeds in the 1980s.

The **Russian Long-eared White** is essentially the German Improved Landrace, and the **Russian Short-eared White** is essentially the German Edelschwein, based on the Large White.

Russian Large White(*Krupnaya belaha*) <Plate 12>

Large white Yorkshire-bred pigs were imported from England in 1880 and continued to come in over the years. From the start, they were developed for Russia, which covers a wide range of climate and feeding conditions. In the early days it was noticed that the English Large White boars on local sows produced highly productive crosses, and there were several more imports of Large Whites from England in the 1920s and again in the 1960s to continue the improvements.

Many breeders and scientists were involved in the development of the Russian or Soviet Large White, and between them they produced an adaptable general purpose breed claiming to be superior to the English in many respects. In 1980 there were 25.554 million of these Large Whites in the USSR and the breed was being widely used in the development of most of the Soviet breeds.

Its type is broadly similar to that of the English Large White. It has a deep, wide chest, a broad, straight back, plump hams down to the hocks, strong legs, and a medium-sized head with a slightly dished face. The ears are thin and elastic, of medium size, and less erect than in the English Large White, tilting forwards. It is of course a white pig and it has the typical Large White qualities such as high productivity, good mothering and high and lasting prolificacy. Strains of the Russian Large White include the BKB-1, KB-V-1, KB-KN, MM-1, UKB-1 and no doubt many more. The **Prisheksninsk** is a meat and lard pig developed from local types in the Vologda region crossed with Large White.

Breitov <Plate 12>

Bred originally on Yaroslavl's collective farms, the Breitov's official history goes back to before the 1917 revolution. Local land owners had imported various breeds - Large White and Middle White from England, Danish Landrace, improved lop-eared pigs from Latvia and Lithuania, Polesians from Belorus and so on - and these had been interbred among themselves and also crossed with native lops. Thus there was a large pool of improved local crossbreds, which were later carefully divided into 16 unrelated groups, subsequently crossed during a deliberate breeding programme to fix desirable traits without inbreeding.

The Breitov's development was dictated by a desire to use locally available feeds - potatoes, roots, clover, chaff and dairy byproducts - with a minimum of fodder grain. It was a lard pig when recognised as a breed in 1948, but was later developed for improved meat quality and is now a general purpose breed. The numbers have fluctuated over the years: in 1960 there were 216,000, in 1969 only 48,000 and in 1980 there were 65,800.

It is usually white, though some have coloured spots on the body, and its well marbled meat is bright in colour with a particularly high protein quality index and palatability score. It is noted for its hardiness and ability to adapt to the climate of north west Russia, consuming large quantities of bulky feeds and with rapid weight gains on low-concentrate feeding. The sows farrow twice a year and often continue to breed until they are five or six years old, but the Breitov cannot compare with the Large White for litter size or litter weight at a month old, nor is its meat quality as good as that of the Landrace. However, it crosses well and is intended for use as a maternal and paternal breed in commercial crossbreeding systems.

The extinct **Kama** breeding group of Solikamsk, Perm, was bred from Breitov and Large White crossed with local short-eared sows.

Murom <Plate 12>

Similar to the Large White in type, the Murom was developed for the Vladimir region from native long-eared sows crossed with the Lithuanian White and Large White. It was recognised in 1957 and there were 56,000 by 1960. In 1980 numbers were down to 16,900. It is white, with the standard deep, wide chest and broad, level back, with an even coat of dense bristles over the body. Its head is light, its face slightly dished. The moderately large ears droop forwards so that they are carried horizontally, shielding the eyes.

Livny <Plate 13>

This white or pied general purpose pig was developed in the Orel region from native lop-eared sows with Large White, Berkshire and (unusually) the Poland China from America. It is a robust, thick sort of pig with strong legs, ample bone, a rough and sometimes wrinkled skin with plenty of hair. Its broad back is sometimes arched, and the relatively short, broad head has a dished face with large, thick ears that droop slightly. Most of the pigs are white, or black pied; some are red pied or wholly black. It was recognised as a breed in 1949; there were apparently 476,000 in 1960 but twenty years later there were only 59,600.

Its robustness serves it well: it is virtually weatherproof and adaptable to a range of feeding conditions. Its meat quality is said to be high, with meat colour the best of all the USSR breeds.

Tsivilsk <Plate 14>

Yet another Large White type, this breed group was developed in the mid 1950s from Large White on local pigs in the Chuvash ASSR. It has a heavier head than the Large White, with a broad forehead, a slightly dished face, rather a long snout, and medium-sized ears tilting forwards. It is white and is used for crossing with Large White.

Urzhum <Plate 14>

As early as 1893, the lop-eared pigs in the Kirov region were being crossed with the Large White. More serious development of the Urzhum began in 1945 and it was recognised as a breed in 1957. It is similar to the Large White in conformation but with more length and depth than breadth to its body, and with massive coarse bone. With strong legs and dense bristles, it is well adapted to local conditions and a useful consumer of bulky succulent feedstuffs. The population in 1980 was much the same as in 1960 at 106,000.

Siberia

The semi-wild pigs in the colder regions of Siberia were described at the turn of the century as "very small, of a slate colour and *mostly bristles*." The Siberian Wild boar (*Sus scrofa ussuricus*) is still found in eastern Siberia, in the Ussuri and Amur river regions, and in Manchuria, China: its colour varies from fuscous to black, with burnt umber to fuscous on the underside and extremeties; typical bristles are 7-10cm long mid-dorsally and 4-6cm long laterally, with a dense, curly underfur varying in colour from smoke grey to burnt umber. There is today a **Minisib** developed from wild pigs (20-25%), Vietnamese pigs (43-56%) and the Swedish Landrace (24-32%), a miniature animal used in laboratory research in Russia.

The native **Siberian** or Tara (*Tarskaya*) in the region around Omsk and Novosibirsk was a primitive, coloured, small-eared type, now extinct; however, it contributed to several prick-eared breeds in the area, some of which survive. One group which disappeared was the **Omsk Grey**, a meat pig developed from a mixture of the local Siberians of Tara, with the Siberian Black Pied and the Kemerovo, crossed with Large White.

Off the coast of eastern Siberia, on the long island that reaches towards Japan's Hokkaido island, is the **Sakhalin White**, bred from local pigs crossed with Large Whites which were imported in 1932.

North Siberian (*Sibirskaya severnaya*) <Plate 14>

A white lard pig resulting from crosses with the Large White, the North Siberian lard pig was recognised in 1942. During the phase in which the crossbred offspring were being interbred, "positive assortative mating" was widely used, with varying degrees of inbreeding but with rigid culling.

The North Siberian is described as having a "harmonious" conformation. It is of medium size, with a broad, straight back and short, strong legs. The face is slightly dished and the erect ears tilt forwards a little. The rather coarse-haired skin is free from wrinkles and there is often an undercoat beneath the long, flexible bristles: it is well protected against cold winters, and also against the mosquitoes and gnats which drive a Large White to distraction in summer. The North Siberian is far better adapted to the harsh climate of the region for which it was developed - Novosibirsk, Krasnogarsk, the Buryat ASSR and Kazakhstan. Immunogenetic tests check the authenticity of its pedigree and there is a determination to maintain genetic similarity within the various lines.

Siberian Black Pied (*Sibirskaya chernopestraya*) <Plate 14>

Known also as the Novosibirsk Spotted or the Siberian Spotted, this breed group is effectively a variety of the North Siberian - a coloured line of types rejected during the development of that breed, to which it is broadly similar in type. However, it is even better adapted to local conditions, especially heat, and it is "zoned" for raising in the Novosibirsk region. It has a rough skin covered with underhair and soft, dense bristles. Typically the black patches on the white are shadow-edged with a ring of white hairs on pigmented skin. Numbers have never been high: there were 4,000 in 1964, 12,000 ten years later, but only 5,300 in 1980.

Kemerovo <Plate 14>

This black pig was originally a lard type, but is now classified as general purpose. Again based on the native Siberian, the infusion in this case included Large White and Berkshire, with a little help from the Large Black, and later (to create more lines and families) North Siberian and Siberian Black Pied as well. It was recognised in 1961 and in 1980 it numbered 53,200.

Black is the standard colour but traces of Berkshire show up in white areas on the body, legs, tail and forehead. Often the pig has a white face and four white socks, with a few streaks of white on the body. It is a densely coated pig with a broad body of medium length and a deep, broad chest and good tough feet. The head is of medium size with a somewhat dished face and small erect ears.

The Kemerovo has proved to be quite capable of withstanding southern Siberia's severe climate: it is hardy and has considerable vitality. It has been widely used in crosses with other Siberian breeds. Part of the Kemerovo population has been mated with Landrace for better meat quality and the new meat-type hybrid was recognised in 1978 as the **KM-1** - which is basically 5/8 Landrace and 3/8 Kemerovo. It is selected for thin backfat and efficient feed conversion.

Kazakhstan

This is the only other Asian republic in the old USSR where there is any significant pig breed - indeed there are two, both in the south east, where the climate is extreme: in summer the day temperatures might climb to 48°C but drop to 5°C at night, while in the winter the temperatures can be almost as low as -50°C.

Aksaĭ Black Pied <Plate 14>

This breed group is still being improved at the Kaskelenski state breeding farm and at the Aksaĭ experimental and training farm in the Alma-Ata region, and is intended for raising locally. It originated from local pigs crossed with Large White and Berkshire, and is now being improved for litter size, meat quality and fattening performance with the help of Large White and Estonian Bacon. There were 11,000 (including 5,000 purebreds) in 1980, and it is used in commercial crossbreeding with North Caucasus, Large White and Landrace boars. It is a black-and-white pig, with varying proportions of the two colours though usually with most of the face white. The face is straight, with a good length of snout, and medium-sized prick ears.

Semirechensk <Plate 14>

This interesting breed, carefully developed for the region's difficult conditions, was the result of mating Large White x Wild Boar with the Kemerovo. The best of the resulting progeny of this three-way cross were interbred, selecting those with at least 75% Large White blood. Interbreeding continued for four or five generations under the direction of the Institute of

Experimental Biology at the Kazakhstan Academy of Science (the breed was initially known as the **Kazakh Hybrid**).

Recognised in 1978, most of the breed are white but some offspring are reddish, dark brown or black pied. The body is moderately long and deep, the chest deep, the back broad and straight, the legs strong. The small ears stand erect, with a tendency to flop forwards a little, and the profile is straight.

It is a thoroughly robust mixture: it has the wild type's disease resistance and strong constitution, and even the whites can stand the region's extreme climate, including the heat. There are fewer cases of respiratory trouble in piglets than in those of the two domesticated parent breeds, and less susceptibility to pathogenic protozoa. The Semirechensk has also inherited the Large White's productivity: it scores as highly and has a higher level of piglet viability and sow hardiness. Numbers have risen sharply since its recognition; there were 4,000 in 1969, 27,000 in 1974 and 43,000 in 1980.

ASIA

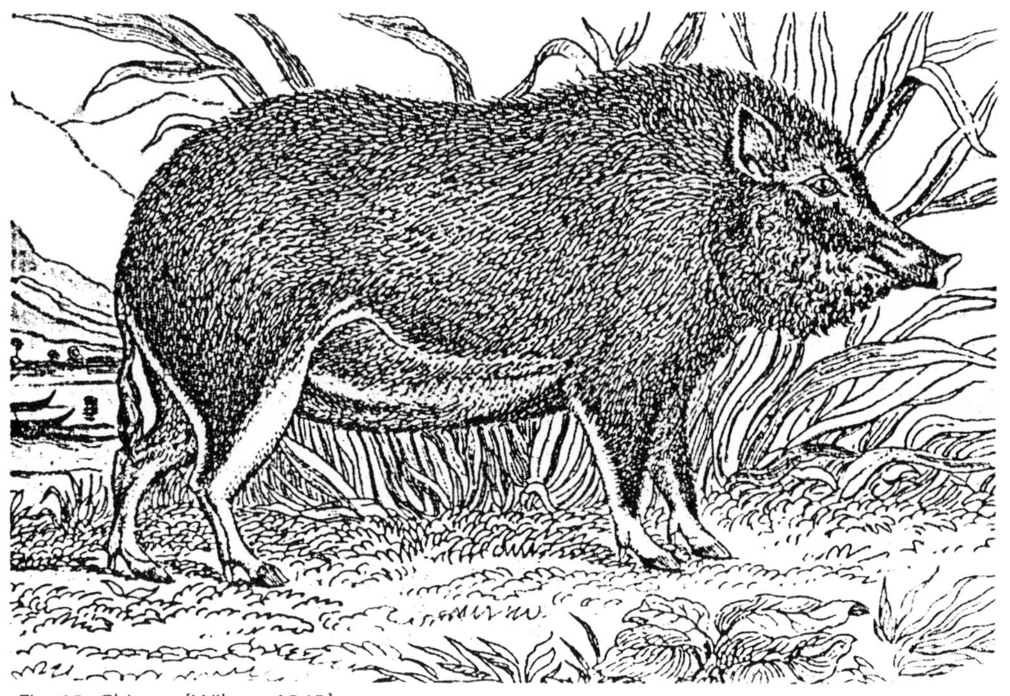

Fig. 18. Chinese [Wilson, 1849]

MAP 3. Pig Breeds of Asia

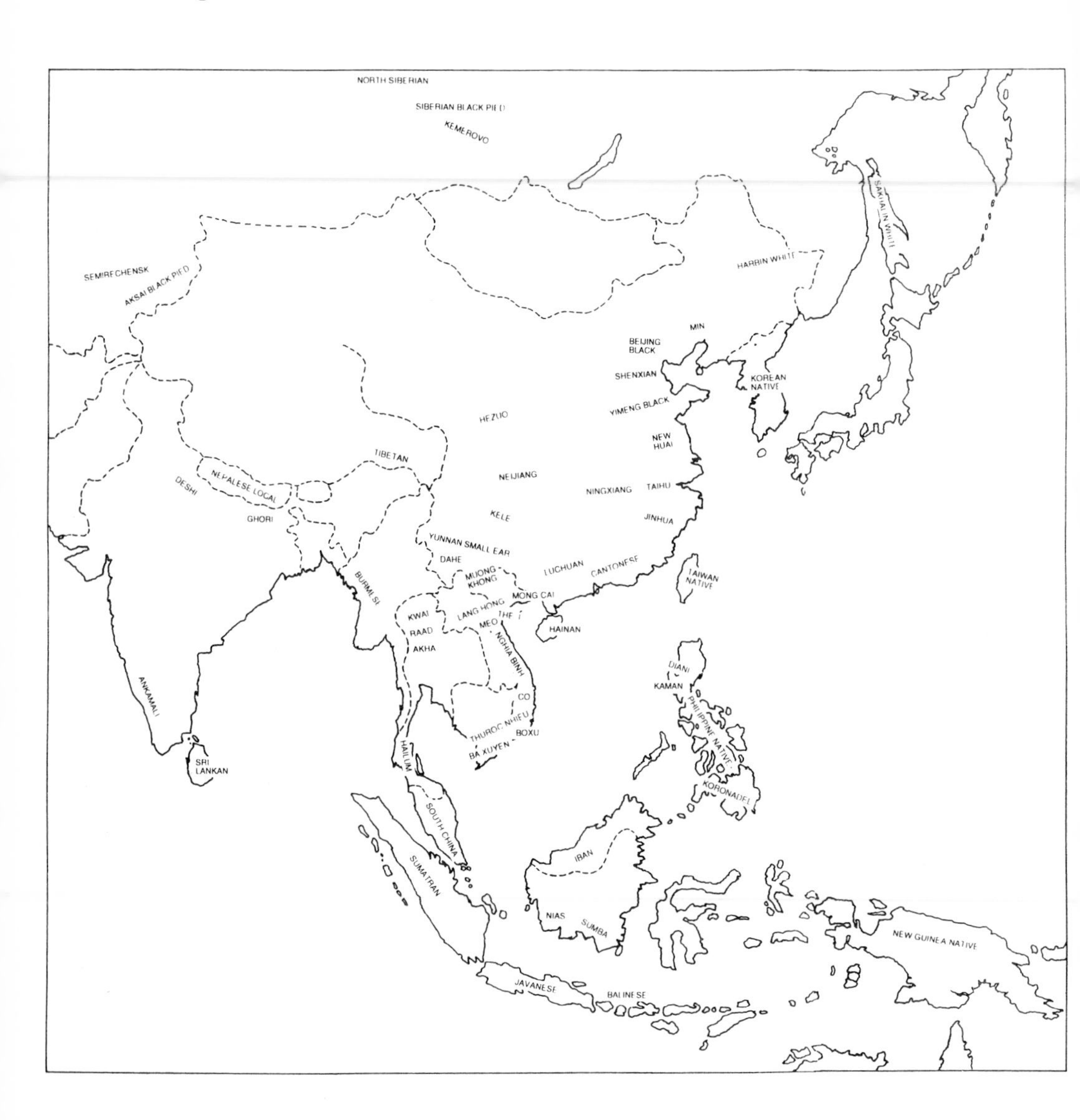

ASIA

Between the many and assorted pigs of Europe and the many more of eastern Asia there is a large area where religious taboos against keeping or eating pigs have been in force for a long time. There are still wild pigs in these areas, and in some of the countries pigs are indeed reared and eaten (as "white beef" in Israel, for example) but pig-keeping is not a tradition, though here and there feral village pigs abound.

Yet pig rearing in the east is very much a tradition and in ways far more closely interwoven with everyday human life today than in Europe. China is the great source of most of the pig types seen in south east Asia and also the source to which European breeders are now turning once again, as they did two centuries ago and as the Romans probably did more than two millennia ago, for new blood to boost their own highly developed pigs.

INDIA

In Hindu society, the pig is despised - or at least that is the attitude to the local scavengers, though these semi-wild animals living on the edge of villages are protected precisely for being scavengers. Such protection is also extended to vultures which, like the pigs, perform an important task in cleaning up unwanted waste.

These generally nondescript pigs are of some interest to the villagers, who can recognise individuals by unusual markings and colours (many have patterned coats) and can claim that some are known to be at least 20 years old. It seems that there are often red animals in this motley collection and their colour leads some to suggest a connection with the **Tamworth** of England: it was the custom for Englishmen on the Indian subcontinent during the 19th century to send young local pigs home as amusing gifts for their friends. Some of these were wild jungle pigs, which are more of a grizzled blackish brown chestnut than red, and it has been suggested that it was a boar of the wild jungle type which Sir Francis Lawley raised at Middleton Hall, near Tamworth in Staffordshire. This boar was widely used as a sire in the Tamworth area but it was said to be reddish. It seems more likely, perhaps, that Sir Francis's pride and joy was not a jungle pig but a feral, a semi-wild red village scavenger. John Nesfield, writing to *The Ark* in 1980 to describe the village pigs of Hindu India, remarked that most of the young were striped at birth - a sign of wild blood or of a very primitive type.

Timothy Broer, working with the American Peace Corps in Kathmandu in 1975, was involved with swine development on a government farm where they used Landrace, Yorkshire and Hampshire. He said that these imports were not despised like the local scavengers: they looked clean, they were bigger and more handsome, and grew fast on commercial feeds. The government at the time was concentrating its efforts on the exotics and had no interest at all in the local swine, even for crossbreeding. Broer noted that the local was not the wild pig (which, with its striped offspring, still ran free in the forests), though it had similarities. It was a very small black pig with short ears and quite prolific: he saw litters of 10. Sometimes they showed signs of crossbreeding as some of them were considerably marked with white. The pigs lived off garbage, including human and animal manure.

Most of India's pigs are nondescripts like the **Deshi** described below but in some places exotics have been crossbred with the native pigs and today large numbers of crossbreds are available. India's official domestic pig population is less than 9 million, for a human population of 823 million.

The lack of interest in the indigenous pigs is such that no one has studied what types there are and what qualities they might have, especially under typical village conditions. Potentially valuable traits remain largely unrecognised, such as conformation, performance, the ability to utilise waste and their disease resistance in a tropical environment. However, the All-India Co-ordinated Research Project on Pigs has made a start on the indigenous breeds and some statistics have been drawn up for a few regional groups. The following figures are for litter size and birth weight.

Region	Litter size (birth weight)
Gangetic Plain:	7.79 (0.90kg)
Tirupati (A.P.):	6.50 (0.70kg)
Jabalpur (M.P.):	6.76 (0.70kg)
Khanapara Dwarf (Assam):	4.5 (0.93kg)
Sikkim:	3.7 (1.07kg)
West Bengal:	5.1 (0.63kg)

The native Indian pig has smaller litters and far lower bodyweights than the exotics when both are raised under intensive systems. Litter sizes for the **Landrace** and **Large White** in 1980 were given as 8.44 (7.35 weaned) and 8.49 (8.20 weaned) respectively.

In Uttar Pradesh, Bihar, Madya Pradesh and Punjab, the local village pig or **Deshi** varies in colour from rusty grey to brown or black and is very small. Down in the south, the **Ankamali** of Kerala, Karnataka, Tamil Nadu and Maharashtra is also rusty grey, or black with white patches, and there is a primitive **Sri Lankan** native which is usually black but can also be grey or tan, or tan-and-grey or tan-and-black. The **Khasi** is a local type in Meghalaya in the north east. The **Ghori** or Pygmy of north east India, Bhutan and Bangladesh is another very small type and has its counterpart in the little black **Nepalese** hill pig, a dwarf primitive which scavenges for wild food as best it can. It is similar to the **Tibetan** pig described in the Chinese section. The black **Pakhribas** of Nepal has been developed at the local agricultural centre in Dhankuta from a combination of the British Saddleback and Tamworth crossed with Hong Kong's Cantonese **Fa Yuen**.

The tiny and extremely rare wild **Pygmy Hog** (*Sus salvanius*) still just survives on the borders of Bhutan and Assam. It used to extend along Nepal's southern borders as well but there is no evidence that it was ever domesticated. There is also a species of Wild Boar (*Sus scrofa cristatus*) known as the Jungle or **Indian Wild Pig** of the Himalayan jungles at up to 4500m; the young are of a rusty colour, changing to dark chestnut brown with maturity, tinged grey at the hair tips, but the coat is sparse, with a mane of black bristles, and there is no woolly undercoat. It is prolific and an extremely active species, quite capable of attacking humans if provoked. In India it is claimed that "all domesticated varieties, except the Chinese, are the descendants of the Indian wild pig. They were bred in India and Turkestan. From there they spread through the Mediterranean region to Europe."

The dwarf **Andaman Island** wild pig is probably a feral population though it has a very long history indeed. There are two distinct populations - one long-snouted and the other short-snouted - and they live in the island forests, forming a staple dietary item for the Onges and Jarawar tribes. Little is known about them and they are now endangered.

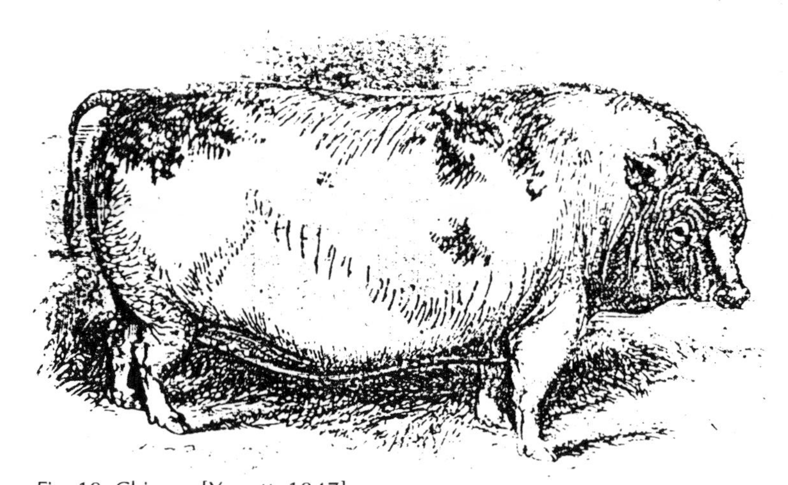

Fig. 19. Chinese [Youatt, 1847]

CHINA

China has appreciated the qualities of its native pigs for several millennia. Charles Darwin, writing in 1868, said that the Chinese claimed to have had domesticated pigs for 4,900 years and that they were markedly different to those of Europe, having wider and shorter heads, dished faces, short legs and considerable fatness.

Environmental pressures in this huge country led to the confinement of their pigs many centuries before population and social pressures did the same to pigs in Europe. Confinement leads to many changes: a reduced desire to wander or root, for example, which in turn makes a more peaceful, docile and frankly lazy pig that converts its food into a lot of flesh and a lot of fat rather than "wasting" its energy intake in foraging for that food. Thus it was that Chinese pigs were already early maturing and easy to fatten by the time England, for example, began to change from the roving herds of long-legged, lean-bodied swine on pannage and pasture, to "proper" and "improved" breeds able to be brought to great weights quickly. To achieve this miracle, the English used the small, fat pigs of China and other parts of south east Asia to cross with their big Celtic swine.

Most Chinese prefer pork to any other meat and huge quantities are consumed. Equally pork is one of the country's main export products, whether as live pigs (3.2 million of them in 1983), or frozen pork or tinned pig meat. The home market's attitude to fat is reflected by the way in which, until the mid 1980s, the thicker the backfat the higher the retail price for the carcass. Then tastes in the cities swung to lean pork and the carcass grading system was changed accordingly. Duroc, Landrace and Large White were used as sires in two-way and three-way crosses to increase the production of lean.

A great deal of research into pig breeds has been and is being carried out in China, and one area of particular interest overseas has been the study of reproductive traits. This showed that the native pigs (and they looked at a diverse range of breeds) were of early puberty (about three months old and 20-25kg liveweight), with high ovulation rates and high prolificacy (21-29 eggs and at least 14-15 born alive in the Taihu), low sterility, high oestral excitability and good maternal instincts. The Chinese also looked at meat quality and decided that the native breeds outclassed foreign breeds for pork colour, marbling, water-retention capacity, lack of PSE meat, fineness of muscle fibre - and hence a greater level of tenderness, juiciness, taste, aroma and palatability.

From 1979 to 1983 a very detailed co-operative project at ministerial level was carried out to study the genotype of ten native breeds representing different agricultural regions, and comparing them with exotics, especially the Landrace. Hundreds of full-time participants were involved in a multi-discipline task force of experts in breeding, nutrition, physiology, biochemistry, anatomy, embryology, endocrinology, disease, meat science, and behaviour. The aim was to justify various claims which had long been made on behalf of Chinese breeds. Xu Zhen-Ying's comprehensive report made intriguing reading and the work continues to evaluate as many breeds as possible, as a prerequisite to their conservation.

Most of China's native pigs are small and black, or black-and-white, while the recently developed breeds include several whites. As well as often being highly prolific and early maturing, the native breeds are adaptable to difficult environments and most have the ability to consume roughage in bulk. The disadvantages of many of them include a high proportion of fat in the carcass (originally much in demand) and consequently a poor feed conversion ratio. It is these, and low weight gains, that the Chinese are now breeding away from, in their projects to develop lean hybrids.

In a land which covers 9.6 million square kilometres and reaches 5,000km from east to west, and 5,500km from north to south, it is hardly surprising that countless different local types of pig have developed to suit the wide range of environments. The climate zones range from subtropical in the south east to exceptionally deep winters in Manchuria; the topography includes mountains and the high plateau of Tibet, deserts, low-lying and fertile plains and river valleys, heavily forested hills and rocky coastlines. Only 11% of this vast area is cultivated, yet most of those who work do so in agriculture of some kind. There are some 2,000 state farms but, in contrast, also 180 million peasant households. Peasants can lease land from the state, to which they contribute according to contractual obligations, after which excess produce is theirs to use or sell as they wish. Sichuan province has led in terms of Chinese pig production for the last three or four decades, followed by Jiangsu. The least developed areas for pig-raising are Tibet, Ningxia, Xinjang and Qinhai.

In 1988 a paper by Wang Ling Yu describing his country's pig breeds (*Pig News and Information*, December 1988) claimed that China produced 500 million pigs a year, and it has long been recognised as the world's largest producer of pigs. It can also boast proudly that it still depends largely on its native breeds, though it imports exotics to create its commercial breeds and has been crossing native with foreign pigs for much of this century. It also uses purebred imported breeds, developed to suit Chinese needs and conditions, and the most influential of these in this century have been the Middle White, Large White and Berkshire from England, the Russian Large White and Kemerovo, and the Landrace.

New breeds are being created or discovered or formalised almost weekly. Many are very similar to each other and fall naturally into the regional groups that are described. Each group has characteristics that are particularly apt for its region; for example, large bellies to make the most of cheap bulky fodder, or splayed feet in marshy areas, or very thick coats in the high plateaus.

In discussing Chinese livestock in relation to environment, it is simplest to divide the land into two main categories: pastoral, and agricultural. The *pastoral* areas, in the northern and western plateau lands, are of high altitudes with a cold, dry climate. These areas are hardly suitable for pigs, though a few rugged local types exist to exploit the environment as best they can. They include the **Hezuo** and the **Tibetan**, which have very special qualities as a result of adapting to the high plateaus.

By contrast, the *agricultural* areas, in the east and south, have a temperate, moist climate and fertile soil, and this is where most of China's pigs are found, producing not only meat but also bristles and valued manure. The north agricultural region has a temperate climate and production is largely of wheat, corn, sorghum and beans; the south, partly in the temperate belt and partly in the subtropical, has rice as the main crop. In both regions, livestock management is more intensive than in the pastoral areas; pigs and sheep are the main small livestock in the north region, and pigs and poultry in the south (other livestock are draught animals of various species in both regions). Three quarters of China's livestock are in the agricultural areas, including 96% of all the pigs - almost the same percentage as of the human population in these areas.

While the great variety of terrain and climate has played a major role in what might be termed "natural selection" for different types of pig in different regions, so too have varying human demands for their produce. The same type of pig might have different local names in different regions and, conversely, several breeds might share a name, so that it is difficult to state how many breeds or types really exist. Work is in hand to sort out the nomenclature and in the meantime this book relies on Ian Mason's authoritative *World Dictionary of Livestock Breeds* (1988 edition). The Chinese pigs are usually divided into six regional types which reflect their characteristics, performance, traditional management, local agriculture, natural environment and history as well as their present distribution. Very broadly, the pigs decrease in size from north to south.

Table 3 gives average sow sizes, litter sizes and backfat thicknesses for the breeds described below as examples of each regional group.

1. North China Type

The pigs of this regional group are in the agricultural areas north of the Huaihe river basin and Qinling Mountains (including North China, North East China, Inner Mongolia, Xinjang), where the temperate climate is dry and cold. The soil is rich in calcium and wheat is the main crop. The pigs here are fed mainly on farm byproducts and other roughage, mostly out on pasture, with limited concentrates. They are usually black with lop ears, and adapted to withstand cold weather and harsh feeding conditions - some have long, coarse bristles and a dense woolly winter undercoat. They are relatively large by Chinese standards, and the back and loin are narrow and level. They have the ability to deposit body fat and are comparatively late in sexual maturity but fairly prolific with an average of 12 per litter, and 14-16 teats.

Min <Plate 18>

(Liaoning, Jilin and Heilongjiang)

The black Min, a meat and lard type with large lop ears, is found in the vast north eastern regions at altitudes of about 240m, where it is particularly noted for its tolerance of cold conditions, its high prolificacy and the quality of its pork. It is a relatively large breed, with a level back, and its black coat has a good covering of coarse, long bristles to protect it in the cold winters of this region, with the extra help of its thicker skin and a thick woolly winter undercoat (the annual mean temperature in the region is only 4.9°C and ranges from 36.4°C in summer to -36.5°C in winter). The pig's ears hang down and, in the case of the sow, so does the belly. The thick skin tends to be wrinkled.

TABLE 3 CHINESE BREEDS - COLLATED AVERAGES

	SOWS							CARCASS	
	Height (cm)	Length (cm)	Girth (cm)	Weight (kg)	Teats	Sexual Maturity (months)	Born Alive	Backfat (mm)	Dressing (%)
NORTH									
Min	87.5	141	130	88.3	14-16	3-4	13.5	32	72.2
Shenxian	60.0		109	75.0	16	3.3	12.0	30-40	65.0
PLATEAU									
Hezuo	44.0		74	32.5	10	3.0	4-7	30	65.0
Tibetan	39.6		61	20.9	10	3-5	6.4	31	66.5
SOUTH WEST									
Kele	54.0		92	63.2	10-12	3-4	8.7	51-72	74.6
Neijiang	61.0		104	90.2	14	3-4	10.6	33-57	67.7
SOUTH									
Hainan					12-14		8-10	70	
Tunchang	55.2		97	85.6	14	4-6	11.3	40-60	72.0
Wenchang	47.2		91	62.0	12-14	4	8-10	70	72.4
Luchuan	51.6		103	79.0	12-14	4	11.5	40-60	69-74
Liang Guang		125	112				10.4	59	
South Yunnan	59.6		105	63.4	10	2-3	11.1	55	74.4
CENTRAL									
Cantonese	60.4		110	68.1	14	3	13.8	39	69.1
Jinhua	65.8		109	74.3	14-16	2.5	13.2	53	72.5
Ningxiang	61.6		114	70.6	14	3	11.5	40	70.0
Daweizi						12.9			
Huazhong		118				11.3	49		
NEW BREEDS									
Harbin White	75.6		132		12-14	5-6	11.3	44	
Beijing Black		145		210.0		4.5	10.1	35	73.2
New Huai	70.6	121			14	4-5	12-13	48	
Sanjiang White					14		12.5	26	
Shanghai White		149		177.0			12.9	37	

In comparative tests during cold weather, the Min could apparently "stay in the open much longer without shivering or squeaking" than other breeds. Sows can farrow in an open shed at 4°C. When put out in hot sunshine, on the other hand, they did not rush to seek the shade but kept cool by being less restless. They also lost less weight than modern breeds when put on reduced feeding (one-third of maintenance diet) but on *ad lib* feeding their daily weight gain is not so high as other breeds. The Min has the knack of storing body fat: it can store 4.6kg of fat in its abdomen.

Min pigs were used (with Landrace) in the formation of a new meat-type breed, the **Sanjiang White**, passing on to the new breed the Min qualities of tolerance of cold, high prolificacy and pork quality. The breed also contributed to **Harbin White**, **Heilongjiang Spotted** and **Liaoning Black**.

Shenxian <PLate 18>

(Hebei)

A variety of the **Huang-Huai-Hai Black** meat pig, the hairy black Shenxian (not to be confused with the Shengxian Spotted of central China) is found in the north at much lower altitudes than the Min (22m), where the mean temperature is less cold (12.6°C) but winter temperatures can fall to -22.5°C and summer ones rise to a very hot 42.7°C. It is smaller than the Min but equally prolific. Its skin is wrinkled, especially on the face of the boar, and the large ears hang over the eyes.

Other North China breeds include:

Bamei (Shaanxi, Gansu, Ningxia, Qinghai)

Hanjiang Black (S. Shaanxi)

Huang Huai Hai Black (N. Jiangsu, Shandong, Shanxi, Hebei, N.Anhui, Henan, Inner Mongolia). Varieties in this group include **Ding**, **Huai**, **Shenxian**.The **Ding** (Dingxian, Hebei) has horizontal or lop ears and possibly some Poland China blood since 1929. The **Huai** (North Jiangsu and Anhui) has large lop ears and was used to create the **New Huai** (with Large White).

Mashen (N. Shanxi)

Yimeng Black (Shandong - named for its distribution in Ling *Yi* and *Meng*yang counties)

Hetao Lop-Ear (Inner Mongolia)

Korean Native (primitive black)

Korean Improved (originally Berkshire x North China)

Penbuk (Korea: North China x local Korean)

There are also several modern breeds in the North, towards the east coast, including **Harbin White**, **Beijing Black**, **New Huai**, and these are described at the end of the Chinese section.

2. Plateau Type

This group is found mainly on the Qinghai-Tibet Plateau at altitudes of about 3000m, where the climate is cold and dry, the vegetation poor and the growing season short. The pigs are on pasture all year, living as best they can on wild plants. They are of small body size and light weight, and have very long dense bristles, small erect ears, straight pointed snouts and strong feet with hard hoofs. They are very alert and are expert at running and jumping. Prolificacy is low (4-7 per litter) and they have ten teats. Their meat has a special flavour.

Hezuo <Plate 18>

(S.W. Gansu province in the Gannan Tibetan autonomous republic.)

This little black pig lives at altitudes of up to 2600m, where the mean temperature is 1.7°C and ranges from 33.6 to -23.8°C. The Hezuo is well protected by a dense coat of long coarse bristles.

It is rather small, or even dwarfish. The snout is slender and tapered; the ears, in contrast with those of the Northern breeds, are small and erect. The combination of face shape, short legs and bristles is strongly reminiscent of a hedgehog.

Tibetan (or Zangzhu) <Plate 18>

In many ways similar to the Hezuo, the Tibetan is even more of a character. It is longer legged, with strong feet, and is exceptionally active: it is adept at running and jumping, and often rather wild, with very quick responses to potential danger. Like the Hezuo, it has a small head, with a long, straight, pointed snout for deep rootling, and small erect ears. It is smaller than the Hezuo and its build is generally skimpy with a narrow chest and light body (about 35kg in mature males), but it has the ability to deposit fat as an energy reserve: its internal and visceral fat is up to twice that of other pigs in proportion to its bodyweight (15%). Its intestines are 36 times its own body length (compared with 28 times in, say, the pigs of Sichuan) and this presumably helps it to make use of the shrubbery on which it browses as well as the stems, roots and hard seeds of wild plants. The meat (what little there is of it) has a special flavour and is marbled.

The black or brown hair coat has dense bristles which, at about 12cm, are two or three times as long as those of other breeds, and also about three times as dense (at 71 per square centimetre) as those of the Sichuan pigs. It is very well protected from the cold and likewise from strong ultraviolet solar radiation. At up to 4800m, the Qinghai-Tibet plateau is very high and temperatures plunge to -30°C in extreme winters, with maximum summer temperatures of perhaps 29°C. The climate is very dry here at 373mm precipitation per annum.

3. South West China Type

This group is mainly found in the region of the Sichuan basin and Yunnan-Guizhou plateau. The climate is subtropical but varies greatly in different places. The pigs are usually black, but sometimes black-and-white or red, and hair colour seems to be influenced by introduced types. They have semi-lop ears, and other characteristics are variable.

Kele <Plate 16>

(Yunnan-Guizhou mountains.)

This is another high-altitude pig (1700-2400m), tolerating erratic weather changes. The winters are dry and cold (minimum -13.8°C) and the summers warm and humid (maximum 32.6°C). Local crops are mainly potatoes and buckwheat but feed supplies for pigs are relatively poor and they share the plateau pasture with sheep and cattle.

The Kele's morphology reflects its environment. It is black, with lop ears hanging over its eyes; the snout is long and straight, the back slightly dipped, the body light and the chest narrow. The skin on the hindlegs is wrinkled and its feet are strong. It is hairier than the Neijiang and has a very thick layer of backfat and a high level of visceral fat (15.6% of carcass weight). The fatness has been deliberately selected for in breeding, as lard is an important part of the local people's diet. Prolificacy is relatively low.

Neijiang <Plate 16>

(Sichuan.)

This black lard/meat pig is comparatively large-bodied and strongly built. It benefits from a mild climate (annual mean temperature 17.6°C, minimum -2°C, maximum 39.2°C) in an area where agriculture is well developed. The Neijiang is well covered: its heavy, creased skin is about 7mm thick, though its backfat is less than the Kele's. It used to be famous for its long bristles (in the 1930s the world's best brush bristles came from China and Russia), its large size and its easy fattening. The snout is very short and snub-nosed, with a roll of fat over the bridge; the lop ears are of medium size. Its back is slightly dipped and the belly low-slung.

It is a precocious breed. Boars are ready to mount at two months and have been found to produce mature spermatozoa at 71-78 days old. Gilts can become pregnant as early as 90 days old, though sexual maturity is on average between 3 and 4 months of age at a liveweight of 40.5kg. Prolificacy is average.

Other South West China breeds include:

Chenghua (lowland Sichuan) - a black, lard/meat pig.

Guanling (central south Guizhou) - black.

Huchuan Mountain - black.

Rongchang (uplands of Sichuan) - white lard/meat type with black eye-rings and occasionally black spots elsewhere, or wholly white; famous in the 1930s for its white bristles, used in brush-making.

Wujin (borders of Yunnan, Guizhou and Sichuan) - small, usually black but sometimes brown; also **Dahe** variety in Yunnan, black or brown.

Yanan (Sichuan) - black, lard/meat type.

4. South China Type

This region is the warm, humid, subtropical and tropical home of the typically fat-wrapped, low-set, sway-backed, pot-bellied and precocious pigs that have found their way to many other parts of south east Asia. The bellies, often touching the ground, have the capacity for large quantities of the abundant local plant material, especially water plants. Most of the pigs first mate at 3-4 months old and have litters of 8-11.

South Yunnan Short-eared <Plate 17>

Also known as the Dian-nan Small-ear, this black pig is in the tropical belt of Yunnan province at altitudes of about 550m, where the annual mean temperature is 21.8°C. It is not as grossly pot-bellied as the true South China pigs, nor is it sway-backed; it has a more solid look to it and the stocky-legged boar has something of the air of a determined hippopotamus.

Hainan <Plate 17>

There is a group of small to dwarf lard pigs with small, upright ears on the tropical Hainan Island off the south coast. The mean annual temperature here is 23.6°C and the precipitation 1603mm.

The long-headed **Hainan** has a smooth skin and a black-and-white pattern: the back is black, the belly, legs and flanks white, and the black head has a white snout or blaze. The backfat is about 70mm thick. The sows are said to be exceptionally good mothers, being extremely careful to avoid squashing the piglets when lying down to nurse them.

There are three varieties of the Hainan. The **Lingao**, with a long tapering snout and very small ears, has a black back and head but the rest of the body (including a blaze on the snout) is white. The **Tunchang**, with black back and head, white body and snout, has a white star on the forehead. The **Wenchang** has similar markings to the Tunchang but a shorter face and is smaller.

Luchuan <Plate 17>

(S.E. Guangxi)

The Luchuan is in the subtropical belt in the Guanxi Zhuang Autonomous Region. It is a variety of the black-and-white **Liang Guang Small Spotted** lard type of Guanxi and Guangdong, and is occasionally black or white but more often white with a black head and back in typical South China fashion.

Other South China pigs include:

Fujian Small Pig (Fujian) - black, or black-and-white; including the black **Huai** in south east Fujian and the **North Fujian Black-and-white**; the **Fuan Spotted** is a rare local variety, and the black **Putian**, grouped with the Fujian Small Pig, is of the Central Chinese type, as are the **Fuzhou Black** and the **Minbei Spotted**, both of Fujian.

Lantang (Guangdong) - lard/meat type with white belly and feet, black head and back.

Liang Guang Small Spotted (Guangxi and Guangdong) - black-and-white group; varieties include **Guangdong Small Ear** and **Luchuan**.

Longlin (N.E. Guangxi) - black.

Wuzhishan (Hainan and central mountains of Guangdong) - black with white belly and feet.

Yuedong Black (east Guangdong).

Xiang (south Guishou, north Guangxi) - miniature, black, usually with white belly and feet; comparatively slow growing; meat fibre exceptionally fine.

5. Central China Type

In this rich area between the Chanjiang and Zhujiang rivers, the pigs are penned and well managed. Some famous breeds have developed as a result, several of interest to European breeders past and present. The most interesting, perhaps, are the **Jinhua**, the **Ningxiang** and the historically famous **Cantonese**.

The region lies in what is described as the middle and south subtropical climate belts but it is temperate or warm, and moist. Agriculture is highly developed (mainly paddy rice) and the area is rich in feedstuffs, especially greens and water plants for pig feed. Most of the pigs are black or pied, with small ears (lop or semi-lop); they are early maturing and quite prolific, and the meat quality is superb..

Cantonese <Plate 16>

(Zhujiang delta, Guangdong.)

Until recently, this black-and-white lard/meat pig must have been China's most widely known breed. Many of the small "improving" pigs that were exported to Britain and America in the 18th and 19th centuries to give western herds the benefit of earlier maturity and better propensity for fattening were from the Canton area, though not necessarily all of the Cantonese type.

The colouring of the Cantonese's coat is white with scattered black patches, especially over the back, rump and head. The patches have broad "blue" edges, where white hairs grow on pigmented skin. Typically of the Central Chinese group, the back is slightly dipped and belly drooping. It is a precocious breed: sows are first mated at 3-4 months old and are prolific, but their milk yield is lower than that of some other breeds. The carcass has rather a high proportion of fat, though the backfat is less than some others of the group. It looks quite a solid pig under its fairly loose, creased skin. The tail switch can be quite bushy and older boars tend to have a light ridge of bristles along the topline. The straight snout is of medium length and the profile is dished. It is easy to imagine the striking contrast when these pigs were introduced into England, where the native 18th century type was long-legged, flat-sided, heavy boned and coarse, with heavy lop ears.

There used to be several Cantonese varieties in Hong Kong but they are probably now extinct. They included the **Fa Yuen**, with black spots on its back, which was being improved in the 1970s by strict culling and better management rather than by crossbreeding, at Kadoorie Experimental Farm; it managed to retain its adaptability to local conditions. Others were the black-backed, white-bellied **Kwangchow Wan** and the black **Wai Chow** or Lung Kong.

Jinhua <Plate 16>

(Upper Fuchun river, Zhejiang.)

The "two-end black" or "black-at-both-ends" lard pig is nicknamed for its colouring: it is white with a black head and a round target-like black patch over the rump and tail. It is a pretty little pig in a compact, dumpy way. The dip in the back is only slight, though the sows do have very low-slung bellies. The medium-sized ears hang over the eyes; the snout is of medium length.

The Jinhua is one of the breeds which have been investigated in recent years by some of the European pig breeding companies - partly for the internationally famous processed Jinhua Ham, which is known for its good flavour and rosy colour. The meat is tender, the skin is thin and the bones are light, and there is a higher proportion of lean than in some other Chinese breeds.

It is also a prolific breed, shedding on average 24 eggs, and the embryo mortality rate is very low. The sows are taller than some of the other breeds in this group. Females are sexually mature at about ten weeks old and have been mated as young as three months old.

Varieties of the Jinhua include the **Dongyang** and the **Yongkang**.

Ningxiang <Plate 16>

(Hunan.)

This black-and-white lard breed is romantically described as being decorated with "black clouds overhanging snows with a silver ring around the neck". It is something of a pampered pig, too, housed and hand-fed all year round. It is less prolific than the Jinhua.

The "black clouds" draped over its back and rump have the traditional silver lining of white hairs on pigmented skin. The neck, muzzle and central forehead are white, with another "black cloud" covering the top of the head, the ears and the cheeks. The Ningxiang has a slightly concave back and hanging belly but, like others in the group, quite a long body.

The **Daweizi** in Hunan is a lard/meat type similar to the Ningxiang. It is black, usually with white feet, and there are large and medium-sized varieties. It reaches puberty at about 116 days (27kg liveweight) and sexual maturity at 123 days. The gestation period is 113 days and the litter averages are 13.45 with 12.9 born alive (gilts 9.78 and 9.39). Litter weights are high at birth and at weaning.

Others of the Central China type include:

Huazhong Two-end Black (Hunan, Hubei, Jiangxi, Guangxi) - white with black head and rump; sows 118cm long, 92.5kg; varieties include **Jianli** (south Hubei), **Tongcheng** (south east Hubei) and **Satzeling** (Hunan) with small lop ears.

Ganzhongnan Spotted (central Jiangxi) - black-and-white.

Hang (Jiangxi) - black head/back/rump.

Leping (Jiangxi) - black, with white forehead/belly/feet.

Longyou Black (Jiangxi).

Wuyi Black (Jiangxi/Fujian, in Wuyi mountains).

Yujiang (Yushan, Jiangxi and Jiangshan, Zhejiang) - black.

Wanzhe Spotted (Anhui, Zhejiang) - black-and-white; varieties include **Chunan Spotted** and **Wannan** (or **Lantian) Spotted**.

Shengxian Spotted (Zhejiang) - black with white feet.

Qingping (central Hubei) - black.

Xiangxi Black (Hunan).

Bamaxiang (Bama and Tiandong counties in Guangxi) - dwarf with black head and rump, nearly extinct.

6. Lower Changjiang Basin Type

The subtropical, low-lying basin of what used to be called the Yangtze river and its coastal strip between north and central China is the home of the precocious and amazingly prolific **Taihu** group of pigs (average litter size 15, 20 not uncommon, usually twice a year). The prime example of the type is the **Meishan** <Plate 15>.

In the mild climate, agriculture is highly developed and intensive. Crop production levels are high and the pigs are well managed and well fed on farm byproducts and water plants, plus concentrates. In general they have black coats, heavily wrinkled skin (especially on the face), long hanging lop ears, and drooping bellies.

There are some very fine piggeries for these precious breeds. One for the Meishan in north Shanghai and another for the Fengjing in south Shanghai, for example, both have immaculate white buildings with tiled, pitched roofs, and sunbathing patios (for the pigs) with plenty of shade from shrubs and pergola-trained climbing plants: a most elegant setting for pigs.

The **Taihu** is by far the most important group but there are some other types in the region, including the **Dongchuan** and **Jiangquhai** in north Jiangsu, the **Hongqiao** of Zhejiang, the **Wei** of south east Anhui and the **Yangxin** of south east Hubei.

The territory of the Taihu group edges that of central China's **Jinhua** and **Ningxiang**, which are also prolific until compared with the Taihu.

Taihu <Plate 15>

The breeds in this group have more similarities than differences: they are black, with heavily wrinkled skin (especially on the face and at the top of the limbs) and big, heavy ears hanging down like those of a spaniel dog. The snout tends to be broad and wrinkled, the back only slightly dipped or almost straight, the belly of the sow (especially when pregnant or lactating) hangs so low that it almost touches the ground. Most Taihu sows have eight or nine pairs of teats and some have ten pairs. Taking the group as a whole, average litter size at the third parity is 15.83 (14.24 born alive, 12-13 at 60 days); average daily weight gain is 439g and FCR 4.00; carcass at 75kg dresses out at 65-67%, with a very variable lean content and with backfat varying according to breed, from about 18mm to 35mm, which is modest for a Chinese breed. They are all small pigs and early maturing.

The group includes the following:

Erhualian (Lower Changjiang basin) - heavy skin.

Fengjing (south Shanghai) - long snouted and short snouted types; sometimes known as the Rice Bran pig.

Meishan (north Shanghai) - black with white feet.

Jiaxing Black (north east Zhejiang) - very high milk yield.

Less important varieties are the **Mi**, the **Shahutou** and the **Jiaoxi**.

Table 4 gives full details, culled from several Chinese sources (performance figures in different environments and systems may vary). As prolificacy seems to be by far the most valuable trait in western eyes, it has been looked at in greater detail in the Breeding section of the introductory chapters.

TABLE 4: THE TAIHU GROUP

	MEISHAN	FENGJING	JIAXING BLACK
Sow av. height (cm)	57.8	69.0	68.3
Sow av. weight (kg)	61.6	69.6	61.3
Teats	16-18	18	16-18
Sexual maturity (m)	2.5	2.5	2.5
Litter size: birth	14.3	15.8	17.5
Litter size: weaned	13.3	13.3	15.2
Backfat (mm)	25	35	18
Dressing %	66.8	66.0	66.6

	JIANGQHAI	ERHUALIAN	JIAXING BLACK
Sow age at puberty (d)	78.25	60.0	
Sow weight at puberty (kg)	11.32	12.6	
Sexual maturity (d)	104.2	120.6	
Eggs shed (sow)		28.0	25.68
Gestation		113.9	114.6
Sow litter born alive	12.05	13.59	14.07
Sow litter weaned		11.52	12.10
Av. no. of teats		18.13	17.33
Piglet birth weight (kg)	0.69	0.79	
Weight at 180 days (kg)	47	47	
Max. growth period (d)	90-120	150-180	
Max. growth rate/day (g)	350	410	

7. NEW BREEDS OF CHINA

Apart from countless native breeds, many "developed" breeds have been created in China during this century by crossing local pigs with one or more exotic breeds, either in a fairly haphazard manner to improve local performance or to a deliberate and controlled breeding programme with a specific aim over several years. By 1983 there were a dozen of these developed breeds and also six exotics used as purebreds in China.

Harbin White <Plate 18>

(Heilongjiang)

This dual-purpose (meat/lard) breed for the north east was one of the earliest deliberately created modern breeds in China. Its development began when the local peasants' crossbred white pigs, apparently of unknown origin, were crossed with the Russian Large White (imported 1896) and the Canadian Yorkshire (imported 1926). Backcrossing and selection over a long period produced a white of the Large White type with prick ears, dished face and a large body size in comparison with Chinese pigs, also rapid growth and the traditionally thick body fat. Boars today average 84.7cm tall, sows 75.6cm, and backfat thickness 44mm. Females are sexually mature at 5-6 months of age.

Beijing Black <Plate 18>

A black meat type, occasionally with white markings, this is quite a bulky-looking pig with short, stocky legs, ears over the eyes, a straight snout of medium length and a bit of a jowl. It was developed selectively from crosses of Berkshire, Middle White and native Beijing pigs, and was approved by the Beijing Municipal Government as a suburban breed in 1982. At a slaughter weight of 90kg, the carcass dresses out at 73.2%, with a lean meat content of 50.3%, eye muscle area 27.5 sq.cm, and backfat thickness 35mm - the meat quality is excellent. The Beijing Black also performs well in a three-way cross of Large White or Duroc boars on Landrace x Beijing Black sows.

New Huai <Plate 17>

(North Jiangsu province.)

A black, lop-eared, dual-purpose (meat/lard) type developed from 1959 based on Yorkshire crossed with the native **Huai** (South China type) in the Lower Huaihe river basin; the progeny of the original 50/50 cross were selectively bred thereafter. The boar stands at about 87cm tall, bodylength about 154cm.

Sanjiang White

(Heilongjiang province.)

This co-operative project began in 1973 and took a decade to produce its new breed: the Sanjiang White was recognised as China's first meat-type pig in 1983, deliberately created to withstand the severe local winters in its region. It was based on 27 bloodlines of the local **Min** in the north east of the country, crossed with Landraces imported from England, Sweden and France - there were 30 sires and 135 dams in the foundation herd, which gave the new breed a very broad genetic background. There were reciprocal crosses between the two parent breeds, followed by selection of F_1 gilts for backcrossing to Landrace sires; thereafter selected offspring from the backcross matings were bred *inter se*. The selection index was based on post-weaning growth rates, backfat thickness and body length at 6 months old. By 1983, seventh generation progeny had been produced and there were about 3,000 sows and 100 boars of the new breed. It surpassed the Landrace for cold tolerance, prolificacy and pork quality. Crossbreds sired by Duroc exhibited high hybrid vigour in performance traits and a leanness in the carcass of 62%; the crosses were free from any PSE symptoms. There is also significant heterosis in performance traits when the Sanjiang White is crossed with Russian White, Harbin White or Large Yorkshire.

The new breed was named for the fertile "Three Rivers" plain of its place of origin - where the Songhua, Heilongjiang and Wusuli rivers meet. It is an area of 1.3 million hectares of cultivated land with more than 50 state farms in what is known as the Big Northern Granary. Soyabean meal and a great variety of farm byproducts are available for meat-type pigs but the winters are very cold (mean January temperature is -20°C and can fall as low as -38°C). The imported Landrace sows were far from happy in such conditions and many proved infertile; the Min, however, is noted for its tolerance of the cold and also for high prolificacy (average 13 per litter) and superior pork quality, though it carries more backfat than the Landrace.

Shanghai White

Another suburban breed, this white was bred in Shanghai from 1978. Parental stock included Large White, Middle White, Russian Large White and the prolific Taihu group.

Other new breeds include:

Hubei White (Hubei province, central China) - from Large White and Landrace on local black Tongcheng; meat type with lop or horizontal ears.

Xinjin (north east China) - from Berkshire x local Min in the 1920s; black with white points like a Berkshire; varieties include **Jilin Black**, **Ning-an**, **Xinjin**.

Meixin - from Meishan with Xinjin.

Heilongjiang Spotted - from Kemerovo and Min (1962-79).

Liaoning Black - from Landrace or Duroc with Min.

North East China Spotted - from Berkshire and Min since 1980.

Fannong Spotted (Hennan) - black-and-white meat type with Yorkshire and Berkshire blood, bred since 1983 at Huangfannong Farm, Sihua county.

Laoshan (Shandong) - meat/lard type from Berkshire and Middle White with local black.

Yimeng Black (Shandong) - meat/lard type from Berkshire with local black in counties of Lin*yi* and *Meng*yang.

Nanjing Black (Jiangsu) - from (1972) Berkshire, Large White, Landrace, Shanzhu (black, lop) and Jinhua.

Shanxi Black (Shanxi) - meat/lard type since 1983 from Yorkshire, Berkshire, Russian Large White, Neijiang (Sichuan) and Mashen (north Shanxi).

Ganzhou White (Jiangxi) - before 1949, Large White with local Ganzhou.

Guangxi White - originally Landrace and Yorkshire with Luchuan of south east Guangxi.

Hanzhong White (south west Shaanxi) - from 1982, including Russian Large White, Yorkshire and Berkshire.

Lutai White (Hebei) - meat type from Russian Large White x Large White.

Yili White (north and west Xinjiang) - meat type since 1982 from Russian Large White x local white crossbreds.

Xinjiang White (central and northern Xinjiang) - originally from Russian Large White x local, with Berkshire and Yorkshire blood.

Taiwan

The main island of Taiwan is mountainous and afforested, with fertile, cultivated, well-watered and heavily populated lowlands on the west of the central ranges. The climate is subtropical, with hot humid summers, mild winters and heavy rainfall. There is a continuous growing season for crops and agriculture prospers, in spite of typhoons, violent summer thunderstorms and flooding, and prolonged winter droughts. About a quarter of the land is arable and 5% meadow and pasture. The agricultural section is declining in importance as the industrial sector grows.

The human population is 19.7 million and there are more than 7 million pigs - virtually all of them of foreign breeds or hybrids. Modern exotics, introduced from 1959 onwards, reflected Taiwan's political history and included Berkshire, Duroc, Landrace, Hampshire, Yorkshire, Minnesota No. 2, Piétrain and the American Spotted - and the sources included Japan as well as the United States and western Europe. The most useful proved to be Landrace, Yorkshire and Duroc for producing three-way meat crosses, but the Hampshire and Spotted were preferred by farmers because of their black hair. The Berkshires, the earliest to be imported, were still being kept after the Second World War for crossing on local **Taoyuan** sows for meat crossbreds. Later it was found that a Duroc boar on Yorkshire/Landrace crossbred sows produced much better progeny for meat production and the three-way cross became more popular. Purebred nucleus stocks of these three breeds and the Hampshire were maintained and constantly improved by selection. In 1952, a Berkshire registry had been established but it lapsed when the three-breed cross developed.

There are drawbacks to imported breeds from temperate areas. The high temperature and humidity deter them from maximum production levels, and also land is in short supply so that livestock rearing is generally a sideline. Pigs are often fed in confinement on smallholdings, with small exercise yards. Feed mills began producing formulated livestock feeds on a large scale at the end of the 1960s (mostly with imported ingredients) and the large swine farms used modern feeding, formulated on the farm, with modern management systems and housing. They also made a habit of sprinkling their growing and finishing hogs with water two or three times a day in hot seasons to reduce heat stress. Today Taiwan is a major exporter of pig meat to Japan. There is also the interesting subtropical system of integrating pig-raising with fish and duck production seen in other parts of south east Asia.

With a monsoon climate similar to that of South China, and with the history of immigration, it is hardly surprising that most of the local pigs are of the South China type. There used to be two small primitives, possibly originating from crosses between the Chinese and the local wild swine: the **Taiwan Small Black**, known as the Aboriginal, and the **Taiwan Small Red**. Both are probably extinct now. The Aboriginal was believed to have descended from a mixture of domestic pigs brought over from the South China mainland by immigrants and the local wild *Sus scrofa taivanus* which had been domesticated by Taiwan's aboriginal people. It had a long, straight snout and very small ears, while the Red had short ears, a slightly dished and wrinkled face, a straight tail and (in the boar) a stiff mane.

The Taiwan native pigs include the **Taoyuan** of the north west, a black or dark grey lard pig with lop ears, wrinkled skin and straight tail, originally from various South China pigs - it is now nearly extinct. Recently extinct types include the **Meinung** lard pig (similar to the Taoyuan but smaller) and the black **Taichung** created from a cross of Taouyan with **Tingshuanghsi** (another extinct type with a larger frame than the Taouyan). The **Lee-Sung** miniature has been selectively bred since 1974 from the Taiwan Small Black, and there is also the miniature **Lan-Yu**, a native small-eared which has been closely studied at the National Taiwan University since the 1970s.

In 1975 six native breeds had been classified, the Aboriginal and five introduced from mainland China (Meinung, Taoyuan, Tingshuanghsi, Small Long-Snout and Large Long-Snout). The Taoyuan was always the most popular of them and the sows were at that time being crossed with Berkshires to produce meat hogs. In the 1960s and 1970s, however, modern exotic breeds were imported on such a large scale that the native types became very rare. The Taoyuan, probably the last of them to survive, was even then only found in tiny numbers in research institutes, while a few Aboriginals remained on the outer islands.

SOUTH EAST ASIA

The Chinese breeds - particularly those sway-backed, hanging bellied, wrinkly-skinned, straight tailed, lardy white-and-blacks of the South China type - have spread during many centuries all over South East Asia. Here, the pig is as important in most countries as it is in China, though its numbers usually take second place to poultry.

European and American breeds have also been imported but these highly developed pigs face considerable climatic stress in the hot, humid environments of South East Asia. Their appetites can become so depressed that they are unable to take in enough energy to maintain body condition, let alone to perform well. The performance figures of any breed must be adjusted according to its context: prolificacy or growth rates which seem, on paper, to be good or poor in the breed's native conditions might become quite the opposite in a different environment.

In some of the countries in this section, there has been considerable research into the indigenous types - for example, with the very active co-operation of the French, the Vietnamese have undertaken detailed studies of their pigs and are able to differentiate several most interesting breeds, one or two of which have found their way to the west. Pigs from IndoChina played an important role in Europe during the late 18th and early 19th centuries when they were used to improve native landraces and helped to create the major breeds of that period. The pigs of New Guinea are integral to village life in a more complex way than perhaps anywhere else in the world: there is the porcine equivalent of a "cattle culture" here, and the pigs themselves have intriguing origins. And throughout South East Asia there are wild species of pig, often unique to an island or two, which in some cases have contributed to the local domesticants - the potential for hybrid vigour in crosses with European and American breeds must be considerable.

Very often the indigenous pigs of this fascinating and diverse part of the world cannot be described as breeds but are of general local types. For that reason, and because of the cultural as well as agricultural context, this section is more of a narrative than a breed catalogue and performance details are necessarily lacking except in the case of Vietnam, where the local research has been more "scientific".

Vietnam

Agriculture is the basis of the Vietnam's economy and in recent years it has included a mixture of state farms, agricultural co-operatives and production collectives. Poultry and pigs are the main livestock by far: poultry number about 100 million and pigs perhaps 13 million. Food processing is a major industry and agricultural products are major exports.

The delta regions of the Red River in the north and the Mekong in the south are cultivated intensively and are densely populated. The climate is subtropical or tropical monsoon.

Since 1980 there has been a series of most useful studies of Vietnam's pigs by combined Vietnamese and French teams, and the 1988 report by M. Molenat, Tran The Thong and Le Thanh Hai forms the basis of much of the information which follows.

Pigs are a source of meat, lard and manure and also, for many families, a source of income. Pig-keeping in modern Vietnam is still largely on family holdings, which represent more than 80% of the national production. The abundant water plants form an important part of the family pigs' diet - hence the value of those "pot bellies" which can be filled with large quantities of such roughage.

Water is exploited in other ways, too, by pig-keepers. For example, families will build bamboo rafts, heap them with soil and plant them with sweet potatoes for the pigs and for themselves. They even collect water snails for the pigs (the snails are cooked before feeding). Imagination is given full rein in securing morsels for the very important family pig.

An increasingly common system, seen elsewhere in south east Asia, is a combination of aquaculture and pig-keeping in a highly efficient energy cycle. The pig house extends over a pond so that the animal manures it direct; the pond thus grows more water hyacinths to feed the pig, and also more fish - partly for human consumption and partly, as fishmeal, for the pig. A similar system embraces the garden as well: the pig manures the garden but its urine still manures the pond and encourages the development of microflora and microfauna which feed the fish.

This is a typical example of Vietnamese ingenuity in making the most of their resources. Pigs can be of considerable economic value to the family: they produce a lot of offspring which, with that ingenuity, can be fed cheaply and in due course sold, though they are also important as the main item on the menu for certain feast days, when the eating of meat is said to ensure future prosperity.

Pig manure essentially feeds the rice paddies, and in turn rice waste feeds the pigs, with the help of kitchen scraps, water convolvulus, water hyacinth, wanter lentils, roots (such as manioc, potatoes and taro) and the foliage of sweet potato plants.

With the private sector producing most of Vietnam's meat, the families tend to be well organised in the canton. Some specialise in keeping one or two breeding sows, which are served by boars brought to the holdings by travelling boar-keepers. The piglets are sold to other families, who rear them to 10kg, when they are bought by fatteners, who take them to 70-80kg, or sometimes by those who specialise in rearing weaners to 25-30kg before selling them on to the fatteners. People might be content with their role, or might seek gradual "promotion" to what they see as a better one, probably as a breeder.

The fattened pigs might be sold to neighbours, or at the market, carried in baskets which are sometimes bottle-shaped like duck nesting-baskets. Peasants might buy a fattened pig, take it to a municipal abattoir to be slaughtered, take the carcass home to butcher it and then sell the meat cuts at the market, or the whole carcass might be sold to a wholesaler or retailer.

The families enjoy keeping pigs and they like the extra income from selling them. They like the idea of having a few pigs in the sty so that there is always meat for anniversaries and feasts. Sty pigs are also "piggy banks": they can be sold when it is necessary to buy new tools, utensils or clothes, and for cash to pay for the children's schooling. Pig-rearing is a form of saving up for occasional necessities and even for little luxuries; there is considerable satisfaction in watching the potential money growing in the sty, and all for not much labour but with plenty of scope for imaginative management. The state is happy, too: the families are its main meat suppliers and their pigs provide manure for the rice paddies when the state cannot afford to import chemical fertilisers.

While the families tend to rear native breeds, the large state and district farms and co-operatives make use of modern breeds and modern methods of management. There is liaison between the two sectors: for example, a district farm rearing 500 sows might distribute young pigs to the private sector, while the families in turn supply a quantity of meat to the state. But more important today is pork for the export market, and for this the traditional family system fails to produce a good enough carcass. However, a co-operative can breed appropriately improved stock and make contracts with smallholders to fatten the animals, under guidance, on behalf of the co-operative, which can then have the pigs slaughtered in good enough condition for export. The big farms wean at 2 months old, when local breeds would weigh 5-6kg and imported breeds 8-15kg. State farms and many co-operatives aim for a slaughter liveweight of 90-100kg.

The traditional pig is killed light to give a carcass weight of about 50kg with coloured meat and soft fat. The fat is trimmed off and used as cooking lard; and even the skin is eaten, cut into fine strips, cooked and salted, and enjoyed with a vegetable mixture. Pork from the indigenous breeds is highly rated: its taste is excellent and the texture of the meat seems to set it apart from that of imported breeds.

The main imported breeds are "**Vietnamese Yorkshire**" (Large White, from Russia and Germany), Landrace and Duroc (both from Japan and Cuba), Hungarian Cornwall (i.e. Large Black) and Red Berkshire. In a minor way there are also the English Middle White, the American Poland China and Hampshire, the Canadian Lacombe, and the Belgian Landrace and Piétrain.

In family pig-keeping, however, there are various disadvantages to the imported breeds. There are problems in feeding them appropriately; there are difficulties with their health, including frequent bouts of pneumonia, spongy feet, fungal sensitivity, susceptibility to parasites in the flood zones and frequent infections of one kind or another; the sows have problems in giving birth outside and lack comparative precocity and fecundity; and the exotics are restless in hot weather, not very adept at free-range living and apparently suffer from deterioration in their sense of smell, their intelligence and their natural instincts. Such problems are best handled in the commercial systems where the breeds are valued for their less fatty carcass and their better growth rates.

The families prefer the indigenous breeds which have always served them so well. In the Mekong delta (one of the great granaries of South East Asia, where the production of rice, pigs and poultry are nationally vital) there is a compromise between exotic and native breeds: the pigs are of new breeds which combine the best of both, such as the **Thuoc Nhieu** and the **Ba Xuyen**. There are other crosses in the Red River delta of the north, where they might use the **DBI** and the **BSI**.

The main characteristics of the native breeds are those shared with the pigs of South China: small size, remarkable precocity and good prolificacy. All in all, Vietnam has a wealth of genetic diversity, with considerable potential for cross-breeding and improving or creating more new breeds.

North Vietnam

Í <Plate 19>

This must be one of the shortest breed names in the world. The pig known as I is of the type found in the West under the more general name of the Vietnamese Pot-bellied pig. It was first exported to Europe and North America for laboratories and zoological collections in the 1960s. It became a popular subject for western wildlife parks and farm parks, and during the 1970s it began to find a very small niche on, for example, British smallholdings. In the late 1980s, it suffered the indignity of becoming a city pet, sometimes kept in apartments and exercised on a lead in the streets as if it were the family dog.

The Í is the dominant type of the Red River delta, where there are about 2.5 million of the breed. It is a small pig: the adults eventually reach 90-100kg and the male is smaller than the female. The black skin is wrinkled, especially heavily about the dished face; the forehead is narrow and the ears small and upright. The back is dipped and the typical hanging belly sometimes sweeps the ground, especially in pregnant or lactating sows. The male has a crest of bristles along the neck and part of the topline. The legs are fine-boned and short and the feet are plantigrade, with all the claws touching the ground - a typical adaptation to swampy land over the centuries.

It is highly precocious. The first heat in gilts is at 3-4 months of age, when they weigh 15-20kg; the oestrus lasts for 3-8 days and the cycle varies from 17 to 23 days. Gilts are usually served at 7-8 months (30-40kg). Boars reach puberty at about 3 months old. The number of teats is modest (mean 10.7) but the breed is prolific, though not as much as some of the Chinese breeds. Gilts average 10.1 in their first litter and sows reach a peak of 13 or more in the fifth and sixth parities. The piglets weigh only 450g at birth and ten times that weight at 2 months old. The growth rate is very slow, and the weaning rate is not particularly good (7 for gilts, 9 or 10 for sows at their peak). However, breeding sows seem to have long, productive lives - most family breeders have Í and Mong Cai sows which have exceeded ten parities without any major problems.

The Í is an ideal smallholder's pig in its native land, happily consuming large quantities of rice bran and of aquatic plants with a very high water content. The carcass is very fat, a trait which is highly valued where the staple human diet is rice.

To improve its performance, the Í has been crossed with Large White to form the **DBI** and with Berkshire to form the **BSI**. Several options had been considered in the search for better performance, including the systematic use of large-breed sires (Large White, Berkshire, Landrace, Duroc, Cornwall), selection within the native Í breed, or the creation of an intermediate race. They chose the third.

The litter sizes of the two new breeds are comparable to that of the Í but birth weights are higher (0.9-1.0kg in the DBI, 0.7-0.8kg in the BSI). The growth rates are far better: at 8 months the DBI progeny achieve 80-100kg and those of the BSI reach 60-80kg, compared with the pure-bred Í's 35-40kg.

Mong Cai <Plate 19>

This north eastern breed is less widely distributed and less populous than the Í: there are about half a million of them in a region vaguely centred on Mong Cai, which is on the Chinese border and on the coast of the Gulf of Tongking (the old Tonquin, from which the "Siamese" or "Tonkey" pigs set sail for England two centuries ago).

The Mong Cai is slightly larger than the Í at 100-120kg. It is a pied breed - white, with black head, white snout, sometimes a white star on the forehead, and black patches elsewhere on the body, often on the rump and like a saddle over the middle of its concave back.

It is another remarkably precocious breed: gilts enter puberty at 2-3 months of age and boars at 2 months. Sows have 14 teats and gilts average more than 11 piglets in their first litter, thereafter steadily increasing the number with each parity to reach a peak of 12.5. The weaning rate is not good (8 for gilts, 9 for sows) but the figures are deceptive: the relatively large loss of young between farrowing and weaning is mainly due to the traditional local practice of deliberately removing the smallest piglets at birth. The average birth weight is 0.6-0.7kg and increases to ten times that weight by 2 months old. Thereafter the growth rate seems to be very variable; weights between 60kg and 100kg have been recorded at 10 months old.

The carcass seems to be a little leaner than that of the Í, with typical backfat thickness of 53-59mm. Some consider that the Mong Cai and its crosses would be the more appropriate Vietnamese genetic type for the future and the breed is now the subject of several studies. In the meantime it also finds a place on many state farms.

The black pied **Lang Hong**, in the same general area, is often described as a variety of the Mong Cai. Its black patches are more randomly distributed; elsewhere the skin under the white hair is a rosy pink. It is not as prolific as the Mong Cai.

Other local types in the north include the **Muong Khuong** in the mountains near the Yunnan border and the **Meo** in the western mountains of the north. There is also a type known as the **Tong Con** just on the Chinese border.

Ha Bac

The province of Ha Bac is the middle region of the north. The local type is a small pig with a broad head, a dipping back and a very well developed belly. Females reach 45kg at 8 months and 75-80kg at 3 years of age. They experience their first oestrus at 3-4 months (the oestrus lasts 3-4 days and the cycle is 22-24 days) and have anything from 10 to 14 teats. Litter sizes also vary. Boars reach only 20-25kg at 8 months; they first mate at 5 months and work as sires for two or three years.

Thai Binh

The local pig in the southern region of the Red (or Hong) River delta is a small, precocious black pied type with large black patches on its white coat. Like others in this area, it is sway-backed and pot-bellied.

Central Vietnam

Co <Plate 19>

This dwarf black pig used to be widespread in central Vietnam but is now restricted to the high plateau regions and mountains, where it runs free-range, finding some of its food in the woods and thickets. It is a thoroughly rustic and active little pig, able to resist disease and look after itself, and its meat is considered to be a delicacy. Its disease resistance is now being studied seriously but its growth rate is very low in local conditions: it takes 2 years to reach a very modest 40kg.

There is also in the central region the white **Nghia Binh** and its black variety.

Tuy Hoa Hairless

In the rich area at the mouth of the Song Ba river on the east coast, the local pigs are white but mixed in type with wide variations in performance. Among them are the hairless pigs of Tuy Hoa, susceptible to sunstroke but able to grow well given good feeding. Local breeders began to select them deliberately and they became a speciality of the region, though not a very practical one: they need careful stockmanship to avoid skin problems such as scratches and cracking.

South Vietnam

Before describing the pigs of the south, it is necessary to pause for a brief excursion into their general history. Once upon a time, there were small, black mountain pigs (**Heo Moi**); the adults weighed 40-45kg and they were sway-backed with large stomachs but were of a lean type that produced good meat. They were raised by families for feasts and ceremonies.

When this type was transferred to the better conditions of the Mekong delta areas, it improved naturally to become a black pasture pig with a mature weight of 60-70kg, a long snout, small erect ears, and the same dipping back and hanging stomach. The sows were very good mothers, very easy to breed, and the meat was excellent. In due course this type was pushed back towards the Cambodian borders and could be described as the **Vietnamese primitive**.

At the beginning of the 18th century, Chinese emigrants led by the mandarin, Mac Cuu, settled in the delta's western zone and built up an important Chinese colony centred on the town of Ha Tien (now on the borders of Cambodia and south Vietnam, facing west into the Gulf of Thailand). This became a trading port for large numbers of junks and commercial vessels from all over South East Asia. At this stage the very small black-and-white **Hainan** pig was introduced into the delta (from China's Hainan Island in the Gulf of Tongking). It adapted well to the saltwater zones and briny marshlands on the delta coasts and the islands of the Gulf, and came to be known as the islands pig (**Heo Hon**), becoming a pig of average size (for the area) with a long body, large head, long snout, and small ears facing outwards. It was white, with some large black splodges over the middle of its dipped back, and four white socks.

Later, another Chinese pig was brought into the delta for the Minh Hai region (An-Xuyen). This type had a massive body, small head, constricted forehead, short snout, straight back and thick, short legs. It was black, sometimes with white spots, and was quite large (90kg at 12 months). They dubbed it the square pig. These two Chinese types adapted well to the salty zones in the provinces of Minh Hai and Kien Giang.

Thus, by the end of the 19th century the Mekong delta's livestock included well adapted but primitive local pigs and two types of Chinese pig, with no doubt a variety of crosses between these assorted populations. The primitive type (small, black, with a sharp-pointed snout, small ears, a dipping back and weighing 60-70kg at 12 months old) was improved more deliberately at the turn of the century with Chinese pigs and the result was the **Sino-Vietnamese** type. About 1920, French planters introduced another element: the Craonnais of the Mayenne. This large Celtic white pig had a long snout, large lop ears, an arched back and rapid growth rates - it reached 90kg at 6 months old. The big white was crossed with the Sino-Vietnamese pigs and the result was known as the **Bo Xu**, a relatively large lop-eared pig. The Bo Xu subsequently became part of a selective development programme which produced two new breeds: the **Thuoc Nhieu** for the sweet-water zones and the **Ba Xuyen** for the salty zones of the Mekong delta - the great granary of South East Asia where, today, most of the pigs are of one of these two breeds or are Large Whites.

Thuoc Nhieu

The Thuoc Nhieu originated from **Bo Xu** sows crossed with Yorkshire (Large White) boars between 1936 and 1956 and with Middle White boars in 1957. The breed now numbers about half a million. It is white with piebald bristles and is of medium size (mature adults 120-160kg) with only a very slight dip in the back, a long body and short legs. The head is of medium size, with a snout of medium length, a fairly straight profile and small erect ears which grow a little forwards. There are two types, in fact: one is short-legged with a rounded body, short snout and broad face; the other long-legged, long-bodied, narrow in the face with a snout of medium length and much closer to the Yorkshire than to the Bo Xu.

Compared with native pigs, Thuoc Nhieu sows have a relatively late puberty (at 6-7 months). However, they are able to come into oestrus during lactation, 10-30 days after farrowing. The oestrus period is 2-6 days and the cycle 18-21 days. Their gestation lasts for anything from 108 to 120 days. Prolificacy is average, at 8-10; growth rates are "acceptable" but the carcass is not always as lean as might be required.

Ba Xuyen <Plate 19>

The **Bo Xu** was crossed with black English **Berkshire** boars between 1932 and 1956 to create the black pied Ba Xuyen for the Mekong delta's salty areas. There are about 300,000 of the breed, which has the Berkshire's characteristic white socks and otherwise has roughly similar proportions of black and white areas on the body, the black splodges (with a rusty tone) being scattered irregularly all over. Adults weigh 120-150kg and the sows reach puberty at about the same age as the Thuoc Nhieu. Likewise they can show signs of oestrus while still suckling. Prolificacy, growth rates and carcass quality are apparently similar as well.

The Ba Xuyen has a head of medium size, with a straight or dished profile and a snout of medium length. The medium-sized ears are upright or grow forwards. The legs are short and the pasterns are almost horizontal, often with all four claws of the hind feet resting on the ground, which is ideal for lagoon life. There are said to be up to five subvarieties but in reality there are just gradations from a low, short, thick type to a heavy, taller one closer to the Yorkshire - as is the case with the Thuoc Nhieu.

Cambodia, Laos and Burma

The land of **CAMBODIA**, surrounded by Vietnam, Laos and Thailand, is mainly fertile lowland around the great lake of Tonle Sap, but three quarters of the country's 181,000 sq.km is afforested. Subsistence agriculture is a way of life for the great majority of the population of some 7 million people. In 1987 it was estimated that there were about 1.3 million pigs.

Pigs have little importance in **LAOS**, a country with a human population of nearly 4 million. The native **Muban** pigs are similar to those of the Philippines: they are short, with dipped backs, drooping bellies, prominent snouts, and a ridge of hair along the shoulders and neck. They are usually black (sometimes spotted) and weigh 40-50kg at a year old. Litter sizes are small: 3-7 at birth, and only 2-5 at weaning.

BURMA, bordered on the south east by Laos and Thailand, the north east by China, the north west by India and Bangladesh, and the south west by the sea, has a tropical monsoon climate and a population of 40 million people, with a little over 3 million pigs. Two local types are the **Burmese** <Plate 19>, with quite a short snout, medium-sized lop ears over the eyes, and a black (or sometimes spotted) pelage; while the **Chin** is a dwarf type weighing only 30kg when mature.

Thailand

Thailand is important in the history of the world's pig breeds: it was presumably the home of the **Siamese** pig <Plate 19> (described in the UK section) that influenced several improved breeds in Europe and American in the late 18th and the 19th centuries. It was sometimes referred to as the Tunkey or Tonky as the pigs were shipped from the Tonquin or Tonguin district. This Siamese was broadly Chinese in type but had rich copper skin under its black hair.

The fertile central plains are the heart of Thailand's agriculture today and also of its industry and its 55 million people. The climate is hot and humid. Agriculture is traditionally the major industry, though it has declined in recent years. The pig population of Thailand is about 4.2 million.

The pigs of Thailand traditionally ranged freely, with minimal supplementary feeding, and remained hardy. They were typical Chinese-type lard pigs and there used to be a few recognised varieties. The **Hailum** of southern Thailand is black with white markings; it was sometimes called the **Hainan** and possibly originated from that Chinese island. In the north was a black pig known as the **Kwai** (which usually means "buffalo"); it sometimes had white legs and white on the shoulders. Another northern type was the black **Raad**, variously known as the Plaung, the Ka Done or the Keopra. Today, however, the types have become almost indistinguishable through crossbreeding and the local pigs are substantially reduced in numbers.

The largest remaining group of native Thai pigs is in the northern highlands, where the hill tribes prefer the old type. Some time ago the indigenous pigs were studied to compare them with other breeds while a commercial pig industry was being established, using imported breeds, but the locals' contribution to the industry became so negligible that the researchers' interest in them faded, though the pigs remained important to the northern highlanders' subsistence economy. More recently they have been studied by combined teams of Australian and Thai researchers.

In the 1960s such statistics as there were showed that the average birth weight of the native hill pigs was 0.73kg and the weaning weight 6.54kg. There seemed to be no difference between the various recognised types, though they did offer higher dressing percentages than imported and crossbred meat pigs.

Various development agencies over the years sought to help the northern hill tribes by improving the pigs' productivity, with only limited success, generally by trying to encourage crossbreeding with sires of imported breeds. The latter had an alarming tendency to die under hill management conditions but some of the crossbred offspring survived and adapted to the traditional scavenging system, though probably with little or no improvement in productivity.

The 1980s Thai-Australian research programme began with a survey to determine the range of factors that limited the productivity of the highland pigs so that a programme to improve them could be designed.

The tribes of the northern hills represent several ethnic groups. In 1980 there were perhaps 330,000 people among them, practising shifting agricultural systems based on growing rice, maize and opium. Most (90%) of the households raised pigs - though the rate ranged from 100% among the Yao and Lisu to only 50% among the Chinese Haw. The average number of pigs per family was 5.2, and an average of 3.2 killed per annum. They were raised mainly for sacrificial ceremonies on the one hand and, on the other, as a form of insurance against possible crop failure or financial difficulty. The pigs were usually sold within the village or to a neighbouring village. Fat was deemed more important than meat, because it was easier to store, but the people generally preferred the taste of meat, and tribes with access to lowland markets (where people could buy fats and oils for cooking) claimed that meat was more important than lard. Meat was salted and hung up in cool, dry air, or it was smoked over the fire or subjected to fermentation.

Most of the hill pigs were free-range, with a chosen few kept in pens from 3-6 months to be fattened for important ceremonies. Feed included rice bran mash, crushed or boiled maize, wild banana stalks and local herbaceous plants. The women usually took responsibility for looking after the pigs. The better fed animals could be slaughtered at a year old but others often took as much as 5 years to reach slaughter weight.

This little native upland pig <Plate 19>, sometimes called the **Akha** after one of the tribes, was black - the preferred colour for religious reasons, though some had white areas on belly and hocks. It was small, usually sway-backed and pot-bellied (but not excessively so), with a rising rump, straight tail, fairly long legs for ranging, long tapering snout, straight profile and very small, semi-erect ears tending to grow outwards towards the horizontal. The boars often grew a mane of bristles on the back of the neck and the withers.

Performance figures were of course very

variable, especially for litter size, which showed a range from 1 to 14, with a mean of 7.1 at birth, and 0-10 with a mean of 5.8 at weaning. The birth weight was equally variable (0.60-1.35kg) and likewise the age at sexual maturity (4-8 months). However, destiny permitting, they seemed to be long-lived: the mean was 12.9 years and many were still alive when 15 years old. Carcass characteristics were closely associated with differences in management, of course, and liveweights did not seem to bear much relationship to age. Naturally the carcasses were fat, by deliberate selection for this trait over many generations.

There had been a rural development project of a different nature during the 1970s, set up in Thailand by a group of companies involved in feed milling, poultry breeding, seeds, fertilisers, and pig and poultry equipment. They established a pig-breeding farm at Sikhiu, north east of Bangkok, in 1973 and by 1986 they had 700 sows in three pure herds (Duroc, Landrace and Yorkshire). These were to supply stock for a new "hog village" in which pig-raising and crop production would be integrated and undertaken by families working with the help of development loans. The site of the village was bought in 1978, some 18km from Kamphaeng Phet. Each farmer was allocated a 4ha holding and there was a central feed mill and a group of permanent staff providing overall management, veterinary services and suchlike. New homes were built for the families and various facilities were provided.

The farmers work with multiplier herds producing Landrace x Yorkshire hybrid gilts to be sold to other commercial producers. Each farm in the breeding-farrowing group aims to produce 600 weaners a year from 36 sows and two boars, and receives a bonus for better weaning weights and litter averages. The growing-finishing farmers have a production goal of 1,000 pigs each a year. The whole family becomes involved in the pig work or in the central services.

Malaysia and Indonesia

West **MALAYSIA** forms the southern tip of the Malay peninsula that hangs like a map tail from the body of Indochina, with Thailand reaching out to link the two. Peninsular Malaysia, with Singapore at its very tip, has a central mountain chain to the west of which are fertile, alluvial plains. East Malaysia is quite a separate land mass: it forms most of the north western part of the large island of Borneo - including Sarawak, Brunei and Sabah: there is an area of swampy coastal plain below the mountainous interior towards the border with Indonesia. Only 3% of Malaysia is arable land; the climate is monsoon, with year-round consistent temperatures (averaging 25-30°C in the lowlands) and high humidity. Two-thirds of the 16.5 million people live in rural areas.

Most of the Malay population are Muslims but there is an ethnic and religious mixture and some are more than willing to raise pigs. The pig population is about 2.2 million - far greater than that of buffalo and cattle (less than a million) or of goats and sheep (less than half a million). Agriculture is no longer the major economic sector, and subsistence farming fails to meet the national need for self-sufficiency in food, even in rice.

The Malaysian pigs are of the same Chinese type found in so many other parts of South East Asia. The Malaysian **South China** is a meat pig, white with the typical black back and head, and there is also a **South China Black**, often referred to as the **Cantonese**. Both these types are in West Malaysia. On Sarawak there is the primitive **Iban** or Kayan pig which is grey, with white feet; it has a long snout, small ears and straight tail.

Sarawak is also the home of the wild Bearded pig (*Sus barbatus*): there is evidence that the species was the most commonly eaten large animal in the area 40,000 years ago and it remains a most popular source of wild meat. This big animal (described in detail in the Wild Pig section) has various subspecies on different islands. The Borneo subspecies, *S.b. barbatus*, remains abundant in parts of Sabah and Sarawak, especially on wildlife reserves, and there are also some in Kalimantan. It is an important food source for hill tribes which have not yet converted to Islam. Another subspecies, *S.b. oi*, belongs to the Malay Peninsula, where it is now rare. The remaining subspecies are in the Philippines, though little seems to be known about them. However, the Bearded pig seems to interbreed with domesticated pigs and produces fertile offspring; clearly they would have considerable natural resistance to tropical diseases and pests, and it is possible that there is a future for such hybrids.

INDONESIA is an archipelago of 13,667 islands scattered from Sumatra (to the west of the Malay Peninsula) to New Guinea in the east, and including the major islands of Java, Kalimantan (the major portion of Borneo) and Sulawesi (or Celebes), along with Irian Jaya (the western section of New Guinea). They are volcanic, mountainous and densely clothed in equatorial rain forest over more than two thirds of the total land area; only about 8% is arable land overall. The climate is predominantly tropical monsoon, with local variations.

Three-quarters of the total human population of 175 million live in rural areas, and 87% are Muslim. On Bali there are 3.5 million Hindus. Otherwise the people are Christian or Buddhist. Agriculture is still a major factor in the economy and the 6.2 million pigs are outnumbered by more than 18 million goats and sheep, 9.4 million cattle and buffalo and 428 million poultry.

As well as the wild Bearded pig on Borneo and Sumatra, there are two other wild species locally: the Sulawesi Warty pig (*Sus celebensis*) and the Javanese Warty pig (*Sus verrucosus*), both described in more detail in the Wild Pigs section. The **Sulawesi Warty** <Plate 19> has in fact been domesticated and is a family or village pig on, for example, the island of Roti. It has also been bred with domesticants of *Sus scrofa* and these hybrids form the common pigs of New Guinea and parts of the Moluccas group. The wild Sulawesi Warty pig has also been introduced to various other islands, including the Philippines. Sulawesi is also the home of a very different species of wild pig: the Babirusa (*Babyrousa babyrussa*), which has proved easy to tame on an individual basis and is a potential domesticant except that its litter size of only one or two is not promising.

The Javanese Warty, which has probably never been domesticated, is considered a crop pest. Its meat is particularly lean, for which it has been hunted over the centuries. The domesticated pigs of Java are a mixture originating from native animals crossed with European breeds (largely Dutch and British). The **Balinese** <Plate 19> is a lard pig, essentially a cross between South China types and the local types which can still be found in the island's eastern mountains. The Balinese has erect ears and is either black, or black with white legs and belly.

The Philippines

There are about 7 million pigs in the Philippines. Today the native pigs are probably all extinct and have been replaced by Landrace, Yorkshire, Duroc and other exotics, and various commercial hybrids.

The **Philippine Native** was black, or black with a white belly like the Balinese, and its varieties (named after their respective islands) included the white-spotted black **Ilocos** and the **Jalajala**. The latter was crossed with the English Berkshire from 1915 onwards to form the **Berkjala**, a black, short-eared lard pig which was already nearly extinct by the 1940s. Native sows in Batangas crossed with the Berkshire and the American Poland China were the basis of the black or spotted **Diani**, while the Duroc cross with the native Batangas was the red **Kaman**. A combination of Berkjala, Duroc and Poland China formed the **Koronadal** of General Santos on Cotabato: it is described as "ash-red" with dark spots, clearly unable to decide which of its parents to mirror.

JAPAN

The volcanic, mountainous islands of Japan linger close to the Korean peninsula. The four principal islands are Hokkaido in the north, the densely populate Honshu (with Tokyo and other major cities), Shikoku and, southernmost, Kyushu. There are more than a thousand islets as well and the total land area is about 372,000 sq.km. The climate is temperate oceanic with warm, humid summers and mild winters in most regions. With much of the land mountainous or afforested, the fertile areas are on the coastal plain.

The total human population is more than 122 million, three-quarters of whom live in urban areas. There are some 5.34 million hectares of cultivated land (11% of the total land area) and the livestock include 11.4 million pigs, exceeded only by poultry (343 million). The consumption of pig meat per capita is very high and much of it has to be imported.

For more than two hundred years, Japan isolated itself from the rest of the world: in 1635 a shogun enforced this national isolation save for a minor degree of trade with China and the Netherlands, until 1854 when it first granted trading rights to the west at the instigation of the Americans. That isolation, and the nature of the land, had a marked effect on the country's livestock. For some 1200 years, under the influence of Buddhism and Shintoism, the Japanese lived largely on rice, fish and occasionally wild meat from forest animals. Meat and milk from domesticated species were simply not part of their diet and there was no demand for them; such livestock as there were undertook working roles, and even these were not originally domesticated in Japan but were brought in by Asian continental immigrants. During the two centuries of isolation, no new livestock were introduced except chickens and horses.

After 1868, the restoration of the Meiji led to the deliberate introduction of western culture and western eating habits. It was now permissible to eat the meat of livestock and to drink their milk, and the governments since then have promoted the importation of improved breeds. Early in the present century those imports included pigs for meat, as well as dairy and beef cattle, dairy goats, sheep, laying hens and working or riding horses. Some of these species were used to improve native animals by crossbreeding, others were retained as purebreds for production, and nearly all the natives soon became extinct except for a few handfuls preserved by chance for future crossing. The public demand for meat far outgrew home production and even in 1977 (when meat production was six times higher than in 1960), 23% still had to be imported. Today Japan still imports large quantities of pig meat, especially from Taiwan and Denmark.

The pigs in Japan are reared for pork production and are now one of the three major species of livestock in the country (the others being cattle and poultry). The breeds include (in order of number of sows) Landrace, Large White, Hampshire, Duroc, Berkshire, Middle Yorkshire, Spotted Poland China, Chester White, British Saddleback, and a large proportion of commercial crossbreds. The Japanese are very good customers for western pig breeding companies and standards are very high.

Although there is some evidence that pig-keeping was carried out in days gone by, today's Japanese pigs owe little or nothing to any native breed or indigenous wild domesticants. The first foreign pigs to be introduced came from England - the white Middle Yorkshire (or Middle White, as it is known in England) and the black Berkshire arrived in the 19th century and remained firm favourites until the fairly recent introduction of the Landrace, which usurped their pride of place. However, the snub-nosed Middle Yorkshire was so popular that a temple and monument were erected to a particularly prolific boar of the breed.

Japan has developed some of its own miniature breeds. For example, the **Ohmini** is a dwarf, bred for the laboratory from miniature Chinese pigs imported in the 1940s with the **Minnesota Miniature** imported in 1952; it is usually black or occasionally black pied. The **Clawn** is another miniature breed from the 1970s, selected for white colour (the name is derived from the initials of the Central Laboratory of White Nipai). It was originally bred from (Landrace x Large White) x (Göttingen Miniature x Ohmini) and is now at Kagoshima University.

And, just for fun, there is the **Inobuta** ("in" indicates "wild pig", and "buta" the domestic pig). It originated from Wild Boar (25%), Duroc (25%) and Berkshire (50%) and the parentage shows in its colouring: Berkshire black with a reddish Duroc tinge.

AUSTRALASIA

AUSTRALASIA

AUSTRALIA AND NEW ZEALAND

The Australian pig population is less than 3 million, compared with 22 million cattle and 149 million sheep. The human population is more than 16 million but the per capita consumption of pork is only about 18kg per annum. New Zealand has more than 64 million sheep and 8 million cattle, with a human population of a little over 3 million, but its pigs tend to be numbered in hundreds of thousands rather than millions. Both countries have some particularly interesting feral pig populations with long histories but in some places the animals are so numerous that they have become major ecological and agricultural pests. One hopes that at least some will be conserved, partly for general interest and partly as a potentially useful gene reserve.

In the late 19th century and the first decades of the 20th, many British breeds were deliberately imported and the Berkshire, Tamworth and Large Black were high on the list of favourites. In New Zealand the Berkshire was one of the country's dominant breeds, used primarily as sows crossed with Large White boars for traditional light pork production, but its demise came in the 1960s with the introduction of the Landrace, which proved more fecund and produced a better carcass. In 1985 only 87 Berkshires were registered in New Zealand and the herdbook total stood at 41,971, compared with 53,365 Large Whites (913 registered that year), 23,676 Landraces (653 that year) and 1,191 Welsh (41 that year). The last ten New Zealand Tamworths were registered, by the Willowbank Wildlife Reserve, in 1983; the last Large Blacks were registered in 1982 (two of them) and the last British Saddlebacks (7) in the same year, though doubtless there are a few unregistered purebreds of all these British breeds scattered about on smallholdings. Meanwhile a new breed came and went in New Zealand between 1940 and 1959: it was the **Lincoln Red**, a meat pig originating from a Large White/Tamworth cross at Canterbury Agricultural College, Lincoln, but the programme was given up in 1959.

The Tamworth had been almost as popular as the Berkshire at one time, and the Saddleback and Large Black to a lesser extent. The coloured pigs in their day had been valued for their ability to graze and to tolerate the rigours of outdoor systems; above all they were popular on dairy farms, where they consumed excess skim-milk and whey, but with the advent of tanker collection during the 1950s and 1960s most dairy farms gave up pig-keeping altogether. Pork and bacon production, relying almost exclusively on whites but with the introduction of coloured Durocs and Hampshires (each similar, in colour at least, to the Tamworth and Saddlebacks respectively) since the mid-1970s, is now entirely in the hands of large and specialised units feeding meal rather than milk.

In the 1970s, Australian Tamworth and Berkshire boars came back to the United Kingdom to boost the bloodlines of what had become rare breeds in their own land. The Berkshires were noticeably rather longer and leaner than the British stock. The Tamworths promptly began to suffer a decline in numbers in Australia: in 1983 there were 10 registered breeders, but by 1987 there were only five. In that year Australian registrations included 1,537 Large Whites, 1,148 Landraces, 631 Durocs, 179 Berkshires, 145 Hampshires, 48 Tamworths, 23 Wessex Saddlebacks and 9 Welsh (newcomers to the country).

Australia, too, has followed the European and American trend towards fewer but much larger pig farms, though in 1991 there were still more than 2,000 units with fewer than 10 sows each. A quarter of the national herd (75,700 sows) are on the top 30 farms but 79% of the units have only 25-100 sows. Most Australian pig farmers grow their own grain and mix their own pigfeed rather than buying from the mills.

Grain and pigs go together in Australia and a lot of both are in New South Wales, where 2,400 pig farms out of the Australian total of 9,000 keep 97,000 sows and produce 1.7 million pigs a year for the bacon and ham market, with about a third for fresh pork. Most are intensive systems on family farms with 50-200 sows, but the biggest, at Corowa, has 25,000 sows.

New South Wales must deal with the major

problem of heat - dry heat - and Australians have become experts at maintaining pig growth rates during the heat of the summer. In moist tropical climates, pigs are frequently sprayed with water to cool them down but the hot, dry climate of New South Wales is countered with plenty of cool drinking water, properly insulated buildings and efficient evaporative cooling systems.

The registered breeds of New South Wales, in order of number of breeders and number of pigs sold, are at present: Large White, Landrace, Duroc, Hampshire, Berkshire, Wessex Saddleback, Tamworth, Welsh - there were no Large Blacks in 1990. The Large White/Landrace F_1 sow to a Duroc or Hampshire sire is the most popular choice, and the use of AI is increasing. The trend, as elsewhere, is towards large breeding companies supplying purebred and synthetic stock. After many years of measuring only backfat, more interest is now being shown in detailed carcass measurements. Pork cuts, traditionally from porkers of 42-70kg liveweight (30-50kg dressed) now usually come from leaner, heavier pigs (dressed weight 60-65kg). Smaller, high-quality hams weighing about 1kg are marketed as Cameo hams.

The Ferals

The first fleet of ships to arrive in New South Wales with Captain Arthur Phillip in 1788 brought pigs with them as on-board fresh meat . They dropped them off here and there during the voyage to become feral and be a future supply of meat for later visitors. Reaching their final destination in Australia, the ships released the rest of their stock to forage and a feral population built up, unchallenged by any indigenous predators. By 1799 the colony's pigs numbered 3,459, some 300 of which were owned by the government, 513 by officers and the rest by settlers. By 1805 there were 20,000 pigs.

That was the start of what became a hefty population of feral pigs. The situation in New Zealand was similar, and some time later even more pigs became feral when despairing farmers simply released them during New Zealand's depression.

Today the ferals are still widespread in Australia, mostly in Queensland and New South Wales but also in significant numbers in the far north of the Northern Territory. There are small, scattered groups in Western Australia and Victoria, and limited small colonies on Kangaroo Island and on Tasmania's Flinders Island.

The island pigs, like so many all over the world, have evolved from shipborne pigs and developed in isolation under the influence of natural selection to form varieties peculiar to their regions. The **Kangaroo Island** <Plate 20> pigs are typically white splodged with black; they have dense hair coats, long snouts, dished faces, small erect ears, low pasterns and strong, healthy feet and legs. They are very small, sometimes even dwarf: the body is 30% shorter than that of a Large White, and the stature 26.5%: the average shoulder height is about 65cm and the length about 137cm, while the body weight is about 98kg. This smallness is probably a combination of inbreeding and low nutrition; they also have only about 6 in a litter, usually weaning 5. But they are well adapted to their environment and are free of disease: they have certain physical characteristics which give them advantages in terms of fitness and vigour. They are descended, it is said, from a British sow and boar released on Kangaroo Island in 1801 from a ship which was refitting at Port Jackson and which was captained by a French navigator, Nicholas Baudon.

These hardy little pigs have also been introduced to life in the laboratory, to which they apparently adapted well, as they did also to intensive systems. The laboratories discovered that, for example, the ferals had higher erythrocyte counts but lower white bloodcell counts than a Large White.

Other ferals have the misfortune to be widely regarded as agricultural pests. They destroy crops, they root up pastures, they damage irrigation layouts and fencing, and it is even claimed that they kill lambs as well as spread disease. In national parks they are accused of disrupting the ecological balance by destroying birds' ground nests and eggs and damaging the habitats of small animals. In their favour (to human eyes), they make good sport for hunters and have also become part of Australia's developing game-meat industry for export.

New Zealand's attitude towards its ferals is similar but local wildlife trusts have taken steps here and there to capture and conserve some of these elusive pigs - for example, on Arapawa Island in the Marlborough Sounds, where the pigs are thought to be of the old English forest type. The **Arapawa Island** pigs are brown-and-black, something like the original Oxford Sandy-and-Black or the unimproved Berkshires and Tamworths. The so-called **Captain Cookers** are the descendants of stock left by the old British sailing ships.

A very different New Zealand pig is the **Kunekune** <Plate 20> or Maori pig. These very small animals (adult sows about 40kg, boars 50kg) used to be kept by the Maoris and are probably Chinese in origin, possibly brought from Polynesian islands with the Maoris more than a thousand years ago, or perhaps by early whaling gangs. The little pigs wandered freely in Maori villages, grazing and feeding on vegetable matter, and following their owners around, taking kindly to a lead and always welcoming a good tickle and stroke - just like the New Guinea pigs. The Kunekune (also called Pua'a or Poaka) has a most delightful nature: it is docile, slow in its actions, easily confined and often a house pet. It is late maturing but seems to fatten on nothing but grass. The colours vary: it might be patched with black and white, or all black, gold, tan or brown, or a mixture of any or all these colours. The face is quite short and slightly dished, with a snubbed snout of medium size and prick ears. Usually there are two wattles ("pire pire") under the jaw. It is not sway-backed; the body is well rounded and short-coupled. The legs are very short and the pig rarely grows taller than 60cm. It is fairly precocious: boars reach puberty at about 6 months of age, and gilts could be mated at 5 months but are best left unmated until a year old. Litter sizes range between 4 and 10, and are typically 5. The pork is said to be very succulent, with a distinctive flavour; however, the name Kunekune means "fat" and in the past its fat was mixed with golden syrup as a substitute for margarine, or was used on its own to preserve dried meat.

Numbers of the Kunekune had dropped to about 50 in 1978, when two men became alarmed at the possibility of extinction. They were already running wildlife farms which boasted some rare breeds of livestock and they bought up the entire population of Kunekunes as the first step in a survival programme. Today there are more than a thousand registered Kunekunes and the number is still growing. Some have recently been exported to the United Kingdom as an ideal orchard pig. In the past they were often crossed with Tamworth or Large White.

Papua New Guinea

This eastern section of the island of New Guinea, close to Australia, has a total area of some 395,000 sq.km on the main island and another 67,000 sq.km over some 600 smaller islands, including Bougainville, New Ireland, New Britain and others. About three-quarters of Papua New Guinea is densely covered with tropical rainforest and only the lowland areas are fertile. The traditional practice has always been shifting agriculture - slash-and-burn, or rather, slash and garden.

It has been suggested that crops like yam, taro and banana were introduced here more than 5,000 years ago and it is claimed that domesticated pigs arrived simultaneously, brought in by Asian colonists. More recently, ships of passing European explorers from the early 16th century onwards would have landed some of their own shipboard pigs on the island as future food supplies, to live and breed as ferals in the meantime. The navigators included Dutch, British and Portuguese - and it was the Portuguese (and the Spanish) who, in the 16th century, introduced the South American sweet potato to South East Asia. The plant spread, probably through the agency of Malay traders, along the chain of islands and eventually reached New Guinea. It provided for both people and pigs (the pigs were, and still are, given the "rubbishy" tubers and the leafy stems), and led to major increases in the population of both. Pigs became the main source of meat protein (apart from fish) but the consumption of them was far from regular: it was, and remains, the subject of occasional but excessive gorging.

There are 1.5 million pigs in Papua New Guinea, and only 3.8 million people. The pigs are in two quite separate classes: the village pig, and the commercial pig which supplies the market for meat. During the 1960s, pig farming was being encouraged by the availability of British-bred pigs from the piggery at Goroka. These pigs, to local eyes, reached enormous sizes and for a while there was something of a boom in local pig enterprises, especially in 1966, but it had collapsed within two years. The cost of housing these exotic pigs was too high, and there was a lack of the protein supplements and management techniques which such refined breeds demanded. They were simply too much trouble.

There is a special relationship between the villagers and their pigs, especially in the highlands: it is one of the very few "pig cultures" in the world, in contrast to the many "cattle cultures". The village pig plays only a minor role in the nutrition of the villagers: it is only killed and eaten for social and ceremonial reasons. The pigs are also highly valued objects of trade. In the highlands, large numbers of them have traditionally been moved along extensive trade routes between communities to be exchanged for durable goods such as axes and shells. Today, however, they are exchanged for cash.

Pigs are involved in many Melanesian ceremonies. They are sacrificed in some places to appease the ancestral spirits and they play central roles at major occasions such as rites of passage (births, the weaning of children, the initiation of boys, a girl's first menstruation, weddings and funerals) or ventures such as house-building and boat-building, and in the festivals at which local men of influence match themselves in prestige competitions. They are also exchanged at peace-making ceremonies after violent disputes.

"Pigs," say the Enga men of the western highlands, "are our hearts!" Highlanders in the Nondugl area in the Middle Waghi claim that pigs are so central to their social and religious life that the animals' place cannot be filled by any amount of money, wives or bird-of-paradise plumes. Among the Siuai of Bougainville's Great Buin Plain, young pigs are treated as pets: they share their owner's cooked food, they are ritually named and baptised, they are given magical treatments for illness, and the women chew up tubers for feeding to weak piglets.

While the men own the pigs, the role of caring for these precious animals is taken by the women, and with considerable pride. They name their animals, share their sleeping-quarters with them (the men sleep separately), fondle them like any other pet and occasionally suckle orphaned piglets themselves.

Huge festivals take place in the highlands at spasmodic intervals - anything from three to ten years apart - and enormous numbers of pigs are killed for these major events: hundreds, or even thousands, are slaughtered, sometimes as much as 90% of the entire local pig population. The animals are roasted and steamed in huge pits, wrapped in banana leaves with vegetables and herbs and placed on fire-heated stones at the bottom of the pit, which is then sealed with branches and leaves. The prestige of the men is directly proportional to the amount of pork they distribute at such feasts, and people gorge themselves on the meat. Then they practise bulimia, by smelling a nauseous species of rhododendron, so that they vomit and can eat more pork. Very often there is an epidemic of "Pig-bel" after these events - it is a severe necrotic infection which leads to perforation of the upper bowel.

Pigs are also slaughtered at times of misfortune or emergency, such as a severe illness, injury, or imminent warfare, when the spirits must immediately be placated with pig sacrifices (but the ancestors are only interested in the pigs' spirits - their flesh is for the living to consume). It is therefore necessary always to have a good supply of pigs at hand in case of such emergencies, and if disasters are frequent there will be no festivals for a long while because there are not enough pigs for the feast. Sometimes, conversely, festivals take place because the pig population has built up through lack of catastrophes requiring sacrifices, and the people need an excuse to slaughter the pigs - which are too important to be slaughtered on a regular basis to meet everyday protein needs. The normal diet is fruit, vegetables, insects and small game, and fish where available, but not pig meat.

This complex system is one way of maintaining the pig population in balance, especially as the animals compete with humans for food from the farm-gardens - a fact which can be a constant source of friction when they invade other families' gardens. Severe depradations are sometimes punished by the blinding of the guilty pig to control its wanderings.

This "pig culture" was not quite so pervasive in the lowland regions, where animal protein was obtained by hunting and fishing. In the lean seasons, domestic pigs and wild pigs were killed for food as well as for ceremonial purposes. In the highlands, too, the tradition of pig-keeping has been eroded in recent years as religious ideas and economic activities change, but pigs do remain important in family life and are still central to the culture of settled groups such as the Huli Wigmen. The pigs also have a valuable role as omnivorous waste disposers on the one hand and producers of manure on the other (the Enga call it "putting grease back into the land") as well as actively helping to cultivate the gardens by rooting. Women take their pigs with them when they go to work during the day in the food gardens - the pigs usually so tame that they simply trot to heel on the way - and the animals turn the soil with their snouts while the women dig. This will have been the pig's habit from a very young age, when it would have been carried to the garden in a basket; sometimes women will build a special pig house in the garden. In the evening, the women call the pigs home for an evening snack of kitchen waste and some sweet potatoes too stringy or small for human consumption, feeding them just enough to ensure that a foraging pig is eager to come home every evening. The pig finds most of its food by foraging during the day for shoots, leaves, tubers, insects and worms - and human manure.

In such a traditional system, quantity has always been more important than quality, and the productivity of Papua New Guinea's village pigs is often low - but then so are the inputs. It was estimated in the 1960s that the mean annual growth rate was 60 pounds and they took four or five *years* to reach slaughter weight. Litter sizes were low, too: four was common, and maybe no more than two or three piglets still alive at weaning.

The prick-eared **New Guinea native pig** is set apart from other domesticated pigs not only by its role but also by its origins. The young are often born striped, like wild pigs, and the adults might be black, black spotted, white, red or grey - indeed they cover the full spectrum of domesticant colours, though most are black. They are neither sway-backed nor pot-bellied; they remind one more of razor-backed wild species than south east Asian domesticants, though their straight profiles are less long in the snout. Their origins are a matter of some debate but it does seem possible that they are hybrids between domesticants (source unknown) and the wild **Sulawesi Warty pig** described earlier. One theory is that the Sulawesi Warty was domesticated in prehistoric times on Sulawesi; it then accompanied settlers and traders to other islands and was in due course blended with the indigenous Wild Boar subspecies of the Moluccas and New Guinea.

The indigenous wild pig of New Guinea is *Sus scrofa papuensis* and there seems to be genetic continuation between it and the domestic village pig. All male domestic pigs are traditionally castrated at 3 months old (so that they will be docile and grow into larger pigs), which means that domestic sires are in short supply. Sometimes one man in a village will keep a stud boar and, for the price of a weaner, will allow other villagers to bring their sows to the boar in due season. More often, though, feral or wild boars are given every opportunity to serve the sows. The wild pigs tend to remain at altitudes below 900m but seem to wander high enough to keep highland domestic sows productive. They are hunted regularly by the Hagerhai tribe in the virgin rainforests of the Shreader Mountains and their orphaned young are raised as tame animals to be slaughtered for ceremonial feasts.

AFRICA

AFRICA

Africa is hardly noted for its pig production. Traditionally, cattle have been far more important livestock, even in areas where there are no Muslim taboos against pigs. Africa's domesticated pigs fall broadly into two groups: the little pigs of West Africa, which are probably of Portuguese origin, and the commercial breeds of southern and eastern Africa, which were originally imported from Europe. The only others are primitive groups in Coptic Egypt and parts of Sudan.

Evidence of domesticated pigs in Egypt goes back some six thousand years, when they were introduced from Syria and Palestine. They were small animals, probably black, with long, slender legs, flat bodies, long necks, twisted tails, long heads with straight profiles and short erect ears. There was a ridge of bristles along the top of the neck and back.

The local pigs of North Africa today are primitive and rare. They are sometimes still seen in Egypt and the Sudan, also in Tunisia and Morocco. They are slender and not well muscled (which is possibly due to poor nutrition rather than breeding) with long, narrow heads and snouts, straight profiles and small prick ears.

Pigs were of no use to the nomadic races of Africa: they were awkward to herd and could not subsist on the scanty vegetation of the deserts and dry savannas. Such pigs as there were would have been domesticants of the Eurasian Wild Boar, *Sus scrofa*. The indigenous African subspecies are the North African, *S.s. algira* (which hardly differs from the European *S.s. scrofa*) and the Nile River, *S.s. sennaariensis*, which some say is not a true wild pig but the feral descendant of domesticants, though not much is known about it. The other wild pigs of Africa are of different species altogether - the Giant Forest hog, the Warthog and the Bush pig - but they never seem to have been domesticated. They are described in the Wild Pigs section.

Pig farming is now developing in many African countries, increasingly with intensive production systems. In East Africa the most common breeds are Large White, Landrace, British Saddleback and their various crosses and hybrids. The pig industry in Kenya began to build up during the 1930s, when they used almost exclusively British breeds for a Kenyan bacon pig based on Large White boars and Large Black, Berkshire and Wessex Saddleback sows. Small primitive domesticants with modest prick ears, straight profiles and tapering snouts are occasionally seen in parts of east Africa. They tend to be reds and blacks, with touches of white, but are now rare.

WEST AFRICA

There is a type of pig which is widespread, though not necessarily numerous, in the coastal areas of West Africa. The type is probably of distant Portuguese origin, no doubt well mixed with pigs from various other sources (including Egypt) over the years since the Portuguese first came to Africa in the 15th century.

The indigenous **West African** pig <Plate 20> is small, with erect ears, a straight profile and quite a long, tapered snout. It is well adapted to local conditions and quite capable of producing a litter of ten or more. Dr N. Pathiraja, a research worker with the National Animal Production Research Institute at Zaria in the 1980s, photographed a **Nigerian** sow <Plate 20> who, in her first three litters, had produced ten, twelve and thirteen young.

They tend to be black, or sometimes the front half is black and the rest white, or there is a white area covering the legs and part of the underside, or occasionally a pig is entirely white. They make a most useful cross with exotic breeds, especially Large White and Landrace. It seems that the best foundation stock for local semi-intensive production systems is based on a synthetic from crossing indigenous and exotic types, but for traditional free-range village pig-keeping the indigenous is probably better bred pure - until it becomes extinct. Both village and commercial pigs can make use of local feeds from tree crops, such as fresh bananas, banana meal, coconut meal and oil palm sludge.

These primitive, dwarf West African pigs have been kept in the hot, humid lowland forests for several centuries, usually as free-ranging village scavengers, south of latitudes 10-14 degrees N. They are almost certainly not true natives, being of the Iberian type, but they appear to be resistant to trypanosomiasis, the disease spread by the tsetse fly which so restricts the type of livestock able to survive locally unless they have been deliberately immunised. There is a noticeable trend towards dwarf livestock throughout this region: the cattle and the goats are also very small.

The West African group of pigs has potential for meat production: they are quite stocky little animals and two varieties have indeed been exploited in this way: the **Ashanti Dwarf** and the **Bakosi** <Plate 20>, both of which can fairly be described as breeds, in contrast to the wide-spread local types of West Africa.

Ashanti Dwarf <Plate 20>

This Ghana pig is usually black, but can be brown or white or pied. It is small (mature female 40-60kg) with a long head, long tapering snout, prick ears and long legs. Average litter 6.5 at birth, 5.5 at weaning. Average weaning age 8 weeks, at 7kg liveweight.

The black **Bakosi** of Cameroon is similar in type, size and performance. It often has random white patches, sometimes quite extensive.

SOUTHERN AFRICA

The indigenous pigs of southern Africa are broadly similar to those of the rest of the continent - long-legged with long head and snout, small prick ears, and often black in colour. Two types have been distinguished: the **Windsnyer** and the **Kolbroek**.

Windsnyer <Plate 20>

(South Africa, Zimbabwe, parts of Mozambique and Zambia).

A long-snouted razor-backed pig of various colours. Typical daily weight gains: 28g (8-16 weeks), 51g (17-24 weeks), 45g (25-32 weeks), with feed conversion ratios of 3.1, 3.6 and 5.0 respectively. The litter size is usually less than that of exotic breeds but the total liveweight of the litter as a proportion of the sow's weight at farrowing is similar (11%). Sow's FCR is as good as exotics; excellent mother, low piglet mortality. The **Kolbroek** of South Africa is short and fat with a dished face, short snout, prick ears; it is of Chinese origin and is usually black or brown.

The history of pig farming in South Africa is a respectably long one. In 1652, for example, the commander of the newly established settlement at the Cape of Good Hope wrote in his diary that a servant had been employed to look after the pig herd.

In 1820 the British arrived, and their settlers found pigs on a small scale. Gradually during the century a pig industry began to develop and most of the produce was converted into bacon, sausages and salt pork rather than eaten as fresh pork. By the turn of the century, most of South Africa's pigs were short-legged lard producers with heavy necks and shoulders, and they were usually black. The Berkshire was among the first breeds to be introduced and was very popular at the end of the 19th century; its numbers decreased sharply in the 1920s, however, and it is no longer registered in South Africa.

Transvaal imported pigs in 1904 for two new government farms at Standerton and Potchefstroom, set up to supply breeding animals to surrounding farmers. The South African Studbook Association was established in 1905 and its first studbook the following year registered 143 pigs. The Standerton herd was liquidated in 1908, however, as the demand for pork was limited and there was a lack of facilities for processing the meat.

There was already a substantial herd of **Large Blacks** at Potchefstroom by 1905 and the breed played a leading role until 1930, after which it declined almost to the point of extinction. Recently, however, there has been a move to revive the Large Black for its docility and its superb mothering of large litters. It is deemed to be too fat as a purebred and its colour is held against it (even in the cross) but the trend has been towards Large Black/Landrace F_1 sows for outdoor systems, in which they have proved to outperform all others in terms of numbers raised on one large unit in Transvaal. When the crossbred sows are put to a Large White boar, the offspring are white.

The **Large White** from Yorkshire was brought into South Africa before the Boer War and became very popular, ousting the Large Black for a while. The First World War led to a greater demand and pig registrations increased suddenly in 1917; the Pig Breeders' Association was set up two years later and the industry began to find its confidence, expanding steadily and then more rapidly as a result of another world war. In 1939 the national herd numbered 466,000 pigs. Twenty years later a few Landrace were imported and quickly became the leading breed. Between them, the Large White and Landrace dominated the pig industry while other breeds such as Tamworth, Middle White, Poland China and Minnesota No.1 quietly faded away like the Berkshire and Large Black.

In 1991 the herd stood at 1.25 million and

the annual total of slaughtered pigs was just over 2 million. Between 1958 and 1991 the pig population had increased at the same rate as the human population. Most of the pigs are in the grain-producing regions and around the larger cities of South Africa. The Transvaal population is about 615,000, that of Cape Province about 306,000, that of Natal 169,000 and of the Orange Free State 163,000. Units have become larger and more intensive and the whole industry is increasingly stable in its production.

The Large White almost disappeared at one stage but has reversed its fortunes in the last decade or so. The **South African Landrace** <Plate 20>, developed from Danish, Dutch and Swedish imports and establishing a herdbook in 1959, had considerable problems with stress susceptibility, which was evident in a large proportion of the national herd, but halothane testing has helped to improve the situation recently: it is considered to be South Africa's "great mother" breed and has played a major role in the country's pig industry.

The two white breeds work together, either in purebred herds or in crossbreeding programmes which make the most of the Large White's high feed conversion efficiency and the Landrace's carcass quality for pork and bacon. Nearly all production is in intensive units, with averages of 19-20 weaned per annum per sow (in two litters). Weaning is at 3-6 weeks. Gilts are usually served for the first time at about 8 months old (at 110kg or more). Sows usually remain in commercial breeding herds for three years and boars for two, though AI is becoming more popular.

Average birth weight is 1.3kg, average weight at weaning at 35 days is 8-9kg, average daily weight gain in high-performance lines is close to 1kg (30-90kg) with an FCR of 2:1. Most are grown to 85-93kg liveweight and marketed as baconers at about 150 days old. Porkers are slaughtered at 60-70kg (about 120 days old) and there is occasional seasonal demand for sucking pigs with carcass weights up to 20kg. Old sows, with carcasses of at least 90kg, become sausage meat.

The white breeds had the pig industry to themselves for many years but in 1980/81 some Americans were imported - the red Duroc and the belted Hampshire - to give a third breed as a sire on the widely used Landrace/Large White crossbred sows. The **Duroc** was preferred: its performance was better than that of the Hampshire and its colour was less of a problem when it was used on white sows (nearly all the progeny are white). The boars are excellent workers but Duroc sows were not good mothers; breeders therefore concentrated on producing high-performance terminal sires, appreciated for being completely stress-free as well as siring strong-growing litters. There is a trend towards selection for improved mothering by the sow in the long term. Meanwhile, semen continues to be imported from the United States of America for breed improvement until the genetic pool is larger.

The **Hampshire** offers the best eye muscle, excellent conformation and low backfat. Good results are claimed for the Hampshire x Landrace F_1 sow but the main use for the Hampshire is as a terminal boar on the Large White/Landrace cross. Colour remains a problem in the carcass.

A very few **Chester Whites** have been imported from the United States as terminal sires, with the advantage of being white. It has been found that the Chester White "nicks" with the Large White to produce an outstanding F_1 gilt and this line is now being purebred in earnest. It is not used as a mother breed (its role in the USA) because the Large White and Landrace are already considered excellent for the job. The boars, like those of Duroc and Hampshire, have excellent bone and seem to be good workers.

There has been a new national pig improvement scheme in South Africa since 1990 to promote performance testing in the industry, to identify genetic potential for improving the national herd, to find high-merit boars for AI, and to ensure that breeding and production methods meet future market requirements. It involves only the breeding companies' pedigree herds or purebreds of notable breeders. There is on-farm boar testing and central progeny testing. Progeny testing began in 1956, boar performance testing in 1965 and sow performance testing in 1975.

Pork has by far the smallest proportion of the meat market in South Africa, with many objecting to it on the grounds of either religion or taste. It is not one of the products South Africans would choose for a family treat and it is, however unfairly, perceived as a fatty food. Thus there is a problem. The industry is such, and the pig itself is such, that production capacity is exceptionally high, especially as smaller and middle-sized producers had almost disappeared by 1983. But the product is not wanted.

AMERICA

MAP 4. Pig Breeds of America

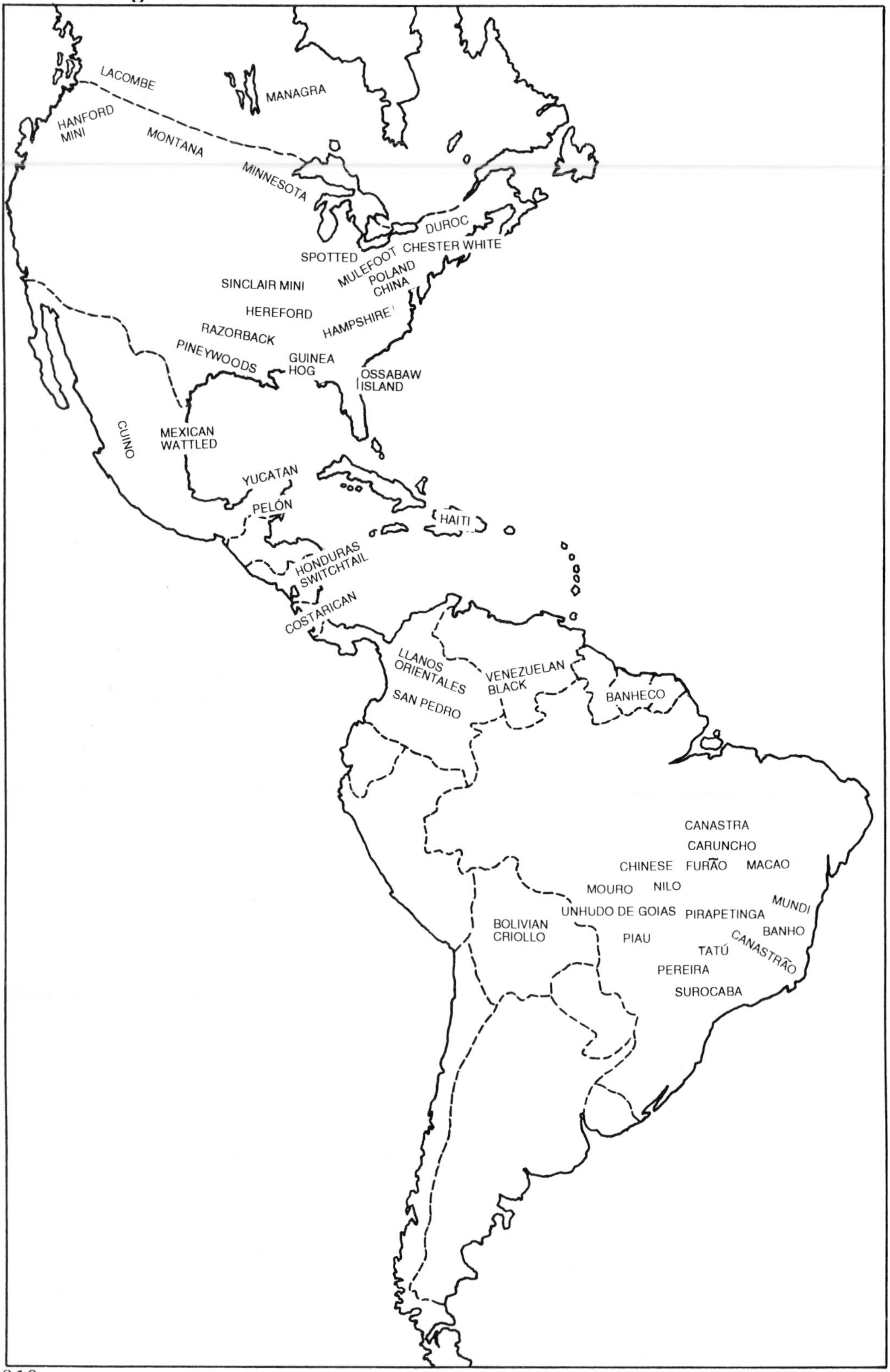

LACOMBE
MANAGRA
HANFORD MINI
MONTANA
MINNESOTA
DUROC
SPOTTED
MULEFOOT
CHESTER WHITE
POLAND CHINA
SINCLAIR MINI
HEREFORD
HAMPSHIRE
RAZORBACK
PINEYWOODS
GUINEA HOG
OSSABAW ISLAND
CUINO
MEXICAN WATTLED
YUCATAN
PELÓN
HAITI
HONDURAS SWITCHTAIL
COSTARICAN
LLANOS ORIENTALES
VENEZUELAN BLACK
SAN PEDRO
BANHECO
CANASTRA
CARUNCHO
CHINESE
FURÃO
MACAO
MOURO
NILO
MUNDI
UNHUDO DE GOIAS
PIRAPETINGA
BOLIVIAN CRIOLLO
BANHO
PIAU
CANASTRÃO
TATÚ
PEREIRA
SUROCABA

AMERICA

CANADA

The population of this large but sparsely populated country is about 26 million people, and there are more than 10 million pigs. The Canadian Swine Breeders' Association was first organised in 1889, and incorporated in 1895. In 1907, 50% of Canadian registrations were of the Yorkshire, with the same ancestral background as the Large White; the rest were divided between seven other breeds.

Traditionally, Canada's pigs have been of British breeds, or were so until the middle of the present century. The first boar registered by the Canadian Yorkshire Club was a Large White imported from England in 1886. From 1940 to 1955 the Yorkshire completely dominated, forming 90% of Canada's pigs. At the time grading standards concentrated on the bacon export trade and thus encouraged a monotypic population of Canadian Yorkshires, of a type that had distinguished itself from the Large White to such an extent that today there is a good degree of hybrid vigour in crosses between the two breeds. There was very little in the way of deliberate development of distinctive strains within the breed, except almost incidentally on a regional basis.

During the 1950s this familiar situation began to change. The Landrace, imported to the United States from Denmark in 1934, was released to the public in 1950 and Canadian breeders set up some Landrace herds, importing more stock from Sweden and Norway when Danish exports were embargoed. The Landrace was first registered in Canada in 1954 and within six years registrations numbered nearly 13,000 and the breed represented 28.9% of the national total, with the Yorkshire reduced to 59.2%.

The Danish Landrace also gave Canada the chance to develop the first breed of its own: the **Lacombe** <Plate 22>. The Canadian Department of Agriculture set up a breeding programme in 1947 at the Lacombe Experimental Farm, with a foundation of (Danish Landrace x Chester White) x Berkshire, the latter for high milkiness, uniform back fat and fullness of ham. The intention was to create a purebred white pig for a high quality carcass; the new breed would then give hybrid vigour in a cross with the Yorkshire. The programme was essentially one of backcrossing F_1 progeny with the Landrace as the foundation male breed, followed by *inter se* matings of the backcross progeny. The final contribution was 56% Landrace, 23% Berkshire and 21% Chester White. Its appearance was closest to the Landrace parent.

The new Lacombe was first registered in Canada in 1958 and two years later the new breed registered 2,214 pigs - 4.9% of the national total; others, in order of population and excluding the whites, were Tamworth (3.4%), Large Black (1.8%), Wessex Saddleback (1.1%), Canadian Berkshire (0.7%) and Duroc-Jersey (0.1%). In that year there were no registrations for the Hampshire or the Chester White, two American breeds which had both figured in the 1950 returns. Over the decade the Tamworth had experienced a sharp drop from 2,987 registrations (7.6%) to 1,524, and the Berkshire an even more dramatic collapse from 1,390 (3.6%) to only 294. The Wessex Saddleback first came to Canada in 1956 but was never very impressive in its new environment, though it did contribute to the **Managra**, a lop-eared hybrid from Swedish Landrace, Wessex, Welsh, Berkshire, Minnesota No. 1, Tamworth and Yorkshire.

Before 1950, the Yorkshire had been the only registered white bacon breed in Canada but now there were three. There was some prejudice against coloured hair and "seeding" of the belly meat of dark-haired breeds but more important was the better carcass quality, growth rates and feed conversion efficiency of the whites under Canadian conditions. The Tamworth graded particularly low and needed 381 units of feed for every 100 units of liveweight gain, compared with 340 for the Lacombe. What is more, the Lacombe reached slaughterweight in 170 days but the Tamworth took 189 days. The Landrace took the prize for the best carcass scores.

The next stage was the reintroduction of certain American breeds in the 1960s, but as slimmer meat-type versions of their former selves. There was simultaneously a new tolerance of non-white pigs in the grading standards and a new attitude which encouraged crossbreeding. The American breeds included Chester White, Poland-China, Duroc and Hampshire.

The Yorkshire and Landrace continued to dominate and the Duroc and Hampshire became increasingly popular, but in the 1980s there were only very small numbers of Spotted. The 1984 registrations of the old British breeds were minimal - 22 British Saddleback, 11 Canadian Berkshire and only 6 Tamworth.

In 1990 the Canadian pig industry was similar in size to that of the United Kingdom and it exported more than 40% of its pig meat, mostly to the United States. Herds were relatively small (many with fewer than 100 sows) and mainly in the wheat-producing provinces of Manitoba, Alberta and Saskatchewan. However, Quebec, the largest producer of pigs, imported most of its grain from the United States, to the dismay of the other provinces. Typical pig units are heavily insulated against the extremely cold winters, in which temperatures often fall to -20°C. The summers can be very hot, with temperatures up to 35°C, and sprinklers are needed as evaporative coolers.

The modern **Canadian Yorkshire** <Plate 21> is a prolific sow with good milking and mothering abilities; carcass quality, growth rates and feed conversion are generally good, and the breed is excellent for crossing. This Yorkshire differs genetically from the Large White, despite their common ancestry, and the carcass quality and liveweight gains of the Yorkshire are better than those of the Large White in Canadian conditions. The **Canadian Landrace** <Plate 21> is prolific, a good milker and an excellent crossing breed with a carcass of as good quality as that of the Yorkshire. The **Lacombe**, a lop-eared and placid breed, is known for good mothering, high quality carcass and excellent growth rates, and performs well in a cross with the Yorkshire; by 1969 it had been exported to the USA, several European countries, Mexico, the Dominican Republic, Cambodia, Singapore and Malaysia.

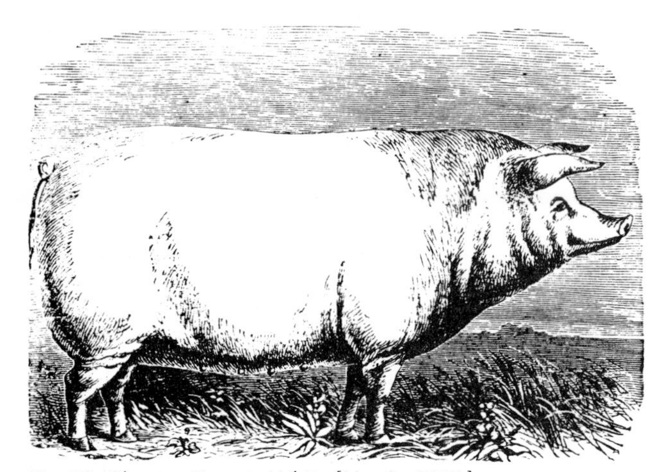

Fig. 20. Chester County White [Harris, 1881]

THE UNITED STATES OF AMERICA

In 1991 the total herd in the United States numbered more than 59 million, a substantial increase from a low point of only 37 million in 1989. By 1996, US producers intend to increase chilled pig meat exports to Japan, for example, by 30% compared with 43,000 tons in 1990, to match the continuing rise of Japanese consumption.

Yet in 1944, the American pig population had been as high as 83.756 million and the country was second only to China as a producer. In 1908 there were 56 million hogs - nearly half the world's population at the time - and the country was exporting a million dollars' worth of lard, half a million each of bacon and ham, and there was still a reasonable trade in that old standby, salt pork. Back in 1879 the hog population stood at 34.8 million and Chicago had taken over from Cincinnati as the greatest swine market and slaughtering point in the world. Those were the days when North America was Britain's major source of bacon, before the Danes began their challenge.

In 1865, according to F.D. Coburn (writing in the first decade of the 20th century), "large size, almost regardless of the time required for its attainment, was in the grower's eye an important object." In the new century, however, "conditions have changed to such an extent that now the old time mammoth is no longer required or wanted." In the intervening years there had been much importation of live pigs, much crossing and selection, and new feeding techniques, the increased use of castration and the more serious study of the whole business of breeding and raising pigs. The tendency towards early maturity had been hugely accelerated and the demand was for pigs that would be ready for slaughter at 15 months old at the most - and would produce flesh rather than the huge quantities of lard for which the American hog was so famous. There had been a steady decline in average liveweights and lard yields between 1879 and 1908.

The main centre for swine breeds and production was traditionally the Mississippi valley, "where Indian corn is grown in greatest abundance and at least expense." The role of the American hog was to turn large quantities of maize into large quantities of lard and meat. As Sanders Spencer put it: "The maize should walk to market." Maize produces very fat pork, which was appreciated by the packers as it did not become so salty, and anyway kept better - an important advantage as American salted pork was often consumed in climates where lean salted pork did not last. The fat was also rendered down as lard for export. What the American pig-keeper looked for in the 19th century was a pig with a wide, fat back, thick neck, heavy jowl and a large volume of lard and of pork for the workers.

Only a modest proportion of all the swine raised for pork were purebreds. The majority, even at the turn of the century, were black, perhaps with a few touches of white on feet, faces and tail tips in the style of the Berkshire. Some actually were Berkshires, some were the similarly coloured Poland China, and the majority a mixture of these two. It seems that spotted black and whites were very rare (indicating that there was little direct crossing of black breeds with white ones) and entirely black animals were also unusual, but it was quite common to cross largely black breeds with red Duroc-Jerseys and Tamworths - the resulting sandy hogs with black spots were described by Coburn as "generally quite satisfactory".

White pigs were not popular at that time: they were said to be prone to sunscald, scurvy and mange. An increasing number of reds had been noticed in markets and abattoirs in the early years of the century. For example, at Indianapolis 17% of the hogs were red or a red mixture and 45% were black; in Omaha 70% were red or brown as they were thought to be more hardy than other colours.

Coburn divided the breeds of his time into large, medium and small. The large included three lard breeds (Poland China, Chester White and Duroc-Jersey), two English bacon breeds (Tamworth and Yorkshire) and most of the contemporary Berkshires which were sometimes for bacon but were raised as lard pigs in the corn belt. The medium-sized, all lard pigs, included the Middle Yorkshire (known in England as the Middle White), the Victoria and the Cheshire, while the small breeds, also all lard types, were the Small Yorkshire or Suffolk and the Black Essex.

In the 1930 census the American breeds included Poland China, Duroc-Jersey, Spotted Poland China, Chester White, Berkshire, Yorkshire, Tamworth, Hampshire (mentioned in passing by Coburn two decades earlier), Essex, Suffolk, Victoria, Kentucky Red Berkshire, Large Black, Cheshire and the Mulefoot (a black pig with undivided hoofs). There were also three new breeds: the Minnesota No. 1 (from Tamworth and Danish Landrace), the Minnesota No. 2 (Canadian Yorkshire and Poland China) and the Hamprace (Black Hampshire and Danish Landrace, later named the Montana

No. 1).

In 1990 the National Association of Swine Records embraced only eight pure breeds: Yorkshire, American Berkshire, Chester White, Hampshire, American Landrace, Poland China, Spotted, and Duroc. In between quite a few breeds have come and gone on the crests and troughs of fashion.

The development of the American pig industry was geared to maize, the staple diet of pigs, especially in the great corn belt where they were turned into the fields to eat cobs straight from the growing plants. The 1919 edition of *Encyclopaedia Britannica* pronounced: "In America nearly all the breeds may be classified as lard-hogs. Bacon pigs fed on Indian corn degenerate into lard-hogs, run down in size and become too small in the bone and less prolific by inbreeding." Thirty years later Charles Wayland Towne and Edward Norris Wentworth wrote in their book *Pigs: From Cave to Corn Belt*: "The lard hog is as characteristically American as the production line in the automobile factory, the six-lane concrete highway, the hundred-car freight train, and the ready-made suit ... It is an American institution, destined to endure until the crops of the corn belt are forced to yield to the synthetics of the chemist - may Providence long postpone that day!"

It was maize, too, that led to a major stage in the development of the pig industry. Plant breeders experimented with hybridisation to produce higher corn yields and the US Department of Agriculture (USDA) realised that similar principles could be applied to pigs to exploit hybrid vigour. In 1937, by the direct authority of Congress, the Regional Swine Breeding Laboratory was established at Ames, Iowa, in a co-operative venture involving USDA and various state experimental stations intent on discovering, developing and testing potential breeding procedures for the sake of greater economy of pig production. They looked at, for example, close-breeding of the Poland China, and at close-breeding of Tamworth x Danish Landrace first-generation crosses to provide inbred stock from which commercial crosses could be raised. They studied different degrees of inbreeding in closed herds and they also investigated standards for production records and testing.

Long before this brave new venture, there had been a lot of pig-breeding and the history of the American breeds is an interesting one stretching right back to the days of Christopher Columbus - or considerably earlier in the case of Hawaii, to which domestic pigs (originally from the East Indies) were brought by early Polynesian settlers by the year 750, via Melanesia, New Guinea, the Solomon Islands, Fiji and Samoa. The full story is told in Mayer and Brisbin's book, *Wild Pigs of the United States*, which gives fascinating background to the many feral pigs still found here and there today.

The Spaniards brought pigs to the Hawaiian islands during the 16th century, and in 1778 Captain James Cook presented Kauai island with a pair of English pigs. Other European stock were added over the years, and as the inhabitants habitually allowed their domestic swine to range freely, there was much mingling of Polynesian and European pigs and a substantial feral population which still exists in the Hawaiian islands today.

The first domestic pigs introduced to the American continent were possibly the descendants of the famous eight said to have been brought by Columbus to Cuba in 1493. His ship had taken on supplies, including pigs and other livestock, in the Canary Islands (Gomera) so that they would have been Iberian in type, and it is claimed that those eight were the progenitors of all the pigs in the Spanish Indies. More pigs were landed in Puerto Rico (1505-1508), Jamaica (1509) and Cuba (1511) and quickly became feral. All too soon they also became a problem for Spanish colonists: they ravaged newly planted crops of maize and sugar cane, they attacked humans and even, it was said, killed cattle. It became the habit of Spanish explorers to capture some of these active ferals as supplies for their various expeditions and it was from this stock that the feral population of the United States must have originated. Mayer and Brisbin give full details of feral pigs in at least 20 states today.

Although the American continent had no indigenous wild species of pig (except the distantly related peccaries), it has been suggested that there were pigs in the New World before Columbus's time. It is also possible that John Cabot, a Genoan who had adopted English nationality, brought pigs direct to the east coast of mainland North America in 1497, when he is said to have discovered New England.

Further south, there were feral hogs in Arkansas in the 1540s which had escaped from an expedition led by Hernando de Soto, and there were others in California in the 1500s after the Spanish arrived, especially on the islands. For example, Santa Cruz, discovered by the Spanish in 1542, became a penal colony in 1582 and six hundred prisoners were abandoned there with a few cattle, horses and swine. They killed the first two species and turned their hides into escape boats but left the pigs to become feral. South Carolina had Spanish pigs by 1526 and Texas by 1542, while Florida's first pigs probably arrived in about 1539 when a Spanish encampment was set up by de Soto, or perhaps even in 1521 when the explorer Juan Ponce de Leon came through. De Soto bought more swine from Cuba to make sure that his Florida expedition did not starve. The true Wild Boar, incidentally, was first introduced here and there in the late 19th century.

The story of the spread of domestic pigs in company with various Spanish conquistadors in the 16th and 17th centuries, and their rapid build-up in new colonies, is told with relish by Towne and Wentworth. Pork and lard were mentioned frequently in conquistador literature and seem to have been almost the staple diet. The Spaniards took the pigs north into what would become New Mexico and Texas, and here they were given to the padres of Texas missions, who record ham and bacon in their supply lists. The Spanish pig, however, was essentially a lard pig, just like the Iberian pigs in Spain today. Writing in the mid 19th century about the history of California, Alexander Forbes said of the pigs of his time in the state's Spanish settlements that they "are reared and fed chiefly for their lard and are of a very good kind derived from the Chinese breed. They are fed in a manner to produce as much fat and as little flesh as possible." These pigs, after an early life of scavenging and rootling in the woods and fields, would be penned at a certain stage and stuffed with maize - as much as they could eat - so that "when slaughtered they are found to be almost all lard to the very bones", often unable to stand, let alone walk.

In 1699, French swine were brought into Mississippi by Pierre le Moyne, Sieur d'Iberville. They thrived and were kept separate from the local Spanish pigs, so that even at the end of the 19th century it was easy to identify descendants of the French pigs in remote parts of Mississippi and Louisiana.

British merchants sent a colonising expedition to Virginia in 1607, and pigs were among the livestock which arrived in Jamestown. Apparently the three sows in this collection increased to more than 60 pigs within 18 months; two years later there were five or six hundred of them. Another group of colonists, sailing for America in 1609, became shipwrecked on Bermuda for ten months but lived well off the feral hogs they found there, until they managed to build themselves a couple of ships, loaded them with pigs and people, and arrived safely in Virginia at last.

Thereafter, Virginia was never without pigs and they multiplied so rapidly that the colonists had to turn them into the woods to fend for themselves. Here they continued to thrive, in spite of wolves, bears and Indians, and spread out at will. By 1627 it was impossible to count their huge numbers. Then, of course, these razorback or woods hogs began ravaging the colonists' new plantings.

The paintroot plant has played a role in selecting Virginia's pigs. White pigs who ate the plant developed pink bones and lost their hooves; black pigs were unaffected. The whites were therefore automatically culled at birth and only black pigs were reared.

The pilgrims from Plymouth, Devon, whose *Mayflower* had landed at Plymouth Rock, Massachusetts, in 1620, were brought livestock by Edward Winslow. The animals were allowed to reproduce for four years and were then apportioned equally among the colonists. More pigs were introduced at intervals until, again, the pig population became too large to be fed easily and the settlers moved farther into the wilderness looking for areas where they could grow corn for their hogs. The New England swine usually ranged freely in the woods, and here too they soon became "innumerable" and had to have their noses ringed because they were damaging the corn fields.

Meanwhile a shipment of livestock, including pigs, reached New Amsterdam with the director of the Dutch West Indies Company. Colonists in Maryland, where the pigs foraged in the forests from the start, were buying their animals from the Virginians or from Barbados. Pennsylvania, which would become a major hog colony, was settled by the Swedish in its earliest days (1638), then the English (including William Penn's Quakers) and the Germans. A few Swedish pigs ran wild and multiplied; they were shot in the autumn to be salted and smoked as winter food, yet by the early 1660s they still numbered several thousand head. Penn was much more methodical: his Quakers fed and sheltered their livestock and were able to export pork and live hogs to the Caribbean islands within a decade of setting up their colony in 1681. The Germans, like the Quakers, were careful with their animals and fattened them on corn to produce high quality pork. By 1700 this Pennsylvania system of finishing pigs on maize became standard practice in New England and the Middle Atlantic colonies. By the 1730s there were stable agricultural and commercial English communities along most of the eastern seaboard, from New Hampshire to Georgia.

Marvellous animals, pigs! Given the freedom of the New World, they made the most of it: they thrived left to their own devices and they thrived under good management as well. In addition to helping colonists to be self-sufficient, they became items of trade, as hogs or as barrelled (cured) pork for export. Even before 1700 Worcester, Massachusetts, was a flourishing trade centre for barrelled pork, soon followed by Boston and Salem. From then until the Revolution, the pork export industry boomed. Virginia specialised in bacon exported to Britain and barrelled pork to the West Indies, Portugal and Madeira: 20,000 barrels were sent to each destination in 1773/4.

After the Revolution came the migration to the West. Naturally the pioneers took a few swine with them, especially that old razorback hog of the woods, well accustomed to using its long legs and foraging for its food with a long and eager snout to fuel its narrow, flat-sided, short-coupled, lean body. Most of the hogs were sandy-brown and covered with rough bristles.

These rough, tough and thoroughly self-sufficient beasts were remarked upon by many a writer visiting the frontier folk, and were noted as the most common of the new settlers' livestock, quite capable of defending themselves against predators and as prolific as ever. One French traveller described them as "of a bulky shape, middling size, and straight eared". They ran more or less wild in the woods but were rounded up now and then by a horseman bearing a few corncobs as bait: he would throw them one or two and then they would follow him home squealing for more.

In 1811 a ship named the *Tonquin* brought the first pigs to the Oregon Territory. It had taken a hundred pigs on board in the Hawaiian Islands, by courtesy of the local king, Kamehameha, and some sugar cane to feed them. They were the first of several shipments over the next few years to supply a carefully developed agricultural system in this fur-trading region, with the encouragement of the Hudson's Bay Company. More pigs came in from Hawaii in 1834 and soon both Oregon and Washington had thriving hog herds.

Those Hawaiian pigs were Asian in character: they had dipped backs, splayed toes, sagging pasterns and blubber-like layers of fat; they rarely weighed more than, say, 125-150 pounds and their litters were small.

Now North America had its razorback woods hogs, its Spanish and Hawaiian pigs with Asian blood, and the European stock from France, Britain, Holland, Sweden and Germany, many of them coarse in bone and skin, often curly-coated, with heavy shoulders and poor hams and inclined or lop ears in the typical old Celtic manner. Colours were random but there seemed to be more whites and spotted pigs than pure black, red or sandy.

This mixture - some of them pannage pigs, some of them graziers and some of them sty pigs - suited their environments and their raisers but were not efficient for fattening. Others were imported to help, and it was these that formed the foundation of the American breeds with a little help from the West Indies, Italy, Africa's Guinea coast, China, Siam, Burma and elsewhere. It was a very cosmopolitan and heterogeneous basis for the national herd.

And then came the sudden burst of livestock improvement in Britain using Chinese, Siamese and Neapolitan pigs to change the big old lop-eared English type into the smaller, earlier maturing and much fatter Berkshires and other breeds, often with short snouts, heavy jowls, thick necks and fat backs - what Sanders Spencer described as "bladders of animated lard". The Americans, keen to retain as much size as possible, crossed the small fat pigs with their large, coarse hogs.

Development of the Whites

One of the improved English breeds was known variously as the **Woburn** or the **Bedford** and had been bred originally on the Duke of Bedford's estate at Woburn Abbey with the help of a large dose of blood from white Chinese pigs. They also became known as the **Parkinson** breed: a pair of the Duke's Chinese-influenced pigs had been entrusted to an Englishman called Parkinson as a gift to George Washington, but apparently the escort sold them instead. The breed quickly became popular and spread through Virginia, Maryland, Pennsylvania, Ohio, New York, Delaware and Massachusetts. They were usually sandy or spotted (often white with brown spots) and the sows were notoriously poor sucklers. As it happened they were exterminated during the Civil War. Of course many a pig had been called a Bedford once the breed became fashionable but most had no right to the name at all.

In the early 1800s, New England's most prominent breed was the **Byfield**, developed at Byfield, Massachusetts, in about 1800 by Chester Forham, who had bought a floppy-eared pig in a local market. The Byfield was a white pig with two varieties: a large pasture type with long, flat sides and flopping ears; and a very different medium variety with obvious Chinese influence in its short, dished face, full jowl, deep chest, broad back, fine hair and refined conformation. It was said to have evolved from the Bedford with Old English and Chinese pigs and, like the Bedford, it was widely used in cross-breeding. It spread to the south and also accompanied emigrants moving westwards to Ohio before 1816. In Ohio it would meet its ultimate fate in helping to create the Poland China, which soon displaced the Byfield.

To confuse matters, there was another **Bedford**, this time named after the English county rather than the Duke. In 1820 one Captain James Jeffries of Westchester purchased a prize-winning pair of these white Bedfordshires (sometimes described as **Cumberlands**). The boar had some bluish or black skin spots (mistakenly attributed to a Berkshire ancestor); he was crossed on some native Pennsylvania sows of the large, coarse, white kind descended from either William Penn's or the old Swedish hogs. The offspring were more refined, with broad backs, plump hams, short legs, fine hair, drooping (but not lop) ears and the boar's characteristic skin spots. A little later, some **White Chinese** pigs were imported from England by Harry Atwood of Delaware County: they were short-legged, sway-backed and pot-bellied, with short faces and drooping ears, excellent feeding qualities, early maturity, and with black, blue and sandy spots on the hair and skin. In due course, the improved strains developed from these Delaware Chinese and the Westchester Bedford crosses were combined with the Chester County White (named after its source of origin in Pennsylvania). This pig had a strong family resemblance to the Lincolnshire Curly Coat, and its early ancestors probably came from Lincolnshire, Yorkshire and Cheshire.

The **Chester White** <Plate 21>proved to be a prolific sow and a good mother. The mature weight was about 450 pounds but boars could reach an average of 600 pounds. The average daily weight gain was 1.36 pounds, and it took three pounds of grain to produce a pound of weight gain.

Then various improvers took the Chester White in hand in Ohio. First, W.K. Townsend of East Haven, Connecticut, apparently imported some **Norfolk Thin Rind** pigs from England, which were black, spotted with white or with a white belt. A Norfolk boar was then mated to a sow of the "Grass" breed (presumably **Irish Grazier**) by brothers Isaac and Kneeland Todd to produce early maturing, quick finishing crosses with a carcassweight of 365 pounds at 9 months old. The Todds migrated to Ohio, taking the pigs with them, and there they crossed the animals again, this time with some hogs originally from Massachusetts which were descended from a similar Grass type sow by a **Byfield** boar. Isaac Todd then introduced a "Large Grass" boar and a so-called "White Normandy" into this mixture and achieved better feeders and good-looking show pigs which quickly raked in the prizes. His son subsequently blended more Chester White into the stock over the next 40 years to produce his **Improved Chester White**.

Another version called itself the **Ohio Improved Chester**, or OIC. This was based on importations from Chester County, Pennsylvania, and was bred for bigger, more rugged and practical pigs than the Todd show type. The Todd breeders, however, changed their breeding policy in the 1920s and gained size as well. By the 1950s, the Chester White was well established in the Middle West, though some claimed its white skin suffered from sunburn and scurf.

Thus the Chester White, it was admitted even by its greatest supporters, was a "made up" breed and even by 1870 Joseph Harris, in his book about America's pigs, quoted Paschall Morris of Philadelphia, who had bred Chester Whites for many years, as saying that "they differ from each other quite as much as any one known breed differs from another." The best of them were "long and deep in the carcass, broad and straight on the back, short in the leg, full in the ham, full shoulder, well packed forward, admitting of no neck, very small proportionate head, short nose, dish face, broad between the eyes, moderate ear, thin skin, straight hair, a capacity for great size and to gain a pound per day until they are two years old. Add to these, quiet habits, and an easy taking on of fat, so as to admit of being slaughtered at almost any age, and we have, what is considered in Chester County, a carefully bred animal, and what is known elsewhere as a fine specimen of a breed called 'Chester County White'. They have reached weights of from 600 to 900 pounds."

Yet, as Morris had explained, they were not consistent. He had often seen offspring from good animals which had long noses "which would root up an acre of ground in a very short time" - they were slab-slided, long-legged, and restless feeders, "resembling somewhat the so-called race-horse breed of the South, that will keep up with a horse all day on ordinary travel, and that will go *over* a fence instead of taking much trouble to go *through* it. They show more development of head than ham, and as many bristles as hair, and are as undesirable a hog as can well be picked up." There was, he said, no such thing as a pure Chester hog, though he earnestly hoped that some breeder somewhere might persevere with deliberate selection to raise what was generally an already high standard and, above all, to give the "breed" a more definite type and character. At that period, although they were extremely popular among down-to-earth farmers, the Chester Whites did not breed true and the impression is that much of the original Quakers' very careful selection and breeding had been wasted.

But improvements were indeed made, without losing the breed's essential ruggedness and size. Today it can be described as reliable and durable rather than stylish. The sow has excellent conception rates and large litters; she milks well and mothers well, and the breed is particularly useful in a cross with Yorkshires and Landraces as the mother of Duroc-sired litters.

Many English breeds came and went between 1820 and 1860 - the black Improved Essex, the Middlesex, medium and small Yorkshires and the Large Black among them - but they proved inappropriate for the efficient use of America's corn. The white **Suffolk**, with plenty of Chinese blood, was early maturing and quick to fatten; it became one of the country's most widespread breeds during the 1850s and 1860s, extensively used in crossbreeding and praised as being easy and cheap to keep, but it was overrated and quietly disappeared in due course. Harris, in his *Book of the Pig*, looked at the English breeds in great detail and devoted only a brief chapter to the breeds of the United States, though his book was written for fellow Americans. He described just three American groups: the Chester County White, the Magie of Ohio (Poland China) and the **Cheshire** or **Jefferson County** pigs of New York, which had recently been winning all the prizes.

The Cheshires were first exhibited as the "Cheshire and Yorkshire", then as "Improved Cheshire" and (in 1868) "Improved Yorkshire" but they were widespread under the name of Cheshire, which confused everybody into thinking that they were an English county breed. There had indeed been Cheshire pigs in England, of the largest and coarsest types then known and described as the "old gigantic, long-legged, long-eared pig, of a large patched black and white colour" which produced a huge carcass of "surprisingly good" and lean meat - in one case a sow's hams each weighed 77 pounds. However, Samuel Sidney had informed Harris that "these unprofitable giants" were almost extinct in England.

It was said that a large sow of the ungainly English type had been taken from Albany to Jefferson County at about the same time as some thoroughbred Yorkshires were introduced into the same neighbourhood from England, and that probably the "Cheshire and Yorkshire" was from a cross of the two, but nobody really knew. Others said that the sows were local ones containing plenty of Suffolk blood rather than Cheshire.

A **Yorkshire** boar had been imported by two local farmers in Jefferson County, on the shores of Lake Ontario where the winters were snowy and cold. It did well at the shows at the close of the Civil War and a pen of Jefferson County pigs won the meatpackers' prize at St Louis in 1870. The Cheshire/Yorkshire type had become more and more like the pure Yorkshire - large and handsome, with finer bones, small fine ears, short snout, well developed cheeks, long and square in the body with good shoulders and hams, and very small bones for such a large white pig. They were nearly as large as the Chester County white, which was coarser in bone, ears and snout. But all that the Jefferson County breeders would say was that their American Cheshire breed was of mixed origin but kept pure sufficiently long to be called a breed. The name Cheshire was officially adopted in 1872.

By 1876 there was only one Cheshire herd in Jefferson County. J.H. Saunders of Iowa, founder of *The Breeder's Gazette*, had tried it out but gave it up, saying it was obviously a local variety of the Yorkshire and was so like the improved Berkshire that it was jokingly known as the White Berkshire. His mockery did not kill off the breed; a breed society was formed in 1884 and in 1905 a thousand purebred animals were registered - by 1910 it was New York's most popular breed and was a white pig with a pinkish skin, in conformation like the Middle White of England, including a dished face with small erect ears pointing forwards. It was of good length, with good hams and shoulders, rather a broad arched back, and legs too light in the bone; it was of medium to heavy weight with flesh of good quality, very early maturing and noted for being a docile pig, though seldom seen outside New York state. Thereafter it went into decline and no herdbook was published after 1914, though the breed remained widespread. By 1930 only 40 remained and it became extinct.

Other local breeds came and went. In 1850 F.D. Curtis of Saratoga, New York, had decided to develop his own **Curtis Victoria** by crossing several varieties selected for their genetic merit, but it did not catch the public imagination and there were no known purebreds by the turn of the century. Quite separately, George F. Davis developed a **Davis Victoria** lard pig in Indiana during the 1870s, from a combination of Chester White, Poland China, Berkshire and American Suffolk, naming his breed after a sow called Queen Victoria; there was a breed society from 1886 for a while but no herdbook was published and the breed was ignored in contemporary textbooks. By 1930 only 94 remained and it, too, gradually became extinct.

Development of the Reds

Red and sandy pigs had existed in the Atlantic coast colonies from the start but not necessarily from separate importations - there were similar red hogs in the Spanish settlements in Mexico and Florida. By 1804 (the earliest definite record, but it could have come much earlier) there was a red or sandy breed brought in by slave traders from the West African coast. It was known as the **Red Guinea** and was described by William Youatt as "large in size, square in form, of a reddish colour" and covered with short bristles which were "smoother and more shiny than almost any other variety of the porcine race". Apparently this breed was mentioned specifically in England in 1767.

The **Tamworth** itself seems to have been a late entrant among the American reds: the first seems to have been imported in 1882 by Thomas Bennett of Illinois, and it also went into Canada in 1888, where it became quite widespread. Thereafter Tamworths in the United States usually came from Canada but to American eyes the breed was too like the old pioneers' razorbacks and woods pigs: they did not like its long legs, long slender body and long snout. Nor did they appreciate that, far from being a pioneer pig, it could not stand being stunted of feed in its youth: it had no resources of fat (even in those days, the proportion of lean meat was unusually high) and would never be profitable once it had been poorly fed. The first cross to other breeds gave an easy feeder, maturing quickly, but a second-generation cross often produced different colours and, more important, different conformations within the same litter.

However, reds and sandies had been known in New England and New York long before the Revolution, shortly after which the big **Jersey Red** hog of New Jersey became well known. It was large and coarse, weighing 500-600 pounds, with some up to 1,000. The name was already in use by 1832, according to some, but not until 1857 according to others, and some said it owed its colour to Spanish pigs imported in or before 1820. It was usually a dark red pig patched with white, and sometimes it was sandy and white.

The next step was to improve the reds and the agent for this was the **Berkshire** from England, which had already been improved itself with the help of Asian blood. The Berkshire had originally been a red or sandy pig with black splodges and large, pendulous ears: its colour did not change into the famous black with white points until well into the 19th century. By 1840 it had developed its prick ears and dished face from the Chinese influence and was the earliest maturing of the British breeds. The Berkshire type had frequently been imported to the east coast even before 1800, though not as a recognised breed: the first importation under the Berkshire name was in 1823 when an Englishman, John Brentnall, brought some into New Jersey, and more were brought in by Siday Hawes of Albany, New York, in 1832. More followed, spreading from New York westwards and southwards. In 1880, a writer said that the Jersey Red bore close resemblance to the Berkshire types of 1830.

The early Berkshire breeders in America, using English and Canadian stock, bred away from the bacon type to produce a meatier pig, and "Berkshire fever" soon set in, until a lack of standards locally led to the breed's deterioration and temporary demise. Its reputation was restored after fresh stock was imported from England in 1865, and ten years later the world's first pig breed society was formed: the American Berkshire Association. It did well in the corn belt, reverted once again to minor breed status, and then bounced back to reach a peak of popularity after the Second World War for its meatiness and its prepotence as an improver; but practical farmers then began to turn to other meaty breeds, with better liveweight gains and litter sizes. For a while the Berkshire lost its superior carcass quality, especially during a phase in which it was excessively selected for a dished face, but it is still well respected in the United States today.

In the 19th century, there were other reds being imported. In 1823 a red boar from a litter of ten, whose sire and dam were probably imported from England, was obtained by Isaac Frink of Milton in Saratoga County, New York, from Harry Kelsey. Kelsey owned a famous trotting stallion and Frink named his red boar in the horse's honour: **Duroc**. The progeny continued the Duroc name and many of them, from common sows, inherited his colour, quick growth and maturity, deep body, broad ham and shoulder, and quiet disposition. The Duroc was smaller than the Jersey Red, with finer bones and a better quality carcass. Its colour was sandy or red.

There were other red elements. In 1837 Henry Clay introduced four red Spanish pigs to his Kentucky farm near Lexington and the type became very popular in Kentucky and Virginia. Red pigs from Portugal were ordered by Daniel Webster, who died before they arrived and the pigs were therefore sold to Solomon Jewett, a well known breeder of Merino sheep in Middlesbury, Vermont, whence the **Red Rock** progeny spread into several southern and eastern states. There is a possible direct connection between the Webster Portuguese pigs and the foundation stock of what became the Duroc-Jersey.

About 1860, the Red Guineas were blended with the red Spanish and Portuguese pigs. Over the years they had also been crossed with local pigs. The mixture lay low for a while until it became well established in the corn belt around 1880.

Gradually, two distinct strains of red pig emerged and, as they did so, the various contributors ceased to have separate identities. In 1872 the breeders of the New York Durocs, the Connecticut Red Berkshires, the Vermont Red Rocks and the Jersey Reds established a uniform standard for their vaguely similar types, though all they really had in common was a touch of red, in many different shades. A breed association was formed in 1883, after which there was no attempt to keep the strains separate, and the new **Duroc-Jersey** began to spread westwards. Thus, once again, the American passion for crossbreeding and combining for greater productivity had led to the casting off of the very breeds whose qualities had been so valuable for their crosses.

The reds had been greeted with ridicule by many: they were coarse, with no style or finish and a "low-bred" appearance - there was lack of uniformity in colour, size and conformation. Gradually they began to shape into a more consistent type and a register of pedigrees was kept, yet Coburn (published in 1909) said that they were still all shades of rusty yellow, rusty grey, yellowish or rusty brown, often close to dirty black, or light or dark sandy colours, or every conceivable variation of red, bronze and copper, though the breeders were trying to select for a "cherry red", whether bright or dark in shade. But they were already known as large, prolific, quiet and peacable, though some strains remained coarse and some carried great weight on bones almost too small to sustain it.

By 1937 the red Duroc-Jersey had become a widespread and thoroughly practical farmer's pig, combining size with feeding capacity and prolificacy.

Development of the Blacks

The origins of Ohio's **Poland China** were not recorded at the time and much was forgotten about its true history. Coburn listened to memories of the days before 1850, from breeders who were still active in the 1870s, and he also looked at scattered and incomplete notes of the earlier period. The breed was not definitely named until the mid 1870s and its breed association was established in 1878, by which time the past had faded into a haze of distorted recollections, but some idea of the breed's development has been gleaned over the years.

The large-boned, coarse, slow-maturing pigs in the Cincinnati hinterland had developed from a mixture of all sorts from New England to Virginia and Kentucky and were notably hardy and prolific. Before 1816 there were only two named breeds in the region: the white **Byfield** (alread described) and the **Russian**, which was usually white, with long bristles, strong dense bones, a long rangy body, long coarse head, thick shoulders and reasonable hams. The Russian was quite prolific with litters usually of 9-12, and able to become very large given 18 or 20 months to grow, but nothing seems to be known of its origins, nor about breeds such as the Calcutta, the Barnitz and the Newbury White, which all came and went during this period. The Byfield and the Russian would provide one of the several random elements of the Poland China.

In 1816 the Shakers of Union Village in Warren County imported a boar and three sows of the so-called **Big China** from a Philadelphia farm. The boar and two of the sows were wholly white, and the third sow was white with some sandy spots superimposed with small black spots. They were probably **Bedfords** of a sort, and they helped to refine local pigs and improve their breeding and fattening traits. It was no doubt the very same breed, calling itself **Spotted China**, that was introduced to Union County, Indiana, some 20 years later.

These Chinas crossed well with the popular Byfields and Russians, and Miami Valley became recognised for its top-quality feeders, but they were far from handsome. They came to be known as the **Warren County** hog. In 1835, some of the new improved Berkshires (black with white points and prick ears) were introduced into the Miami valley and were used extensively on the Warren County hogs. There was also some talk of Neapolitan blood. The Big China itself gradually lost its identity under this onslaught of crossing and its name quietly disappeared.

The final element was the white, thin-coated **Irish Grazier**. In its home country this was a variable type; but a thoroughly self-sufficient one, well able to look after itself on backyard grazing and dairy wastes. It was big in bone and slow to mature but large numbers were brought in by Irish immigrants in the early 19th century. It became very popular, especially in the south, though it gradually disappeared between about 1870 and 1900, having served the purpose of several breed developers in the meantime. In 1839 a Cincinnati meat-packer, William Neff, brought into Ohio's Miami Valley from Ireland a boar and some sows of a particularly meaty strain of the Grazier, with long bodies, strong muscular backs and full hams. These, too, contributed to the improvement of the Warren County hogs and by the early 1860s the "breed" was known as the **Poland and China**. The supposed Polish element was a very minor influence from the progeny of a hog obtained from Asher Asher (the nearest that the locals could get to pronouncing his name), a Polish-born farmer near Monroe in Butler County, south west Ohio, whose pigs naturally came to be described as Polands.

Many breeders tried their hand with the Poland China, especially from the late 1850s to the early 1870s, and the breed began to spread. By 1872 it had become known as the Poland China officially - over the years it had acquired many nicknames, including the Butler County, the Warren County, the Miami Valley, the Poland, the Poland and China, the Great Western, the Shaker, the Union Village, the Dick's Creek, the Gregory's Creek, the Magie, the Moore and no doubt several others. It was time to end the confusion! Harris (1870) quotes an essay on the agriculture of Butler County, Ohio, by the Hon. John M. Milliken who wrote that no county in the United States had produced so many hogs of superior quality as his own county and that of adjoining Warren county. He did his best to trace the history of this highly esteemed local pig but, even so much nearer the time of its evolution, he could only say that as early as about 1820 "some hogs of an improved breed" were obtained and then crossed upon the local Butler county stock and that among the supposed improved breeds there were the Poland and the Byfield - both of them "exceedingly large, of great length, coarse bone, and deficient in fattening qualities." To make up for its deficiencies, the Poland and Byfield cross was "bred with an esteemed breed of hogs then becoming known, and which were called the Big China". Later William Neff imported fine stock from England, including some Irish Graziers which were "white in color, of fair size, fine in the bone, and possessing admirable fattening qualities. Berkshires, about the same time, were attracting much attention, and both breeds were freely crossed with the then existing stock of the county." This had produced excellent results and thereafter the breed was developed by selective breeding with no admixture of any other breed. But he admitted that "they can scarcely be said to have a well-established, distinctive name. They are extensively known as the 'Magie stock.' They are sometimes called the 'Gregory Creek hogs', but more generally they are known as the 'Butler County stock'. It will be doing no one injustice to say that D.M. Magie has bred these hogs as extensively and judiciously as any other man in the county." The writer also admitted that the hogs of neighbouring Warren County had assisted in the formation and establishment of what he wanted to call the Butler County breed.

Harris used the heading 'The **Magie** (Ohio) Pigs' when quoting this writer and said that evidently the Butler County farmers knew how to raise and fatten hogs (he reproduced the writer's tables of slaughterweights for the breed) but that it did not follow that there was necessarily any special merit in the Magie breed, and that "they may be the best breed in the world, but the fact that the credit of the breed is awarded to the county, and not to individuals, does not indicate any special and decided characteristics."

So this pig of many names had quite a chequered history of development in a fairly random manner subject to various genetic influences. That lack of uniformity remained a characteristic of the breed, in that several different breed associations were formed from time to time, breaking away from the "official" herdbook formed in 1878 (and later called the Ohio Poland Record).

It also kept changing type. Before 1870 the Poland China was large, coarse and spongy-boned, with heavy drooping ears, and was spotted with black and white in equal proportions. Then they began to breed it for increasingly more black on the body until it became coloured like the Berkshire, with medium to small ears which still drooped. Until 1895 it was of the early maturing type needed for lard. It had originally been developed in response to the need for pigs which would help market the crops from the new corn belt, which had no readily accessible market as grain because of huge transport problems. Nor was there refrigeration for fresh meat, and pork was much more successfully salted or pickled or smoked than beef or mutton. With river transport available for salt pork, especially fat pork, to good markets in the southern states and the West Indies, the Poland China had found its niche.

Then it began to change shape in response to changing demands. From 1895 to 1912 it was quite large, short-legged and deep-bodied; by 1923 it had become of the extreme "big type" and very long in the leg; after the Second World War, with the development of vegetable fats and the consequent drop in demand for lard, it began to be bred for a leaner carcass and by the early 1940s it had reverted to a medium type but was the heaviest American breed. By 1950 it was black with white nose, forefeet and tail tip, a straight profile, drooping ears, a very broad arching back, good hams and short legs. It was an excellent grazier and a dry-lot pig too, rivalling the Chester White for early maturity. It had tended to overfatten until the years of the Great War, when it became large and slow to finish for a while. After 1935, however, it had become one of the best breeds for a meaty carcass, and the modern Poland China is lean and meaty, a consistent winner of carcass competitions.

Meanwhile the **Spotted Poland China** was being developed from the old spotty type that had been common in the breed before the development of the black type in the 1880s. (One of the original Big China sows of the Shakers had a few spots on her.) Three men from Indiana made a habit of bringing home some Ohio boars and sows from time to time and crossing them with their own pigs in the counties of Putnam and Hendricks, and they developed their own breed with large black spots on white. It became a rugged, useful and profitable farmer's pork producer. Two Gloucester Old Spots were imported from England to boost the breed and create new bloodlines, a move which was not popular with some purists but it did achieve its aim. A record association was formed in Indiana in 1914 to promote the Spotted pigs as a separate family and the breed was known as the Spotted Poland China until 1960, when the association changed its name to the National Spotted Swine Record and voted to call its breed the Spotted Swine, or simply Spots.

The story of the black-and-white belted **Hampshire** breed is less clear than most. Its belted pattern was well known in southern England's New Forest region in the county of Hampshire, though that local pig was not given the county name (it became the **Wessex Saddleback**). Some say that English pigs from Hampshire were brought into Massachusetts during the 1820s by a Boston ship-owner named Mackay; it is unclear whether these were belted pigs but **Mackay** hogs achieved some popularity in the state. It should be noted that the American breed did not acquire the name of Hampshire until the turn of the century.

The Mackay was sometimes known as the **Thin-Rind**. In 1835 Major Joel Garnet brought belted Thin-Rind pigs with him from Pennsylvania when he settled in Kentucky, and they became popular in that state. They were taken thence to Illinois and were often known as the **Rhinoceros** hog as well as the Thin-Rind. Other names for the saddlebacks included Belted, Ring Middle and Ring Necked. An American Thin-Rind Record Association was formed but it was decided that the name was misleading and it was changed to the American Hampshire Swine Record Association in 1904, when it was said that "the breed known in England as Hampshire is, however, of a different type, being black."

it is unclear whether Garnet's pigs were related to the belted Norfolk Thin-Rinds imported from eastern England. However,the belted Essex was not the same as the famous little **Black Essex** which owed its character to a hefty infusion of Neapolitan blood; this improved English breed did come into the United States in 1820 and was most popular among smallholders at the time - it was early maturing and gave excellent results for minimal inputs, especially a large proportion of lard. It was never widespread or commercial but an **American Essex** herdbook was published in 1890, though there were only three volumes: it was simply too delicate and too fat for America at the time and by the 1920s it was already fading. When almost extinct in the late 1960s, it was revived briefly at the Texas A&M University as the **Guinea Essex**, a miniature experimental breed.

Development of the American Yorkshire

The **Yorkshire** is one of the USA's two major breeds: its population expanded very rapidly after the Second World War. Highest numbers today are in Illinois, Indiana, Iowa and Ohio, but it is found in almost every state. The modern type is muscular, with a high proportion of lean meat in the carcass and a relatively thin layer of backfat. It has long since been bred away from the originally imported bacon breed.

The first Yorkshires from England probably came into the United States about 1830, and were introduced into Ohio by 1840, though not necessarily under the name of Yorkshires. The early type was large and white with enormous drooping ears and with wattles dangling from its throat. In about 1850 it was improved by crossing with other breeds but for a while it seems that the breeders were only interested in maintaining its considerable size, an aim in which they succeeded to the detriment of other qualities. Specimens weighing about a thousand pounds were sometimes displayed. At this stage the breed was confined to the northern states and Canada to produce a meatier carcass for Wiltshire-cure bacon exported to England in large quantities. Some of the original American breeding stock came in from Canada.

The Yorkshires which came to Minnesota in the early days possibly originated in Lincolnshire, around Louth, and perhaps had felt the Bakewell touch in their breeding during the 18th century.

In 1893, an American Yorkshire Club was organised as a stock company based in Minneapolis. Its first herdbook was published in 1901 and the first Yorkshire registered in the United States was the boar, Clover Crest A, imported from Canada to Minnesota by officers of the Club. The early volumes included Middle Yorkshire and Small Yorkshire but they were listed separately as distinct breeds. The first registered sow was called Thomas Hester and had been bred at the Clover Crest farm at White Bear Lake, Minnesota, by the Wilcox Company. Illustrations of the Clover Crest animals show dish-faced pigs that are more like Middle Whites than Large Whites, but the Middle type never became well established in the United States, though it was a better fattener. The compact Small type, generally known as the Suffolk, was the earliest to mature, and a good feeder and quick fattener, always fat and "chuffy" on fair keep and never growing to any great size. The most strongly influenced of the three types by Chinese stock, it was too fat for good bacon, nor was it particularly fecund nor a good milker, and it was never of any consequence in American pork production.

Imports continued apace and the breed was rapidly spreading: it was in 39 states by 1910. The fifth volume of the herdbook in 1915 registered 5,299 Large Yorkshires (and but a handful of the Small and Middle types). During its first 64 years, the Club registered 200,000 Yorkshires but between 1957 and 1972 it entered another 500,000 into its record books. In the meantime the breed's fortunes had varied. For example, during the First World War pig fat was in great demand - not just for food but also for the production of ammunition. Suddenly all the recent American breeding *away* from the old lard hogs was reversed, and muscle was rejected in favour of lard. Just after that war, however, the lard market was already disappearing and unfortunately many Yorkshires of the period still had a great deal of Middle and Small Yorkshire blood, betrayed by very dished faces and plenty of lard. Registrations became static and the breed faced a quarter of a century of depression. In 1935 only 150 were registered, but after that nadir they slowly picked up again. After the Second World War, they still lacked in growth rate and were also often not as good as they were promoted to be, and disappointment in performance kept their numbers down. Then, in 1947, fresh blood was imported in the form of the English Large White to save the American breed from itself and a year later the Club's secretary retired after a record-breaking stint of 45 years in the job. An invigorating new era commenced and farmers began to find the Yorkshire more to their liking as breeding stock, at a time when many farms' pig herds were lacking in litter size, good mothering sows, good frame and carcass length - exactly the qualities the Yorkshire could supply. Still a little hesitant after their earlier disillusionment with the breed, some did try it again and this time they were not disappointed. From then on the big white's numbers grew solidly. Improvements and importations continued, including an entire English herd purchased from Ontario in 1955, the year in which the Club presented President Dwight D. Eisenhower with a Yorkshire barrow to help him recover from a heart attack. The pig duly had its photograph taken at the White House, which was quite a publicity coup for the breed. By 1981, registrations were running at more than 220,000 a year and the American Yorkshire now proclaims itself as "the Mother Breed ... and a whole lot more."

Experimental Breeds

Minnesota

A group of new breeds and lines was bred over many years by the University of Minnesota and the Minnesota Agricultural Experimental Station.

The **Minnesota No. 1** <Plate 22> was claimed as the first livestock breed ever to have been developed by adhering strictly to scientific principles. Those principles were the use of a combination of crossbreeding, inbreeding, and selection on the basis of detailed performance records. The latter was inspired by the Danish method of improving its Landrace, and indeed the Danish Landrace was one of the two breeds deliberately chosen as the basis of the new pig for their special qualities: the white Landrace for high standards of fertility, mothering, efficient feed utilisation and superior carcass, and the red English Tamworth, described at the time as having been "long famous for high fertility, good mothering ability, and for the production of lean carcasses." The development programme lasted from 1936 to 1946.

The foundation stock was chosen on the strictly practical grounds of performance, with no attention being paid to "fancy" points, and preference was given during the programme for red animals. The Minnesota No. 1 became a remarkably uniform type and very prepotent in the crosses - it was intended for use in cross-breeding in commercial hog production. Carcasses were superb, with a large yield in the prime cuts, low fat, and excellent streaky bacon.

The breed was red with occasional black spots, a body about 2 inches longer than most American pigs of the time, with a level rather than arched topline. It had a light jowl, slender neck, rather narrow shoulders and full hams: the overall impression was of a V-shape. The legs were short, the bone small and the skin was thin. The snout betrayed the Tamworth: it was rather long, but trim. The ears could not quite decide on their origins: they were somewhere between the erect ones of the Tamworth and the drooping of the Landrace. The final proportions were 52% Tamworth, 48% Landrace.

The **Minnesota No. 2** <Plate 22> was created between 1941 and 1948 from the Canadian Yorkshire (40%) and the Poland China (60%). The original first generation of the cross were all white, as white was dominant, but the aim was to produce black-and-white spotted pigs and the final result was spotted in the same way as the Gloucester Old Spots. The ears were erect, the topline level, and the length was the same as No. 1 but looked less because of a shorter snout.

The **Minnesota No. 3** was a splendid combination of European and American breeds, deliberately chosen to establish a highly heterogenous gene pool. Each breed was chosen for certain qualities. The Welsh (13%) was similar in type and performance to the Landrace; the Gloucester Old Spots (31%) was a minor British breed recognised for its foraging ability and ruggedness in difficult environments; the Large White (12%, and in fact the offspring from an imported Large White boar and a Gloucester Old Spots sow) was chosen for carcass merit and prolificacy; the Minnesota No. 1 (6% - from Danish Landrace and Tamworth) added high fertility, good growth rates and mothering ability; the Minnesota No. 2 (5% - from Canadian Yorkshire and Poland China) produced a lean carcass; the black-and-white **San Pierre** (5% - from Chester White and Berkshire) offered high fertility and heavy birth weights; and the Poland China (21%), from a synthetic "C" line with low fertility and survival as a purebred, gave a lean carcass in the cross with the No. 1. As well as all these, there was the **Beltsville No. 2** (6%), a hybrid from Danish Large White, Duroc, Danish Landrace and Hampshire.

The initial combination of these breeds was somewhat complicated and it is hardly surprising that, to quote the team involved, "Wide variation in superficial traits (e.g. hair and skin colour; head and body type; size, shape, thickness and set of ears) have been observed during the early generations."

Most of the animals showed a resemblance, in head and body type, to several of the parent breeds but some new types also appeared. For example, although none of the original stock displayed the belting factor, it did appear (with variable frequency) after the third generation; and there was even a gilt in that generation with longitudinal striping in her coat, which appeared in varying degrees in each subsequent generation. Ears appeared in various sizes and carriages, too, but although there was considerable superficial phenotypic variance, actual performance variance was not so great.

Not content, they went on to combine Nos. 1, 2 and 3 in the **Minnesota No. 4** but the experiment finally ended during the early 1970s.

Miniatures

In the meantime, between 1950 and 1961, Minnesota also investigated minituarisation and managed to reduce the body size of the **Minnesota Miniature** by at least 29%: it weighed 172 pounds at 12 months old. This small spotted pig for medical research was selectively bred at Hormel Institute, St Paul, by crossing four distinct feral strains to form the basic herd: the **Guinea** (13%) from Alabama, the **Pineywoods** (49%) from Louisiana, the **Catalina Island** (16%) from California, and the **Ras-n-Lansa** (22%) from Guam. The new pig was also known as the **Hormel Miniature** and is now extinct in the USA but was the origin of two other miniatures, the **Göttingen** of Germany and the **Czech**.

Pigs, to their misfortune, have many similarities with humans and are therefore a popular subject for medical research; ordinary pigs, however, are too big (and smelly) for laboratory handling and several miniatures have been developed for such work.

The **Sinclair Miniature**, for example, was developed for USDA in Missouri from the Minnesota Miniature and the **Pitman-Moore Miniature**, the latter having been selected (1969-73) at the University of Iowa's College of Medicine from the **Vita Vet Lab Minipig**, a light grey bred from Florida Swamp pigs (1948 onwards) at Marion, Indiana. And there were more, like the **Hanford Miniature**, developed from 1958 onwards at Pacific North West Laboratory in Washington state from Pineywoods ferals and the **Palouse**, which had itself been bred between 1945 and 1956 at Washington Agricultural Experimental Station from Danish Landrace (65%) x Chester White (35%).

The **Yucatan Miniature** <Plate 24> was selectively bred for smallness from the local pigs in Mexico's Yucatan peninsula, in a programme commencing in 1972 at Colorado State University. It is a grey, hairless little pig which has also been used in Hampshire, England, to develop the **Froxfield Pygmy** <Plate 22> by crossing the **Yucatan** with **Vietnamese** potbellied pigs.

Beltsville

USDA was also involved with pig development at the Agricultural Research Centre in Beltsville, Maryland, to synthesise new character combinations of greatest economic importance to producers. The **Beltsville No. 1** <Plate 22>, bred between 1934 and 1951, was based on the Danish Landrace (75%, for bacon - descended from stock originally imported from Denmark in 1934) and the Poland China (for growth rate, plump hams and black colour). The population was deliberately inbred and a herdbook was opened in 1951 for this black pig with white spots, moderately large drooping ears (but not over the eyes) and typical Landrace conformation - a long body, good hams, and not much trace of the "American arch" to its back. Sows had at least 12 teats, and yearling weights for male and female were 400-600 pounds and 350-500 pounds respectively.

The **Beltsville No. 2** was another inbred mixture (1941-52), this time from Danish Large White (58%), Duroc (32%), Danish Landrace (5%) and Hampshire (5%). It was a red pig with a white underside, occasionally with black spots, and it had short, erect ears.

The **Maryland No. 1**, bred at the Maryland Agricultural Experimental Station between 1941 and 1951 as an inbred line, was based on Danish Landrace x Berkshire, backcrossed first to the Berkshire and then to Danish Landrace, and then bred *inter se*; the proportions were 5/8 Danish Landrace and 3/8 Berkshire. It was a black pig with white spots and erect or semi-erect ears.

Hamprace

The Black Hamprace, later called **Montana No. 1** <Plate 22>, was developed between 1936 and 1948 at Miles City, Montana, from Danish Landrace (55%) and **Black Hampshire** (not belted), crossed reciprocally and backcrossed to both. It was a solid black pig with a small, narrow head and medium-length ears which were erect or slightly drooping. The **Red Hamprace** was a red line (with black spots) which occurred during the formation of the Montana No. 1.

Modern Breeds

American Landrace <Plate 21>

White, lop-eared. Originally from Danish Landrace (imported 1934) and Norwegian Landrace (1954). Breed society formed 1950. Heavy birthweights, ease of breeding, good mothering. Good for cross with Yorkshire.

American Yorkshire <Plate 21>

White, prick-eared. Second most popular breed. Large and long, well proportioned. Face slightly dished. Originated from large white English bacon type. Now found in almost every state, highest populations in Illinois, Indiana, Iowa and Ohio. Sow is very fertile, produces large hearty litters (average 11 born alive) and is excellent mother. Boars renowned for early sexual maturity, prolificacy, prepotency, and siring quick-growing crossbred offspring. Average 21-day liveweight more than 120 pounds (many herds more than 140 pounds). Modern type very muscular, with high proportion of lean meat in the carcass and low backfat.

Chester White <Plate 21>

White, semi lop-eared. Reliable, durable and hardy, outdoor or indoor systems. Originally from early 19th century English imports such as Cumberland, Lincolnshire Curly Coat, Bedfordshire, old Yorkshire early 19th century. Named for Chester County, Pennsylvania. Breed society 1884. Once a practical lard pig, now meat, and no longer so popular. Large litters (especially in crosses) at birth and at weaning - higher average than other American breeds, even outdoors (11.67 born alive, 9.50 weaned). Sow milks well, good mother. Useful for crossing with other whites, Duroc etc. - plenty of hybrid vigour.

Duroc <Plate 21>

Red, semi-lop ears. Leading breed in United States and major breed in many other countries, especially as terminal sire or in hybrids. Origins from Duroc of New York with Jersey Red of New Jersey and others, combined 1860, breed society 1883; known as Duroc-Jersey until 1934. Colour varies from light gold (almost yellow) to almost mahogany; "cherry" red favoured. High daily weight gains, good feed conversion rates. Terminal sire adds growth, strength and robustness to litters from crossbred white sows. Strong legs. Meat taste and appearance good, fattier than some (lean 58.79%, intermuscular fat 3.66%, subcutaneous fat 12.20% in purebred, fat levels slightly higher in crossbred - UK figures); marbled for succulence and tenderness; low PSE and DFD. Some prejudice against colour (deep-rooted hairs in carcass - slaughterhouse must skin carcasses, also of small proportion of crosses); also against past reputation for being too fat and for boars lacking aggression. Some doubts recently about performance of crosses.

Hampshire <Plate 21>

Black with white belt, prick-eared. Well muscled and lean meat breed. Originally from imported English 19th century (possibly from county of that name in England); breed society 1893. Useful as stress-free sire on stress-susceptible meaty Belgian sows; has been used in several European countries as alternative to Duroc. Greatly improved in recent years; boars more aggressive now. Active breed, good rustlers and grazers. Good carcass quality: minimal backfat, large loin eyes; but not the best for processing. Feed conversion efficiency can be as good as 2.0. Average litters 9.2 farrowed, 7.9 weaned. Shiny black with white belt and forelegs; ears originally erect, now rather heavier, and face longer, straighter and more narrow than many - production considered more important than fancy points. Past names have included Mackay, Norfolk Thin Rind, Ring Middle, Ring Necked etc. Widely exported; ranks fourth in United States.

Spotted <Plate 21>

Whitish with black spots, heavy drooping ears. Originally from Poland China and local spotted, boosted in 1914 by Gloucester Old Spots. Breed society 1914, when still known as Spotted Poland China. Major breed in United States, based in Indiana. Also known as Spots. Active, tough, durable and thrifty: excellent outdoor pig. Boars aggressive breeders; sows look after themselves and their litters. Stocky, big-boned, quite heavily built, thick and muscular, with strong legs. More level on topline than some American breeds. Snout of medium length; ears of medium size falling forwards above the eyes. Heavily patched with black splodges (proportion of black varies, and less emphasis now on even, "round" spots.) Practical farmer's pig rather than producer of top quality carcass, though latter is improving.

Minor and Rare Breeds

Fashions come and go, and pig breeders are always quick to respond to them, whether in the show ring or in the marketplace. In the old days, the former was often more important than the latter, but the situation today is reversed. The biggest changes in American pig breeding since the 19th century (suggests Bruce Kalk in the March 1991 issue of the American Minor Breeds Conservancy *News*) have been: (a) from smallholdings with a few pigs for household consumption, to commercial production for distant markets; (b) from lard types to bacon types; and (c) relocation of the industry from the eastern seaboard to the mid west.

The American Minor Breeds Conservancy (AMBC) conducted a census in 1985 to determine which breeds of livestock were in danger of extinction. In the case of pigs, they designated as "Rare" those breeds with less than 500 registrations a year and as "Minor" those with less than 2,000 registrations a year. They also established a "Watch" category, for breeds whose registrations over a 25-year period had shown a steady decline or where registrations were less than 5,000 per year. Breeds with a limited number of bloodlines or limited geographical distribution were included even where numbers seemed relatively high. In addition there is a "Feral" category for stock known to have been running wild for at least a century with no known introductions of outside blood. The breeds were all from those which had been recognised in North America since at least 1900, or which arrived later but were part of a very small world population.

AMBC categorised four pig breeds as Rare, of which two are English breeds (Gloucester Old Spots and Large Black, both also rare in their own country) and two were American (Guinea hog and Mulefoot). The Tamworth, another English breed rare in its own country, was categorised as Minor, and the Ossabaw Island hog as Feral. Two breeds fell into the Watch category: the American Berkshire and the once ubiquitous Poland China.

The **Gloucester Old Spots** <Plate 22>, a large-framed and lop-eared spotted pig, was imported in small numbers in 1985 to Bloomington, Illinois, as a low-input outdoor breed - it was traditionally an orchard pig in England and a renowned mother, but has to be carefully fed to avoid becoming too fat at slaughter. Originally with as much black as white on the coat, the English type today is usually white with only one or two black spots. It is now rare worldwide.

The **Large Black** <Plate 22>used to be widely used in England as an outdoor breed and has often been crossed with whites. A few came into Canada in the 1920s but it has never been numerous in North America. In 1985, however, fresh importations were made to Illinois: Ag-World Exports considered this big, all-black lop-eared breed to be hardy and productive in difficult outdoor conditions. It is also a docile and friendly pig.

Poland China <Plate 21>

Black with white points; drooping ears. Of mixed origin (e.g. Byfield, Russian, Big China, Irish Grazier); colour influenced by Berkshire. Herdbook 1878, united breed society 1946. Developed in south west Ohio and neighbouring states; once the most widespread and popular of America's lard pigs, now with low ranking though beginning to increase in United States (rare in Canada). Large, hardy, meaty carcass, trimmer than it used to be when size was more important than quality. Has frequently changed shape and size over the years. Not outstanding prolificacy or mothering ability or rustling; not very adaptable to intensive systems. Usually black with white legs and white on face and tail tip; sometimes dark with spots.

American Berkshire <Plate 22>

Black with white points, erect ears. The longest history of any breed in America: originally from English imports of a world famous breed, first to North America 1820s. Excellent outdoor pig, careful mother and good suckler, hardy and adaptable, not as prolific as larger commercial breeds. Carcass quality used to be famous (sweet, lean pork), now less so but getting leaner, and growth rates improving. Thrives on good pasturage but also adapts to confinement. Good-looking, consistent, economical; sound legs and feet; thick rump and wide loin; males 500-750 pounds, females 450-650 pounds. American type more muscular and leaner than the current English type of Berkshire. Originally refined by the Neapolitan and thus thinner skinned and generally less coarse than Poland China. Short head, dished face, medium-sized ears erect but tend to droop in older animals. Black with four white legs, white tail tip and white on face - splash of white elsewhere allowed in United States. Colour and hardiness appreciated in hot, sunny regions worldwide.

Tamworth <Plate 22>

Red, prick-eared. Introduced from England in 19th century as bacon producer, subsequently most importations from Canada. Slow maturing, very lean outdoor breed, very hardy and active, an affectionate and intelligent pig and can be quite a challenge to confine. Long in body, legs and face; good sound feet. Medium to large size, not fat - good lean meat, though American tendency to breed away from bacon type for a meatier animal shortened and thickened the Tamworth and it tended to lay down more fat. Used to have excellent fecundity but litter numbers now smaller, though good mothers. Ginger coat (golden red to dark red). Useful cross for hybrid vigour - genetic distance from most other breeds. About 2,000 registered in United States in 1985; now rare in Canada and critically rare in home country. A pig with great character and potential.

Mulefoot <Plate 22>

Black, prick-eared. Syndactyle, i.e. hoof is fused rather than cloven. Known at turn of century in south west United States, some in Texas, Lousiana and Arkansas, and a few in Missouri and Indiana, and said at the time to be common in parts of Old Mexico; origins unclear. Syndactyles have been described elsewhere and in much earlier times - for example, by Aristotle in Greece, Darwin in Britain, also in Sweden. National Mulefoot Hog Record Association formed by Indiana breeders in 1908. Called **Ozark** hogs in southern Missouri and northern Arkansas, and *Casco de mula* in Colombia. By 1910 there were two breed societies and more than 235 registered herds across the country, and also in Canada. Now one of the rarest American breeds; last registry closed in 1975 and only one small herd known to exist (in Missouri) that conform to the original breed standard, though there are lots of other mulefooted animals as syndactylism is seen quite often in pigs. Originally a hardy outdoor pig on high forage diet for bacon and lard, with no particularly remarkable economic traits though claimed to equal other breeds but with greater vitality; said to resist all diseases including cholera. Suggestions that the "mule foot" characteristic might be helpful in solving problem of splaying feet among confined herds. Medium sized pig, black, often with white markings or points. Soft hair coat. Often with wattles on lower jaw. Said to be fairly gentle and used to fatten quite easily, achieving 400-600 pounds at two years old.

Red Wattle

This tasselled pig, sometimes called the Red Waddle, looks something like a Duroc or perhaps a Tamworth/Duroc cross, but with a pair of wattles (influenced by a single gene) hanging from the neck. The Red Wattle was quite a stable breed but has at least three different registries in the United States and is also recorded in the Canadian Swine Registry - it is not clear which of these record the original breed, or whether populations with nothing in common except the wattling gene are included regardless of other characteristics. The AMBC no longer considers it to be a breed.

Hereford <Plate 22>

Red and white, semi-lop ears. Possibly originally from Chester White, Duroc, Poland China and Hampshire up to 1920; breed society 1934 in Missouri. Only 670 registered in 1981. First bred by R.U. Weber of La Plata, Missouri, who refused to co-operate with other breeders and none of the present Herefords trace back to his herd, which was based on common sows in Macon, Adair, Knows and Shelby counties to Duroc, Chester White and Ohio Improved Chester. The first sale was in 1920 and it proved a popular breed largely because of its colour. John Schulte of Norway, Iowa, led a group in early 1920s to re-establish the type using Duroc and Poland China, selecting for type and colour. Foundation stock established 1934 and breed society formed. Fairly popular in the 1940s but soon waned as its performance was only moderate - colour had been the main selection criterion, though Weber had aimed for a good early-maturing butcher's animal, fattening rapidly and economically. Schulte's group in theory also looked for conformation and superior feeding qualities, and they managed to acquire the sponsorship of the Polled Hereford Cattle Registry Association in Des Moines, Iowa, to set up their National Hereford Hog Record Association in 1934, based on a hundred selected animals from several herds in Iowa and Nebraska.

Colour is the hallmark of the breed: red with white head and ears, white legs and belly and white tail tip, similar to the markings of Hereford cattle - hence the name. No known connection with the county of Herefordshire in Britain, though Loudon (1825) said that there used to be a large, useful breed in that county and published an illustration of a heavy-shouldered, lop-eared and long-snouted pig of the old English type, looking similar to his illustration of the old Hampshire but less sprightly, and with no trace of the white-faced Hereford cattle markings.

It has proved difficult to obtain details of the present Hereford, though it is claimed to be prolific, of quiet disposition, a good suckler weaning large litters, maturing at an early age and able with care to reach 200-250 pounds at 5-6 months of age. They are said to be good rustlers, easy to confine in pastures or lots; they are also said to be prepotent, crossing well with other breeds.

Guinea hog <Plate 22>

Black, red or sandy; small erect ears. Probably first imported from Guinea coast of West Africa in slave ships, to United States by about 1804; also in England (18th century), France, Spain. Became a common homestead pig in southern states, but numbers dropped sharply with collapse of lard market and trend towards commercial pork production; a rare breed today. Originally red or sandy, large and square, with long tail and pointed ears; hardy grazers and foragers produced lard and pork on pasture and mast.

The Guinea is now small (15-20 inches tall, 150-300 pounds fully grown) and usually black and hairy. Easy to care for and very gentle, useful for backyard pork production. Investigations in hand to establish relationship between modern and historically documented Guinea hogs.

Ferals

There are probably about three million feral pigs in the United States, and very full details of many populations are given by John J. Mayer and I. Lehr Brisbin, Jr, in their invaluable book, *Wild Pigs of the United States: Their History, Morphology, and Current Status* (1991, University of Georgia Press), which includes a comprehensive survey, state by state, of wild-living domestic stock, the Eurasian Wild Boar and hybrids of these two groups. Returns were received from a very wide geographical spread. In several states the animals are hunted by sportsmen; in others they have been used to breed stock for research laboratories.

With such diverse origins and long periods of random breeding, the ferals show a wide range of colours - including every colour and pattern seen in domestic swine. The most common is all black, closely followed by all red or brown, then black-and-red or brown spotted, and then black-and-white spotted. The least common are tricoloured spotted, and red or brown with white points; red or brown with a wide white belt is also relatively uncommon. In between were whole whites, black with white belt, black with white points, red-and-white spotted, brown-and-white spotted, and various combinations. None of the pigs of domestic origin showed the grizzled colouring of the true Wild Boar.

Razor-back <Plate 22>

At the turn of the century there were some "wild" razor-backed hogs in the Colorado River delta near the borders of Arizona and California. They had sharp tusks and long legs; they were said to be as "fast as horses, shifty as jackrabbits and, when cornered, ferocious as tigers." The tusks of old boars were scimitar-shaped, razor sharp, needle-pointed and enormous - quite a formidable foe. There were not many of them at the time as they had gradually been killed off by Mexican hunting parties for meat. They were said to be descended from domestic hogs taken there in 1886 for a colonisation scheme which was subsequently abandoned. There was also a popular (if unlikely) local belief that these "wild" pigs had interbred with the peccary or javelina and that it was this breeding which had given them their suppleness and their murderous tusks.

Razor-backed hogs were generally found in Arizona, New Mexico, and the swamps of Texas, Louisiana, Arkansas and Florida in the early years of this century but they were clearly ferals: they did not resemble the European Wild Boar. The old razor-backs had been the thoroughly hardy and useful woods pigs which accompanied pioneers as they headed west from the settlements of the eastern seaboard. Ungratefully, these tough and brave old foragers were in due course rejected for "improved" breeds and were dismissed as coarse and illbred. At a state fair somewhere in the Deep South many years ago, the senior hog judge was casting his professional eye over a fine entry of Poland Chinas, Duroc-Jerseys, Hampshires, Chester Whites and such like. To the consternation of all, he awarded the supreme championship to a pen of multi-coloured razor-backs because, he explained, "In this here state, sir, if'n a hog cain't outfit a bar and outrun a man, he ain't fit to *be* a hog!"

There are still plenty of razor-back ferals in the United States, as described in Mayer and Brisbin, though the term is mainly used now to describe the feral hogs of Arkansas, where they are found in the south and in the Ozark National Forest. There have been free-ranging domestic pigs in the state since some of de Soto's swine escaped in the 1540s. From the early years of the 19th century right up to the 1950s it was common practice for farmers in the state to let their domestic pigs range freely, especially in what are now national forests and the large areas owned by paper companies. Many of the present razor-backs have a feral history stretching back several generations.

Ossabaw Island <Plate 22>

Ossabaw is an island of about 35,000 acres some 15 miles south east of Savannah, Georgia. Mrs Eleanor Ford West, resident on the island, knows its feral pigs well and they have also been closely studied by Mayer and Brisbin.

Tradition has it that the animals' ancestors were originally introduced by the Spanish in the 16th century, and this is confirmed by Dr Brisbin, who explains that the early Spanish explorers had on board pigs of the typical mediaeval European village type: small, with heavy hair coats, long snouts, prick ears, and an innate ability to scavenge and survive. Many escaped as the Spanish expeditions crossed south eastern states and they became feral in the bottomland hardwood swamps and forests, where their descendants remain today.

Until the early 1900s (or in some places much later) it was common practice to run domestic hogs in the same forests to fatten on acorns, so that most mainland ferals are now an amalgamation of the original Spanish type with modern domestic breeds. But some of the coastal islands remained free from any significant number of domestics or of human influence in general, and Ossabaw is one of the most notable examples. Here for many years the island's owners protected the habitat and its flora and fauna, including the feral swine.

The animals' main characteristics relate to their need to survive in such circumstances. The most immediately noticeable is the small size; they are almost the smallest in the world, with an average length of 95/96cm and average weight of 21.9/24.0kg, the smaller measurements being those of the males. Similar island dwarfism is seen elsewhere - think of the ponies of the Shetland Islands in Scotland. However, the Ossabaw pigs will grow larger when managed in captivity for traditional production.

The study of the pigs' behaviour has provided several interesting insights. For example, they tend to be very aggressive (except for a few who have become tame around Mrs West's home), especially the boars when sows are ready to mate, and sows with young. It has also been noted that the sows will eat deformed or sick piglets in their own litters.

The Ossabaw pigs' adaptation to periods of famine is to become the fattest wild-living mammals in the world at certain times of year - with backfat up to 8cm thick. They also have unique fat-metabolising enzymes which release enough energy from stored fat for the pigs to survive when times are hard. Associated with this is a form of low-grade, non insulin-dependent diabetes, and the pigs have been used since the early 1970s at the University of Georgia and elsewhere in the study of human obesity.

Over the centuries, only a few domestic hogs have reached the island but they have not had a singular genetic effect on the indigenous population. The pigs are not managed, but the population is controlled by trapping safely with corn-baited traps so that the pigs can be taken to a mainland stockyard at intervals to prevent numbers growing out of hand. It has to be admitted that they do damage the environment; and they destroy the nests and eggs of loggerhead turtles. More than 900 pigs were taken off Ossabaw in the first eight months of 1990 and the aim is to maintain a balance of 500-800.

Most of the animals are solid black and there are also reds, red spotted with white, white-and-black spotted, red-and-black spotted. Mrs West has observed that the bristles of the Ossabaw ferals are different from those of domestic pigs: they have split ends. Brisbin remarks that the bristles are unusually long, averaging 6.8cm on the spine and 4cm on the flank of the boar (6.2cm and 3.7cm on females).

In 1986 the AMBC established a studbook for the Ossabaw Island pigs, taking into captivity three males and three females as foundation stock, and in 1988 collecting eight more to avoid inbreeding.

Brisbin and Mayer point out that feral hogs, globally, are probably the most widely distributed of the wild-living swine morphotypes: they occur in every major realm except Antarctica. In the United States today, there are feral populations in 16 states; there are also, as a result initially of deliberate introductions, free-living Wild Boar (*Sus scrofa*) in New Hampshire and Tennessee, and Wild Boar/feral hybrids in several states.

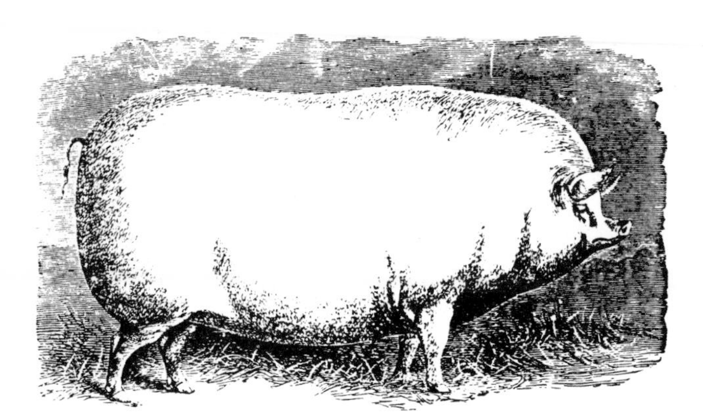

Fig. 21. Jefferson County [Harris, 1881]

LATIN AMERICA

It was in the Caribbean that European pigs made their earliest landings in the New World. These first arrivals were of Spanish and Portuguese origin, accompanying explorers' sailing ships partly as on-board supplies of fresh pork, partly as stock to be left as a food resource for future voyagers, and partly to accompany mainland expeditions as walking larders. The pigs came from Mediterranean lands and found themselves in tropical and subtropical climates; some, though of the same origins, had already become acclimatised by several generations of life on the islands off the African coast where the ships had taken on supplies for their great Transatlantic adventures. The shipboard pigs were a mixture of large Celtic stock and smaller Iberian types, which already had Chinese blood in their veins.

In the Caribbean today there seem to be two main types of native pig, and contrasting ones at that: the most common bears a vague resemblance to the Eurasian Wild Boar in that it is hairy and long snouted, with strongly pigmented skin, while the other (in the words of J.S. Wilkins) looks like "a pigmented, very fat Middle White" and is used for lard production in a few areas where vegetable oils are not available for cooking; it is clearly a partly Chinese pig.

The character of the pigs of five centuries ago is still evident in Latin America. Like the contemporary Spanish and Portuguese cattle, those original pigs found their niche in the New World and exploited it, multiplying at an amazing rate, with the freedom of a whole continent in which to range. They are now considered native to the Americas, superbly adapted to a wide range of local environments, but, like native pigs the world over, they have been threatened by a new wave of European pigs in the present century - pigs which are considered superior for their "improved" breeding. Yet the native pig of Latin America holds its own in Brazil, at least in crosses if rarely pure now, and to some extent in Central America as well. The natives and their crosses form types rather than breeds on the whole and the main ones seem to be the black hairless Pelón group of tropical regions, the miniatures of the Mexican highlands, the small wattled pigs of dry regions, and the Celtic and Iberian groups of land races. Some of the old types are very small and have become the chosen subject of those who breed pigs for laboratory research.

The largest Latin American pig population is in the largest country - Brazil. There were nearly 25 million pigs in Brazil in the 1930s (out of a South American total of 30 million) and today there are perhaps 32 million. It is the home of a wide variety of breeds, old and new. Here the native pig has been taken in hand and improved, whether by selection within the type or by crossing with others. It is only in a few regions - especially Mexico, southern Brazil, Argentina and Chile - that imported breeds play a major role in commercial pig production systems, though only in Mexico and Brazil is the pig industry substantial. Mexico, for example, had a pig population of fewer than 4 million in the 1930s; today it is about 19 million.

Nearly every pig-keeping system seen in Europe and North America has been adopted somewhere in Latin America, including in one special case the old American practice of transporting abundant corn in the form of pig meat. In some of the lower valleys of the Andes, the fertile land has been producing high yields of maize for centuries and it proved easier to feed it to pigs, who could then walk out over the ridges, than to take the grain out by pack mules. This practice continued in southern Bolivia well into the 1970s.

In the Latin American context as a whole, pigs are more efficient than any other red-meat livestock at producing meat from cheap feed - pasture, crop residues, industrial by-products and household garbage. Nor does a pig need much space, and the combination of these factors makes it the ideal backyard source of protein for the family, with the added bonus of plenty of offspring each year for sale or barter.

In 1971, in a report to the FAO's Third Ad Hoc Consultation on Animal Genetic Resources, in Copenhagen, Sr Jorge de Alba (manager of an important demonstration farm in Mexico) drew attention to the "inefficiency" of Latin American pig production. At the time the total number of pigs alive in any one year in the entire region was estimated at about 100 million - almost as much as the total pig population in Europe. More than half the animals were in Brazil, which in some years reported even higher pig populations than those of the USA (60 million). Brazil, however, sent only 10 million pigs a year to market, while the USA sent more than 80 million. Latin America as a whole killed out only about one fifth of its pig population, and produced about 1.5 million tonnes of dressed pork, while Europe's production was about 10 million tonnes.

Although the Latin American pig population could be described in marketing terms as largely inactive, it was acknowledged to play an important role in the peasants' survival economy, to which the native animals were so well adapted. It was difficult to improve productivity either by introducing commercial breeds and systems or by "improving" the local pig. Only in Brazil was any attempt being made to increase the productivity of the natives, and de Alba pointed out the paradox: it appeared that as pig production improved technically, it moved away from the stress elements (nutritional and environmental) that made the native pig so valuable. But it seemed that nobody had done any proper research into the native pig's qualities.

There was little point in improving the native into a more productive but also more demanding pig unless there were the means and incentive to use the better feeding it would require to achieve that higher productivity, and consumers willing to pay the higher price for pork from pigs that had required higher inputs. In Mexico, it worked: the national income level had risen and with it the demand for pork and lard, to such an extent that, with the help of trade barriers against cheap pork imports, producers could achieve good returns in spite of their feed costs being at that time among the highest in the world. But temporary booms do not create a solidly based pig industry, and every pig farmer in a commercial system knows full well how the industry experiences fluctuations from boom to depression in almost predictable cycles. It is a shaky foundation from which to expect careful breed improvement, especially when it entails a completely different way of life for those who keep pigs.

BRAZIL

Pigs are important livestock in Brazil and it is here that the native types have been deliberately developed into true breeds. The European influence is there, too, especially in the south where generations of German and Italian settlers have reared Large White, Landrace and Duroc. Brazil has large numbers of imported commercial breeds which include, as well as these three, Wessex Saddleback and Hampshire. The Landrace was originally from Swedish stock imported in 1955, later supplemented from German, Dutch, Belgian and Danish sources.

The main native breeds today are **Macau**, **Caruncho**, **Moura**, **Canastra**, **Pirapetinga**, **Piau** and **Nilo-Canastra** and there is a good history of their conservation in Brazil. A national research programme for genetic resources was set up in the country in 1974 and it include animal genetic resources in 1981, with particular emphasis on the rapidly disappearing criollo cattle. A few years later the programme was broadened to include pigs and other livestock of local breeds, i.e. those which originated with animals introduced by settlers and which, over several centuries of natural selection, had acquired adaptive and productive traits for Brazil's diverse ecological conditions. The programme set out first to identify and record populations of genetically diluted populations, then to establish characterisation of the germplasm (by bloodtyping and cytogenetics) and to evaluate productive potential, meanwhile conserving the breeds by means of breeding nuclei and the freezing of sperm and embryos where appropriate.

The pigs identified as being in danger of extinction were (in order of rarity) Pirapetinga, Canastra, Caruncho, Moura, Macau, Nilo and Piau. There had been a marked decrease in the population of local breeds in general since the establishment of an industrial structure based on well developed exotics which were crossed with local pigs. The latter were raised by smallholders in low-input extensive systems with low production levels, but the survival rate of the native breeds was very high.

By 1989 EMBRAPA had started its survey to identify nuclei of the local breeds with the help of other organisations and had already drawn up a census of Moura, Caruncho, Piau, Nilo and Canastra. There were private nuclei herds of all except the Pirapetinga, and official herds of all except Macau, Nilo and Canastra. The next step was to study their production potential and to investigate how the fast-growing science of biotechnology might help to conserve what remains of some of the old breeds.

The original pigs brought into the country were primitives from Portugal and from Spain. No doubt there were also some Dutch introductions, especially into Pernambuco, Paraiba and Rio Grande do Norte. The native stock divided broadly into three main types:

IBERIAN (originally from the **Alentejana** or Transtagana): probably a hybrid between Celtic and Asian.

CELTIC (originally from the **Galician** and **Bisaro**): large, late-maturing, from European Wild Boar.

ASIAN (originally from **Cantonese**): small, short-eared, with ample storage capacity, good for fattening.

With a long period of slave-trading between Brazil and Africa, it is more than likely that a few African pigs would have made the voyage too.

By the 1940s the principal types were **Canastrão**, **Canastra** and **Tatú**, broadly representing the three main groups (Celtic, Iberian and Asian respectively). Variations of these types, and products of their random crosses, included Pereira, Piau, Caruncho and Nilo. The Canastrão was the largest and was raised mainly in Minas Gerais. By the 1950s the main breeds included Piau, Tatú, Pereira, Nilo, Pirapetinga, Canastra, Canastrão, Caruncho and Estrélo de Goias, derived from those colonial Portuguese imports. Many of the native pigs were (and remain) simply local primitives of the lard or *banha* type.

It was during the 1960s that they began to be crossed with imported breeds (largely American) so that it became quite difficult to trace the proportions of native and exotic blood. The exotics faced many problems. Brazil has three major climatic zones based on median annual temperatures: subtropical, tropical and equatorial. When temperature and humidity are high, European pigs are under considerable stress. They prefer temperatures in the range of 16-21°C, in well ventilated buildings; above this range, stress increases and both health and performance suffer. Native pigs, however, tolerate high temperatures and also the direct effects of solar radiation (white exotics often suffer from sunburn). Thus exotic breeds, especially whites, are generally confined in ventilated housing, while the native breeds, crossbreds, coloured and synthetic lines can be reared on pasture.

The native breeds which persist can be grouped within the three main types according to original source:

IBERIAN: Canastra

CELTIC: Canastrão and varieties (e.g. Pereira, Junqueira)

ASIATIC or TATÚ: Macau, Nilo, Pirapetinga

There are also those which derive from crosses between the groups or are of uncertain origin, including Nilo-Canastra, Caruncho and Sorocaba in the Asiatic/Iberian group and Moura and Piau in the Celtic/Iberian group. Nearly all are essentially lard types.

Canastrão <Plate 23>

Minas Gerais and Rio de Janeiro.

Largest native breed (200-220kg), of the Celtic type, originally from the black, white or pied **Bisaro** of northern Portugal. Something like the Large Black: usually black, sometimes with white spots. Thick skin, often wrinkled in the adult, abundant short hairs (sometimes curly). Quite a heavy jowly head, with broad snout, concave profile, large lop ears extending forwards over two-thirds of the face, long neck, often with wattles. Late developing (fattens in its second year). Sows fairly prolific, and good mothers, with at least 10 teats. Young reach 18kg at 3 months, 85-95kg at 12 months when they are at least 60cm tall (the strong legs are quite long) and 80cm in length. Fat and bacon producers.

The first colonists brought Celtic pigs of the type known today as Bisaro, Beiroa and Calega, and these three came together to form the Canastraõ. It was probably named for the Serra de Canastra, in Minas Gerais, where many pigs of this type were raised.

There are regional varieties, including a red (which was crossed with Duroc in trials during the 1930s). The **Junqueira**, for example, was developed by a family of that name which improved their Canastraõ by crossing with English breeds. The **Capitão Chico**, or Maranhão, was another variety. The local names for Canastrão varieties include **Zabumba** (in Bahia and Sergipe), **Cabano** (in Paralba and Goias) and the red or **Vermelho** of Goias.

Pereira and Moura <Plate 23>

São Paulo.

The Pereira is possibly a cross between Canastraõ and the Iberian type Canastra, perhaps with some Yorkshire blood, or perhaps mainly Canastra with some Duroc input. It was bred originally by Domiciano Pereira Lima of Jardinopolis. It is a dappled pig, usually grey roan (or black), sometimes with red spots. The loose skin forms folds; the abdomen is well developed, the body deep and the back and loin are broad - it shows a good aptitude for meat production and makes a useful cross with American or English breeds. Average birth weight is 1.097kg and the pigs reach 88kg at 12 months old and 140kg at 24 months. Average litter size 6-8. The broad head has a wide forehead and concave profile, with large semi-erect ears; the legs are short and strong. It has been improved by selection at the government's Santa Cabriela experimental ranch in Sertãozinho.

The **Moura** or Mouro appears to be the same breed, developed for the south from Canastra, Canastrão and Duroc as a meat and lard type with a blue roan or occasionally red roan coat: the grey skin is often covered with a mixture of black and white hairs. It has a medium-sized head with a broad snout of medium length, and semi-erect ears whose carriage is between that of the Duroc and the Landrace; the back and loin are broad, the back slightly arched. There were only 200-300 according to EMBRAPA's 1989 survey but numbers were increasing.

Piau <Plate 23>

Paranaiba river basin in the south west.

The name Piau suggests speckled or painted, and almost any pig with dark spots is called a Piau. The background colour might be white, grey or sandy and the spots, usually black, might be round or irregular. There are large, medium and small types in this group of pigs, some of them the result of crosses with exotic breeds which have been given regional names like Goiano, Francano, Triangula Mineiro and so on. A more fixed and older type is the **Caruncho Piau**, and its new red variety, the **Sorocaba**, which have separate entries below.

In the 1940s the Piau was deemed to be either a variety of the Canastrão or of the Canastra, or a cross between the two, with American blood (mainly Duroc and Poland China). It was found largely in São Paulo, Minas Gerais and Goias and it was a yellowish-white pig with black spots. It had some enthusiastic supporters, who claimed it was the best of the native types, easy to rear for meat or fattening easily for lard as well. From 1939 it had been selectively improved as a proper breed, initially at the São Carlos experimental ranch by A. Teixeira Viana, who produced medium and large types.

The head is of medium size with a straight profile and medium-sized ears either of the Iberian type or small and erect like those of the Asiatic type. It is cream or sandy with black spots, with 70-80% of the body the lighter colour (some are dark roan with black spots) and the smooth hair is evenly distributed over the body. It is a rustic breed, averaging 7.5 pigs reared from each litter (some sows have been known to give birth to 14 in a litter), and could usefully be crossed with exotic breeds for more meat. The weight at birth is about 1kg; it reaches up to 150kg at 12 months, and is considered to be a meat and bacon breed. In 1989 the population was more than a thousand.

Caruncho <Plate 23>

São Paula and Minas Gerais.

This is something like a small Piau; some say, however, that it is a variety of the Asiatic type or Tatú. It is small, with a spotted coat of sand with black patches and smooth hair; the skin is smooth and black. Some pigs are white, black and red-yellow. The head is small, with a short, wide, dished and jowly face, often with wattles under the throat like many other Brazilian pigs; the snout is short and broad, and the ears are either of the small, erect Asiatic type or medium-sized Iberian type - typically the ears point outwards.

It is a lard pig, reaching 90-100kg when fattened, with a deep, rounded body, thoroughly hardy and tranquil by nature. It numbered fewer than 200 in 1989 but the population was stable.

Sorocaba

The Sorocaba is a red variety of the Caruncho deliberately bred to exploit the Caruncho's rusticity by combining it with the lean meat and bacon of the English Tamworth and the precocity of the American Duroc, in the proportions of 3 parts Caruncho, 3 parts Tamworth and 2 parts Duroc. It is a large, red pig with a head and ears of medium size. There are no wattles and the ears are semi-erect. The topline is straight; the legs are of medium length and fine-boned. Boars, when fat, reach 480kg. The typical litter size is 8-9 and the ideal slaughterweights are 40kg for home eating or 75kg for commercial outlets. The backfat depth depends on feeding but is usually 20-30mm; the meat is well coloured and fine grained. The Sorocaba consumes 3-4kg of feed for every 1kg of meat produced.

It is a very hardy breed, essentially a pasture pig, and able to convert grass and legumes efficiently into meat. The sows are good mothers, hardly ever losing a piglet. The colour comes through strongly in the boar's crossbred offspring, 50% of which will be red if the sows are, say, the spotted Piau or the black Nilo.

Canastra <Plate 23>

This widespread Iberian type has a name misleadingly similar to the Celtic type Canastrão and it also has various names in different regions, such as Meia Perna (which means "half leg"). The **Maxambomba** of Minas Gerais and Goias is probably the same. Nationally it is heterogeneous and some are more like the original primitive types introduced from the Iberian peninsula long ago - for example, the **Furão** or Vara variety.

The Canastra is thought to have descended from the Portuguese breed known as Alentejana or Transtagana, and it shows many Iberian characteristics. It is possible that the Alentejana type was crossed in the Canastra's past with the black Berkshire of England.

The Canastra is usually black, though some individuals are spotted or red, and has an abundant coat. Compared with the Canastrão, its head is smaller and lighter, with a subconcave profile, a broad and rather short snout, plenty of jowl, a short, broad neck and medium-sized ears held horizontally. It is a medium-sized pig (adults weigh 150-160kg), with a broad back and a great aptitude for fattening as an important producer of grease, though it is less fat in crosses with improved breeds. It is precocious and fecund, rearing 8-10 per litter, and is useful for extensive or semi-extensive systems, but there were fewer than 200 in 1989.

Canastrinho <Plate 23>

This term is used to denote the third group of Brazilian pigs, those with Asiatic ancestors introduced by Portuguese colonists. They gradually developed into regional varieties of similar conformation but with differences in, say, colours or ear carriage. They are derived from various Asian sources; some were Chinese (often Cantonese), some Siamese, some of Macau (the Chinese port held by the Portuguese from 1557 and the oldest European settlement in the Far East) or of Cochin China (Vietnam).

As a group, these Asiatic pigs are small, with short, compact bodies, well developed stomachs (they are often pot-bellied and sway-backed) and short, slender legs. They are gentle by nature and ideal for smallholders for domestic consumption, particularly as lard producers. Some are prolific, some are not. Some are black, perhaps with a few white spots on the snout or feet and body, while others are red or speckled; some have very fine hair, others are quite hairless; some have wrinkled black skin. The ears are small, short, narrow and erect in most varieties.

An alternative name widely used to cover several local names for the Asiatic type, which is found over a vast area, is **Tatú**, and other local names include **Macau** <Plate 23> for the Cantonese type, also **Nilo**, **Bahia** (in the north east), **Perna-Curta** ("short legs"), **Carunchinho** and others, many of them black hairless house pigs. There are also varieties such as the **Nilo-Canastra** or Tatú-Canastra, the **Pirapetinga**, the **Mandi**, and the **Orehla de Colher** ("spoon-eared"). The name Tatú refers to their armadillo-like heads. They are all good for extensive systems.

The **Macau** (or Macao, Tatú or Bahia) is typical: it has a small to medium-sized head, short snout, broad cheeks and small erect ears which might flop over at the tips, like those of a collie dog. It is black, almost hairless, and with a dipping back. The belly tends to drag on the ground when fattened, or when the sow is pregnant or lactating. Adults reach 70-90kg and are of the lard type. The sows produce rather small piglets but they are able to make good use of cheap, bulky feeds and are very amiable. There were fewer than 500 in 1989.

Pirapetinga <Plate 23>

Minas Gerais.

This pig has been known in the Mata zone for a long time, especially among the estates of the Pirapetinga river. It is clearly of Asiatic origin (some say it is simply a variety of the Tatú which has developed separately in adaptation to its local environment) and is thought to have been introduced in colonial times. It is of medium size, with very fine bones and a good length, its back tending to curve low into a dip. The head is of medium size, with wrinkled skin, a straight profile, broad forehead, protruding eyes and medium-sized erect ears. The skin can be black or rosy - it sometimes looks like iron grey over pink - and is hairless (it looks rather like a rhinoceros!). A rustic breed, and long lived, it can be raised on pasture and makes use of a wide variety of feeds, fattening easily. It is an active and vivacious pig, though a lard type, and can produce good bacon with plenty of grease. Average litter size 6.3 (4.6 weaned), birth weight 1kg; grows to 70-90kg at 12 months of age and 120-140kg at 24 months.

In a series of trials raising the Pirapetinga and the Piau with exotics (Poland-China, Duroc and Berkshire) under the same conditions, the exotics had a higher number of piglets born dead or mummified than the natives. The Piau had much higher post-natal survival rates than any of the American breeds but the Pirapetinga only outclassed the Poland-China in the number weaned. The EMBRAPA survey in 1989 found fewer than twenty pure Pirapetinga pigs.

Nilo <Plate 23>

The Nilo is a small hairless pig of the Asiatic type but best known in its cross with the Canastra - the **Nilo-Canastra**. A similar type exists in Portugal.

The Nilo-Canastra is a black pig with fine, smooth, soft black skin. A little white on the legs or snout is tolerated. The profile is usually straight and the face is broad between the eyes, with a medium-length, slender snout, erect ears pointing forwards, and large slightly prominent eyes. The neck is short, without wrinkles; the body is blocky, broad, long and deep, often sway-backed, and the legs of medium length. Average height 65-75cm; adults can attain weights of 180-200kg. It is a rustic breed and the improved type can be quite precocious, with good, rapid growth; they do well on pasture with supplementary rations. The average litter size is 6-8, average birth weight 0.8-1.0kg. Excellent quality lard and bacon. Crosses well with English and American breeds. The 1989 population was more than 500.

OTHER SOUTH AMERICAN COUNTRIES

Argentina, with its close British links over the centuries, used to be a major exporter of pig meat to the UK. By 1944 Argentina was killing 4 million pigs per annum, 30% of which were Duroc, 30% Poland China, 10% Berkshire and the rest of no particular breed. Today there are still the same number of pigs in Argentina as in the 1930s - four million. Argentina is cattle country.

Venezuela is also largely cattle country but there is an efficient and rapidly growing private pig-farming sector. In 1971 the annual production was about one million animals; by 1975 production was at 1.33 million per annum from the 1.8 million pigs in the national herd; by 1980 the production had jumped to 1.7 million, yielding 70,000 tonnes of pig meat in that year, which met the demands of the home market in full. This was a period during which substantial government resources had been allocated to agricultural and rural development.

These producers are, of course, companies and larger farmers with the money and technology to invest in commercial breeds and intensive systems. By contrast, as elsewhere in Latin America, there are diminishing numbers of subsistence farming families who keep a few pigs, usually of the local type, but many of these people have joined the migration into urban areas.

The **Venezuelan Black** is a group of often semi-feral pigs found on the llanos of Venezuela and Colombia and also on the savannas of Tabasco. The vast plains of the tropical llanos of the Orinoco stretch across Venezuela between the Highlands of the north and north west and the great river to the south, beyond which are the Guyana highlands that cover half the country.

Rather than being household pigs, these tall, strong black criollos often fend for themselves, rooting up tubers and rhizomes in the more sandy areas and quite capable of defending themselves against jaguar attacks. They are not completely wild: there is an annual round-up during which most of the males are castrated and then released so that, in the following year, they can be taken to market, often reaching more than 90kg. It seems that they are no more difficult to load on to a truck than any other pig and just as noisy about the whole business. They have longish hair and are quite long in the snout.

This type is the typical criollo of Colombia and Bolivia as well as Venezuela, though the common Colombian is equally often grey and hairless.

In Bolivia, the British livestock specialist Dr John Wilkins (with the British Tropical Agricultural Mission in Santa Cruz for many years) produced a report in 1983, with Ing. Luis Martinez of CIAT. It described typical pig-keeping in Bolivia's lowland villages and revealed the complexity of traditional systems. The area under study was flat land subject to periodic flooding and high humidity. Most of the local farmers lived in the villages that were strung out along a single and deteriorating north/south road, and the northernmost were frequently isolated when the river's spate prevented vehicular access. Most of the pigs were kept in the villages rather than on farms, in a system of small-scale subsistence production which combined scavenging with backyard breeding. For much of the year the pigs were free about the village, their scavenging supplemented with kitchen waste and with maize and cassava from crops that were either unfit for human consumption or were unsold because the road to the markets was impassable. In the run-up to the harvest, the pigs were penned or tethered to protect the crops and were sometimes given purchased rice bran.

Most villagers possessed only one or two sows, which usually mated with free-ranging boars in a haphazard manner. Young pigs were sold at 4-5 months old. There had been attempts to persuade the villagers to become specialist producers using imported sows but very few were interested.

The pigs were an assortment from natives crossed with improved breeds and the subsequent indiscriminate breeding of their progeny. The true **Bolivian** criollo (black, with longish hair and a long, narrow snout) was locally rare, and the colours of the village pigs <Plate 24> included, in order of frequency, brown, brown spotted with black, brown with a white saddle, black with a white saddle, white with brown or black patches, and wholly white.

The prime reason for keeping pigs was to make up for the lack of banking facilities. Pigs were bought after harvest, when surplus funds were available; they were fed on what would otherwise be wasted crop products, and they were sold when cash was needed, perhaps to hire field labour. One result of this system was that pigs frequently changed hands: of 140 sows included in the 12-month study period, 55 were sold, 12 were slaughtered for home consumption, 17 simply died, and 6 were shot by neighbours for damaging crops just before the harvest. Sows were usually sold within the village, but young pigs (except gilts for breeding) were sold outside and only 2.6% were slaughtered for home consumption.

Farrowing details from 185 litters showed the average litter size to be 7.6 but only 974 of the 1,404 piglets born were still alive at two months of age (a mortality of 31%) and a further 110 died before five months of age (a mortality of 11% of weaned piglets). There was a marked difference in the survival rates on a geographical basis: the most southerly fared much better (with a mean of 6.4 surviving per litter at five months) than the most northerly (only 2.7 surviving per litter).

The results for litter size at birth were surprisingly good in view of the presumably low level of nutrition. The piglet losses were affected by several factors. Hog cholera was locally endemic; foot-and-mouth disease also occurred, and high internal parasite loads were engendered by a combination of high temperature and humidity and the system of management. It was noticeable that sow productivity was in inverse proportion to the distance from the source of veterinary advice and pharmaceuticals.

Yet this system could produce more than ten piglets for sale per sow per year and made their owners a satistactory profit from a short-term investment. The conclusion drawn was that the introduction of exotic sows would not automatically improve fertility and could indeed be counterproductive in view of the problems of access to vaccines, parasite controls and advice. Fertility was not as much of a problem as piglet mortality before and after weaning. Exotics would be even more susceptible to parasites and diseases, and the inputs would therefore be higher even before feeding was taken into account. Wilkins and Martinez rightly concluded: "Both production and profit can be greatly increased in a practicable manner by modifying and not revolutionising the present system of peasant pig production." And that meant conserving the native pigs, not displacing them with expensive exotics.

CENTRAL AMERICA

Most of the native pigs of Central America are slow to mature, with low litter numbers, and many are very small types but they are superbly well adapted to their difficult environments. Brazil is really the only Latin American country to have native breeds in the formal sense; other countries have native pigs that fall into different racial groups but cannot truly be called breeds.

Pelón <Plate 24>

(Mexico to Colombia.)

This black, hairless group of Iberian pigs, well able to survive in adversely hot climates, includes the typical household pigs of tropical Central America. They are very like the Black Iberian group in Spain. The name varies in different regions: the word Pelón means "hairless" and the type is known as **Pelón Tabasqueño** in most of Mexico, or **Birish** in Yucatan, and **Pelón de Cartago** in Costa Rica. It is present in every country from Mexico to Colombia but is most common in the Gulf of Mexico and Yucatan, and in Costa Rica and El Salvador.

An excellent scavenger, with the capacity to make use of bulky, low-grade feeds, it is often fattened as a lard pig on fruit wastes, especially bananas, though for most of its life it survives and becomes plump on handouts or whatever it can find. Boars reach about 90kg, sows about 80kg.

The Pelón's black skin is usually smooth, though some individuals become wrinkled, and has almost no hair. The medium-sized ears are floppy and the snout of medium length. Size and performance vary immensely according to circumstances but the average litter size seems to be 6, and the average birth weight in one of the few studies concerning the Pelón was 1.38kg, with an average weaning weight of 8.78kg. A notable quality of the type is that losses at birth and up to weaning are negligible.

Yucatan Miniature <Plate 24>

Mexico's Yucatan peninsula is hot and arid. The local type of Pélon is smaller and is slate grey, with a shorter snout. It is raised for lard and meat and is noted for its exceptional intelligence and docility, qualities which attracted the attention of laboratory workers in the United States who needed easily handled pigs for medical research. In 1960, they set to work to miniaturise some Yucatan stock by selective breeding and have succeeded in reducing the mature weight from 75kg to 30-50kg - the goal is 20-25kg. These grey, hairless Yucatan Micropigs (a registered name) are in proportion: there is no dwarfism, nor is there any reduction in breeding ability. They have the additional bonus of being almost without odour.

Cuino

(Mexico.)

Up in the Mexican highlands there is a group of true miniature pigs, weighing 10-12kg at the most. They are probably the smallest domesticated pigs in the world and are Chinese remnants but do not have the dipped backs so often associated with the pigs of south east Asia. The colours include black, spotted and yellowish.

F.D. Coburn, whose book *Swine in America* was published in 1909, was earnestly advised that this pig of Old Mexico was the product of "crossing a ram and a sow". It was claimed that a ram was traditionally kept with sows from the day it was weaned, the sows being of any kind but usually the typical razorbacks that were common ferals in the southern United States and Mexico. The progeny of "this rather violent combination" was said by a Mexican resident to be "a pig - unmistakably a pig - with the form and all the characteristics of the pig, but he is entirely different from his dam if she is a Razor-Back. He is round-ribbed and blocky, his short legs cannot take him far from his sty, and his snout is too short to root with. His head is not unlike that of the Berkshire. His body is covered with long, thick, curly hair, not soft enough to be called wool, but which, nevertheless, he takes from his sire. His color is black, white, black and white, brown white. He is a good grazer and is mostly fed on grass, with one or two ears of corn a day, and on these he fattens quickly. The Cuino reproduces itself and is often crossed a second and third time with a ram."

Whatever the truth of its parentage, the Cuino was the most popular breed in the state of Oaxaca in the late 19th century, because of its propensity to fatten on very little. Ignoring imaginative tales of ancestral rams, the genuine Cuino was still very popular in the 1920s in the corn-growing areas of the highlands and had adapted to being fed almost entirely on maize. It was probably first imported from China during the 15th century at a time when there were regular galleon trips between Acapulco, the Philippines and the rest of east Asia.

This miniature was ideal for its environment and fitted in well with the local economy, which fluctuated with the success or otherwise of the corn crop. The region is dry and there are periods of successive crop failures, during which the feeding of a large pig would have been a serious strain on a family's resources. The Cuino, though, was much less demanding and could survive during the lean years, ready for fattening in the good.

The name Cuino was applied to all small pigs, whether or not they were the true miniatures. There were plenty of them in the 19th century but they began to disappear as improved pigs moved in from North America and some of the last of the miniatures were photographed by Jorge de Alba up in the mountains of Sonora and Chihuahua (where the dogs are also tiny). They were considered for use in medical research but the idea was dropped when it was discovered that they were far from prolific, usually producing only two or three in a litter. The true Cuino is possibly already extinct.

Mexican Wattled

There are pigs of assorted colours in Mexico known locally as Cerdo Coscate. They are notable for their wattles. The pigs are quite small, usually no more than 60kg when mature. They are very hardy and active, and are adapted to their dry environment: they are strong in the leg and back and well used to ranging widely to find scarce food. Most are red, or black spotted.

Honduras Switch-tail

In the central mountains of Honduras is a small native pig, weighing up to 50kg, which is traditionally brought down from the mountains to fatten in the valleys. These pigs have good, hard feet, which is a great asset during the migration when the herd might have to walk for several weeks under the watchful eyes of the swineherds. Jorge de Alba saw such a herd heading towards Choluteca Honduras on the fortieth day of the journey: the pigs were moving at a brisk pace, picking up berries and fruit as they went, and also catching insects along the river valleys. They looked not only healthy on such a regime but were also clearly gaining weight. Their most striking characteristic was a tail about 30cm long with a hairy tassel, which the pigs switched to keep the flies away. The type is probably now extinct.

CARIBBEAN

The delicate balance in use between native pigs and imported breeds is well illustrated in Haiti by a situation which could have occurred in any region of Latin America and could be a useful lesson worldwide. Traditionally, almost every family kept at least one pig, of the **Haiti Creole** type <Plate 24>. This native scavenger required very little capital outlay or attention: it was good at foraging on wasteland and utilising crop residues; it provided manure and a popular meat for the household; it was the family's "bank", acting as a major source of ready cash in times of need. With a handful of such pigs, the family could also set up a little cottage industry in processed pig meat for sale from roadside stalls and at markets.

In 1978, it was discovered that African swine fever was present in Brazil, the Dominican Republic and Haiti. The epidemic hit hardest at the small farmers who did not have the larger commercial producers' resources to minimise the risk of infection. In Haiti, 30,000 pigs were dead within a month. By April, 1980, the total was 300,000 and another half a million pigs had been sold off at low prices to butchers who were spreading the rumour that the government was about to order mass slaughtering.

The rumours were correct. USDA opted for a policy of the total elimination of the island's creole pigs as a means of controlling the disease and every single pig was slaughtered. USDA the noffered to restock the island with commercial American breeds and tried to encourage farmers to set up the type of modern pig units to which the imported pigs were best suited, which meant that only a few farmers could afford to keep any pigs at all. Those that could soon found themselves in trouble because of a lack of experience in intensive management.

Some of the Haitian and French non-government organisations suggested that it would be more sensible to use hardy creoles in extensive systems. The French set about designing the perfect breed to suit the economic, cultural and environmental conditions in Haiti, aiming for a rustic type of pig but more prolific and productive than the eradicated local type. The project began in 1986 and the foundation they chose included 65 creole pigs (*porc planche*) from Guadeloupe and 89 **Sino-Gascony** <Plate 15>, a first-generation cross between the old black Iberian Gascony breed of south west France and two Chinese breeds, the Meishan and the Jiaxing Black. The rare Gascony was hardy, robust and black-skinned (a useful trait in the tropics) and a notably good mother. The small Chinese pigs were known above all for their high prolificacy. This project is now at the stage of monitoring various combinations of these breeds <Plate 24> to find which is best for the family small holdings of Haiti.

The **Guadeloupe Creole** <Plate 24> was decended from 15th century Spanish pigs which became feral and over the centuries, mixed with introductions such as Large Black , Yorkshire, Duroc, Hampshire, Normand and Craonnais. The result was a polymorphic population displaying a whole gamut of colour - black, spotted, grey and so on. The type is rustic and sexually precocious, with typical litters of 7 or 8 at birth, and the sows are excellent mothers. Liveweights at 140 days range from 25-85kg and the carcass is relatively fat, but the meat is much in demand locally for its good quality.

In Guadeloupe, the French produced improved pigs suitable for local conditions by combining the precocity, maternal qualities and rusticity of the Creole with the good growth rates and conformation of the Large White and the prolificacy of the Chinese Meishan, Jinhua and Jiaxing Black. They have had the sense to exploit the thoroughly adapted native pig rather than to replace it with unsuitable exotics, and are continuing that process in Haiti as well. And that, perhaps, is the message of this book: that the irreplaceable value of the indigenous pigs should be recognised and that they should, wherever possible, be saved from extinction. Even if their qualities seem irrelevant today, they may well be vital in the future.

APPENDICES

APPENDIX 1

THE PIG BREEDING COMPANIES OF THE UNITED KINGDOM

After the Second World War the pig farmers of the UK found that, like poultry farmers but in contrast to cattle and sheep farmers, they were without subsidies. Although it was uncomfortable for them at the time, it turned out to be a blessing in disguise in that they had to be particularly efficient simply to survive. Both the pig and the poultry sectors turned disadvantage to advantage.

They began to specialise and the breeding of parent stock became a separate function from the rearing of pigs for meat. It had long been the practice for livestock farmers to bring in replacement males so that they avoided inbreeding within their herds. The next step came when a small group of breeders improved their stock to a high degree so that producers could also import replacement females from them. For large-scale producers, this was an important step in increasing efficiency.

Then pig farmers took a long, hard look at their outgoings and decided that feed costs were a major consideration. They realised that a good understanding of pig genetics could save the industry's bacon, so to speak: they needed to breed pigs with the highest possible feed conversion efficiency - a factor which is highly heritable. They also needed excellent growth rates, and at the same time were aware of the rapid changes in public tastes away from fat and towards very lean meat.

In the early 1960s, the UK pig breeding industry was still dominated by pedigree breeders, some of whom seemed to have more interest in the show ring than in the market place. Many commercial producers felt that the industry had become bogged down and that even the pig-breeding schemes of recent years had failed to meet the needs of commercial farmers or of consumers. A new spirit of initiative became apparent as some breeders began to form co-operatives or companies with the objective of supplying improved breeding stock (male and female) to commercial pig farms, and in some cases to work directly with retail outlets as well. The key to their success was the production of hybrids.

The stories of some of those pig breeding companies are outlined below and some of their products, which have been widely exported, are illustrated in <Plate 5>. Their emphasis on hybridisation might send a few shudders down the spines of purists, especially those whose concern is for the future of rare breeds, but many appreciate that it is in the companies' interests to ensure the survival of as many pure breeds as possible: they are their seed corn for the future.

There are, broadly, two types of pig breeding groups: substantial companies deeply involved in research and development on the one hand, and co-operative groups of farming families actively producing breeding stock for others, often with the guidance of a geneticist.

Pig Improvement Company (PIC)

In 1962 a group of half a dozen farmers in Oxfordshire decided to pool their resources and set up a company, on a 400-acre disused airfield at Fyfield Wick, to produce their own disease-free replacement stock of gilts and boars for intensive systems. They based the project on a boar performance testing model which combined feed conversion efficiency, individual growth rates and ultrasonic backfat scanning. Their foundation stock of breeding sows was based on Large White, Landrace and Welsh.

The nucleus herd formed the basis of the company's selection and crossbreeding programmes but PIC soon began to scour the world for useful breeds. For example, in 1968 it introduced American **Duroc** genes into its breeding programme and in the 1980s it turned to China and the **Meishan**. The intention was to find different products for different national markets and to work with large numbers of pigs so that recording and testing was on an acceptably large sample. PIC kept dam and sire lines separate, concentrating on the reproduction performance of gilts and sows, and on the progeny's growth and carcass characteristics through the boar lines.

Within seven years of its establishment, PIC found itself supplying a tenth of all the replacement gilts sold in the UK. It also had associate companies in France and Germany, and was involved in a huge scheme to ship a substantial order for breeding stock to revitalise the entire Bulgarian pig industry. Its major F_1 hybrid gilt, the **Camborough** (named after Cambridge and Edinburgh, two vital sources of support and advice) had been introduced in France in 1965/6 by setting up a "clone" arrangement. The company soon entered similar schemes in Italy, Canada, Germany and Mexico, usually providing the stock and the knowledge to a partner who supplied production facilities and marketing.

In 1970 the feed company Dalgety invested in what was by then a highly successful breeding company stretched to its physical and financial limits by its rapid growth. In 1967 it had sold 600 boars and 6,000 gilts (only five years after its inception) and it would increase both those figures a hundredfold, worldwide, twenty years later. It now has wholly owned companies in the United States, Germany, Spain, Portugal, Denmark and Mexico as well as in the UK, and associated companies in fifteen other countries, with agents in five more, so that it can tailor its product to suit local needs. More recent projects have been launched in Cuba, China and the Ukraine, supplying stock and providing technical back-up with production, veterinary and distribution support.

After initially selecting within and crossing between its original breeds, PIC has since added several major breeds and is investigating many others. In 1972 the UK's boar licensing scheme ceased and PIC was free to introduce crossbred boars, a system widely used in the USA and France. At the time of writing there are 25 basic lines producing four main gilt products and about 14 specialised boar products. The best known are: the **Camborough** parent gilt (Large White x Landrace, or vice versa), which is now hyperprolific; the **Camborough Blue** outdoor hybrid gilt (Saddleback with Camborough blood), which tended to be too fat and was replaced for the UK market by the leaner but equally prolific **Camborough 12**, an outdoor type crossed to PIC HY or Large White boars for large litters of strong, heavy pigs grading well at heavier weights. The PIC boars include terminal sires such as the 200 (free from the halothane gene), the 300 (lean at bacon weights with ad lib feeding) and the 400 (meaty with high killing out % and hybrid vigour). The HY boar was developed originally in response to German and French demands for well muscled boars on the Camborough bacon-type gilt and is a careful combination of Large White/Landrace, Piétrain and Belgian Landrace.

Masterbreeders

Masterbreeders (Livestock Development) Ltd. was created from a very different basis - it was the result of a merger in 1979/80 between two pig breeding companies which were wholly owned subsidiaries of the UK's largest pig meat manufacturer, Wall's Meat Company, and the largest animal feeds company, BOCM Silcock.

Initially run by Unilever, Masterbreeders became a private company in the mid 1980s but maintained strong links with both its progenitors, which contributed to its research and development programmes. Its pig improvement programme had started in 1957 with a detailed evaluation of the merits of the country's major pig breeds; it later concentrated on separate sire and dam lines of Large White, Landrace and **Westrain** (which originated from a combination of Piétrain and Wessex Saddleback) and also acquired a **Duroc** herd.

Under the guidance of geneticist Dr Rex Walters, the company developed what it described as "fast tier genetics". It also produced a pregnancy detector for pigs, and the Walsemeta pig service indicator. By 1972 Masterbreeders AI Limited, a separate company, was providing 64% of all UK pig inseminations, and in 1978 it designed a major AI station in Spain. Similar arrangements were set up in other countries, including for example South Korea in 1987. The service was developed from that of Walls, which had started it in 1962 as a method of reducing the genetic lag in nucleus and multiplier herds.

Stock from Masterbreeders has been exported to many countries. As well as purebred Large White, Landrace and Duroc gilts and boars, the products included: the improved white **Mastergilt** hybrid (from Large White and Landrace, with good qualities in farrowing, conformation, constitution and docility); the hardy blue **Sovereign** gilt (based on Westrain and Landrace, which were originally used in the formation of what was initially marketed as the **Monarch** blue gilt for economic production in very rugged conditions); the improved white **Sterling** hybrid gilt, containing Duroc blood for a rugged constitution; and the **Meatmaster 555** terminal sire from whites and Duroc for progeny with a high lean content.

National Pig Development Company (NPD)

This Yorkshire company was established in 1969 by the Curtis family, who began a breeding programme in the 1950s. Initially it was known as the Northern Pig Development Company but it became one of the largest pig breeding companies in the UK and changed its name to reflect the scale of its influence.

At the time of NPD's establishment, the Pig Industry Development Authority (PIDA) had become part of the Meat and Livestock Commission (MLC) and the word went out: hybridise for heterosis. Initially NPD had one pure-breeding pedigree Landrace herd within a traditional mixed farming system and undertook painstaking recording and lengthy progeny testing, sending animals for central performance testing in common with other pedigree breeders. It implemented a selection programme with the MLC's help, testing and crossing the UK's two official and prolific white breeds - Landrace and Large White - to produce the **Manor Hybrid**.

NPD continued with its own performance testing, with the emphasis on feed conversion, growth rates, carcass quality and the relationship between feed and lean. They began to test females as well as boars, and tested individuals and batches on feed conversion. It was a period when the whole pig industry was struggling to survive: the UK was not then in the European Common Market and NPD found itself having to pay a subsidy to Brussels when it began to export its new Manor Hybrid. But in a way the struggle built the company's strengths and made it that much more determined to breed thoroughly tested hybrids on the criteria it had already chosen. Detailed testing remains the foundation of company policy today.

The company stayed faithful to Landrace and Large White, both of which were prolific, and the programme became more complicated as it began to produce a specialist terminal sire line, hardy outdoor females and lines selected for improved reproductive performance and meat quality. It developed the **Hamline**, a synthetic white or coloured meat sire (but a registered breed) bred to produce a larger ham by carefully introducing Piétrain, Duroc and Hampshire to the Welsh, Landrace and Large White, to combine the ruggedness of the North American pigs with the efficiency of the British. The outdoor **Manor Ranger** gilt is a first cross between the Hamline and the Landrace, giving colour for an outdoor pig.

In the mid 1970s NPD set up an overseas division. It established a network of nucleus and multiplier farms in other countries - in Africa, for example, and Canada, Holland, Italy, Japan, Spain and the Philippines, all supplied with original UK stock adapted to the different climates and management systems. It continues to export its breeding stock to other European countries (especially France) and to the Far East and South America. It has just started a major and ambitious project in the United States. In the UK it owns and manages eight nucleus breeding units and multiplier units, retaining control to ensure strict implementation of its selection principles, the regulation of health status and the maximisation of quality control.

NPD has actively pursued the industry's research into increasing prolificacy with the help of Chinese breeds and in the early summer of 1992 it announced the new **Manor Meishan** hybrid <Plate 15> - the UK's first commercial Meishan crossbred. It is one quarter Meishan, one quarter high-litter-size Large White and one half high-prolificacy Landrace and is said to be capable of producing more than 30 pigs per annum. It boasts early sexual maturity, at least 14 teats, high farrowing rates, docility and mothering ability, though growth rates and feed conversion efficiency are slightly reduced - but this can be improved in that it crosses well with Large White or Hamline boars, from which the progeny can grade to all slaughter weights. Current MLC trials show averages of 59.5% lean, 9.4mm P2 backfat (at 72.2kg) using NPD's lean boar lines to counteract the inherently poor Chinese carcass characteristics. MLC eating quality tests suggest a third more marbling fat and reduced drip loss.

The Meishan was introduced into the UK in 1987 for a co-ordinated breeding research programme involving four of the breeding companies and the government.

Cotswold Pig Development Company

The story of this research-based company goes back several decades. In the 1930s John Angell began poultry farming in the Cotswolds and by the 1940s his Ardencote herd of Large White pigs had become established and was proving its worth in the show ring. In the 1950s Angell became president of the National Pig Breeders Association (now the British Pig Association) and was much involved in the association's establishment of Britain's first pig progeny testing station, at Selby in Yorkshire, which was later taken over by PIDA.

In 1961, realising the importance of applying to pig breeding the scientific principles already being used in poultry breeding, Angell and a local feed company formed the Cotswold Pig Development Company. Its gene pool was founded on selected animals from several breeds and in due course the company bred and marketed the **Cotswold**, said to be "the world's first proprietary mammal".

Ten years after its inception, the company was acquired by the Lincolnshire-based Nickerson Group, whose activities already included plant breeding and duck breeding (Cherry Valley ducks) using soundly based genetic principles to improve efficiency. By the mid 1970s, new pig facilities had been established in Lincolnshire using the same principles of genetic selection in the production of pig breeding stock. By the 1980s, Cotswold stock was being exported to at least thirty countries but the company continued to develop its own technology in its search for genetic superiority - including AI, and the statistical technique known as BLUP (Best Linear Unbiased Prediction) to analyse data on individual pigs and families, for accurate comparison in different geographical situations.

By 1990 the company's total population of breeding sows numbered more than 4,000. The company's stated aims in 1992 were to create the maximum possible genetic improvement and to transfer that improvement to customers through the ability of Cotswold products to produce pig meat of the highest quality at low cost. That meant high growth rates for lean tissue, large litter size, good yields of quality lean meat, and physically sound stock; it also meant remembering that, ultimately, consumers' demands decide what should be produced. The company has achieved notable improvements since the early 1960s, a time when a good bacon pig took 200 days to reach slaughterweight and would have an FCR of 3.7 and a backfat measurement of 25mm; today on a commercial unit the average Cotswold pig can reach slaughter weight in 160 days at 2.25 FCR and 12mm backfat.

In common with others, the company had begun with only Large White and Landrace stock, which were kept as closed populations and improved. In 1986 the Large White type line was divided into separate sire and dam lines, to allow more rapid and acurate selection for different traits, and in 1987 a new group nucleus scheme made its debut using the company's own AI station and its innovatory BLUP system. Dr John Webb, previously with the national Animal Breeding Research Organisation (ABRO) at Edinburgh, became Cotswold's geneticist. The hardy red Duroc was introduced during 1987 into the outdoor lines the company had already developed, and in 1991 it exhibited what was probably the world's first *white* Duroc in response to UK prejudice against colour in the traditional "crackling" on a pork joint.

The Duroc contributed to the company's hardy, prolific and docile outdoor **Cotswold Gold** gilt, bred for maternal ability and lean growth on free-range systems, but also for intensive ones, especially where robustness is needed. Other products include the white **Cotswold Platinum** hybrid gilt, a first cross with maximum hybrid vigour, and a range of terminal sires, especially the **Cotswold 16**, selected over 15 years for growth rates, FCR and lean content, the **29** (F_1 cross of unrelated lines) and the **90**, which combines the qualities of the 16 with the Duroc's ruggedness. The highly prolific **Meishan** is being assessed to see if its prolificacy can be incorporated into the company's breeding programme.

Cotswold pigs have been exported to some 36 countries, the main overseas markets being in the European Community, the Far East and North America.

Peninsular Pigs

This breeding company is unusual in that it has formed a direct link with major retail outlets. It is essentially market-led, with close co-operation between the breeding company, the pig farmers, the retailers and the processors. The emphasis is firmly on eating quality and on the concerns of consumer rather than only those of the producer.

The company was originally formed in 1973 by six pig breeders in south west England (its headquarters remain at Frome, in Somerset) who were using Landrace and Hampshire. It now retains a nucleus herd of more than 400 breeding females including Large White (for outstanding FCR and daily liveweight gains), Landrace (for carcass characteristics, low backfat, fine bone structure and the milkiness of the sows), Hampshire (for the lean percentage of the loin and rump, its good flavour, and also its robustness, hardiness, strong legs and good mothering) and Duroc (for the outstanding eating quality of its marbled, succulent meat, and also its robustness). These supply the company's multiplication farms which, in turn, supply parent gilts to customers at home and abroad. The company's hybrid outdoor female, the **Hampen**, benefits from Hampshire and Landrace genes.

Peninsular has long been involved in outdoor pig systems: it established an outdoor herd in 1979 largely in the interests of pig welfare, but also for economic reasons and because nobody else seemed to be doing it. Public concern for animal welfare agreed with Peninsular and in the late 1980s the company was already in a good position to supply the growing demand for meat from outdoor stock. It has reached an agreement with ASDA to supply welfare-friendly "conservation grade" pork, for example.

It had also been concerned that modern pork had become "bland". In 1981 it began to discuss this problem with the giant retailer, Marks & Spencer. A scheme was developed and was in production by 1985. That year Peninsular Pigs abandoned indoor systems and continued to progress as outdoor breeders and producers in co-operation with M & S. By 1991 all M & S fresh pork in England, Wales and Scotland was produced from the Peninsular programme, and all the pigs were bred in outdoor systems. The basis of the M & S pork was the **SPM** pig from a Duroc boar on a Hampen gilt, the robust progeny of which are large-eared tan-and-whites (often belted), bred deliberately for fresh, tender, succulent pork, rather than being immature baconers used for pork. The initials SPM were derived from the three main elements of the programme: processors Scotbeef (who lease Peninsular boars to selected farmers rearing sows, and then process their pork), breeders Peninsular Pigs (who sell breeding stock to Scotbeef), and retailers Marks & Spencer (who buy the meat already wrapped by Scotbeef). M & S has no financial investment but controls the programme from breeding to packing.

Newsham Hybrid Pigs

This company, like NPD, is based in Yorkshire - at Malton. Its stock is based on Large White and Landrace in various lines and combinations and it has also introduced some improved lines of Duroc and Piétrain. The key factor is the pig's efficiency at converting feed into lean meat and the company builds on the tried and very successful traditional backcross system of Large White x (Large White x Landrace) by using the other breeds to ensure flexibility in meeting changes in public tastes, whether in meat or in animal welfare.

Whilst acknowledging that Large White and Landrace are ideal terminal sires for markets such as bacon production, Newsham has selected these traditionally dual-purpose breeds as the basis of their female crosses and is therefore emphasising their reproductive performance. It has developed a **High Conformation White** from the Large White, as an efficient and heavily muscled terminal sire to produce carcasses with a high lean percentage. The Duroc, effectively a dual-purpose breed, has been selectively bred by Newsham so that it retains its characteristic robustness and strength but is also more lean and efficient than its American ancestor. Newsham's Duroc cross females are prolific, maternal outdoor sows and their offspring have the well known Duroc meat marbling. The company also offers a "quality lean" terminal sire (Duroc and HCW) and a "high lean" hybrid boar for coloured gilts.

The company has been using the Piétrain as a terminal sire, and crossbred boars (Piétrain with HCW or Large White) for continental markets. It has companies in Germany and the United States and, with the recent appointment of agents for Japan, Thailand and the Philippines, Newsham Hybrid Pigs now operates in 18 countries.

The company offers its own purebred Landrace, Large White, Duroc, Piétrain and High Conformation White boars, and Landrace and Large White females. Products include two basic crossbred parent females: the **Line 21** gilt, (traditional Large White/Landrace cross) and the **Line 32** outdoor gilt (Improved Duroc x Landrace). There are also threeway and fourway crosses.

Premier Piglink

Premier Pigs was established in 1965 by leading Large White and Landrace breeders and was enlarged in 1991 by a merger to become Premier Piglink, based in Cambridgeshire. The nucleus herds include Large White, British Landrace, Welsh, Hampshire and Duroc. There are multiplication units in Holland as well as the UK and it has supplied breeding stock to more than thirty countries. It specialises in the genetic division within the breeds for female lines and meat lines, and is unusual in having the **Welsh** as a major female line for sow longevity and for a higher rate of pigs born alive per litter.

It has concentrated on its separate male and female lines for more than fifteen years and has achieved high sow fecundity in the females, with maximum economy of production and carcass quality in its **Meatline** terminal sires. Specific Meatline sires include the **Hampline** hybrid based on the Hampshire, with good libido and strength, heavier litter weights and weaning weights, high percentage of lean, low PSE (for the butchery trade), the **Euroline** (selected from Large White lines for meat carcasses to suit the EEC classification system, with high ham and loin yield and low fat), and the **Norline** (selected from superior specialist meat lines in Large White and Landrace for long lean carcass and low fat). The hybrid gilts include the **Premier** and also the **Tribred**, a very hardy and prolific "blue" outdoor gilt from nucleus grandparent Tribred x nucleus Welsh landrace, which is crossed to Meatline boars for pork, cutter and bacon production.

APPENDIX 2

SOME OF THE EXTINCT BREEDS OF THE WORLD

EUROPE

CZECHOSLOVAKIA
Rychnov

FRANCE
Amelioré
Bayeux
Bigourdain
Boulonnais
Bourdeaux
Breton
Bresse
Cazères
Charolais
Corrèzze
Craonnais
Dauphine
Flemish
Loches
Marseilles
Miélan
Montmorillon
Piégut

GERMANY
Bavarian Landrace
Bronze
German Berkshire
German Cornwall
German Land Pig
German Pasture
German Red Pied
Güstin Pasture
Hoya
Meissen

HUNGARY
Ancient Alföldi
Bakony
Szalonta

ITALY
Abruzzese
Apulian
Bastianella
Borghigiana
Catanzareze
Chianina
Cosentina
Faentina
Forlivese
Friuli Black
Fumati
Gargano
Garlasco
Lucanian
Lagonegrese
Maremmana
Modena Red
Murgese
Parmense
Perugina
Reggitana
Riminese
Romagnola
San Lazzaro
Valtellina

POLAND
Large Polish Long-eared
Polish Marsh
Polish Native
Pomeranian Large White
Small Polish Prick-eared
White Prick-eared

ROMANIA
Transylvanian

SPAIN
Andalusian Blond
Asturian
Baztán
GalicianLermeña
Galician
Majorcan
Vich
Vitoria

SWEDEN
Old Swedish Spotted

UNITED KINGDOM
Black Essex
Black Suffolk
Cumberland
Dorset Gold Tip
Large White Ulster
Lincolnshire Curly Coat
Manx Purr
Old English
Small Black
Small White
Yorkshire Blue and White
(and many other 19th century)

YUGOSLAVIA

Bagun
Black Mangalitsa
Krskopolje Saddleback
Šiška
Šumadija

RUSSIA AND THE STATES OF THE FORMER U.S.S.R.

Alabuzin
Chausy
Dnieper
Dobrinka
Don
Ievlev
Imeretian
Kalikin
Kama
Kartolinian
Krolevets
Lesogor
Meshchovsk
Moldavian Black
Omsk Grey
Podolian
Polesian
Rossosh Black Pied
Siberian
Slutsk Black Pied
Ukrainian

ASIA

HONG KONG

Fa Yuen
Kwangchow Luan
Wai Chow

TAIWAN

Meinung
Taichung
Taiwan Small Black
Taiwan Small Red
Tingshuanghsi

AMERICA

UNITED STATES

Beltsville Nos.1 and 2
Cheshire
Jersey Red
Kentucky Red Berkshire
Maryland No.1
Miami
Minnesota Nos.2, 3 and 4
Ohio Improved Chester (OIC)
Palouse
Pitman-Moore Miniature
Red Hamprace
San Pierre
Suffolk
Victoria
Vita Vet Lab Minipig

APPENDIX 3

SOME SYNONYMS

The formal breed name (*vide* Mason) is shown first. The given synonyms do not include those which are recognisably similar to the formal name, nor the name in its native language where it differs (these are given with breed entries), nor the almost interchangeable "Yorkshire" and "Large White". The main Index cross-references the synonyms in alphabetical order to their formal breed names.

Alentejana: (Red) Portuguese, Transtagana
American Essex: Greer-Radeleff Miniature, Guinea Essex
Andalusian Spotted: Jabugo Spotted
Apulian: Mascherina
Baltaret: Marsh Stocli
Basque Black Pied: Béarn
Beijing Black: Peking Black
Belorussian Black Pied: White-Russian Spotted
Bentheim Black Pied: Wettringer
Bisaro: Beiroa
Black Hairless: Guadiana
Black Iberian: Andalusian Black, Extremadura Black
Black Mangalitsa: Lasasta ("weasel"), Syrmian
Black Slavonian: Pfeifer
Borghigiana: Fidenza

British Lop: Cornish White (Lop-eared), Devon Lop(-eared), Devonshire White, Lop White, National Long White Lop-eared, White Large Black, White Lop
Cantonese: Dahuabai (Large Spotted White), Guangdong Large White Spot, Large Black White, Macao, Pearl River Delta
Casertana: Napolitana, Pelatella
Chianina: Cappuccia (Hooded) d'Anghiari, Casentino
Cosentina: Orielese
Cuino: Mexican Dwarf
Dutch Yorkshire: Edelwarken
East Balkan: Kamchiya
Edelschwein: German Large White, German Short-eared, German White Prick-eared
Extremadura Red: Andalusian Red, Red Iberian
Fengjing: Rice-bran pig
Forest Mountain: New Lesogor
Friuli Black: San Daniele
Fumati: Brinati
Galician: Celta, Santiaguesa
German Berkshire: Black Edelschwein
German Landrace: German Long-eared, German White Lop-eared
German Pasture: Hanover-Brunswick, Hildesheim
Ghori: Dome, Pygmy
Guinea hog: Gulf pig
Hampshire: Belted, Mackay, Norfolk Thin Rind, Ring Middle, Ring Necked, Saddleback, Woburn
Hereford: White-faced
Iban: Kayan
Iberian: Mediterranean
Jianli: Kienli
Jinhua: Two-end-black
Krolevets: Polesian Lard
Kunekune: Maori
Large Black: Cornwall, Devon, Lop-eared Black
Large White: Grand Yorkshire, Large English, Large York, Yorkshire
Lee-Sung: Taiwan Miniature
Lucanian: Basilicata
Majorcan: Balearic
Mangalitsa: Hungarian Curly Coat, Wollshwein
Maremmana: Macchiaiola (forest pig), Black Umbrian, Roman
Miami: Warren County
Middle White: Coleshill, Middle Yorkshire, Windsor
Minnesota Miniature: Hormel Miniature
Montana No.1: Black Hamprace
Montmorillon: Poitou
Munich Miniature: Troll
Old Swedish Spotted: Black-White -Red Spotted
Oliventina: Raya
Oxford Sandy-and-Black: Plum Pudding pig
Parmense: Black Emilian, Reggio
Pelón: Black Hairless of the Tropics
Piau: Carioca
Pineywoods: Gulf pig, Swamp hog
Preštice: Bohemian Blue Spotted, Pilson, Plzen, Saaz
Pulawy: Golebska
Raad: Plaung, Ka Done, Keopra
Resava: Vezicevka
Romagnola: Bologna, Castagnona, Moor
Rongchang: Bespectacled White, Jungchang White
Semirechensk: Kazakh Hybrid
Siberian: Tara
Siberian Black Pied: Novosibirsk Spotted
Siena Belted: Cinta, Montagnola
Small Polish Prick-eared: Local Short-eared
Small White: Middlesex, Small Yorkshire (and many others)
South China Black: Cantonese
South Yunnan Short-eared: Dian-nan Small-ear

Subotica White: Bikovacka
Šumadija: Milos
Taiwan Small Black: Aboriginal, Small Long-snout
Tamworth: Staffordshire
Taoyuan: Lung-tan-po, Chung-li
Tatú: Bahia, Macao
Tibetan: Zangzhu
Tunchang: Denchang
Turopolje: Zagreb
Vich: Catalan
Vietnamese: Annamese
Vitoria: Álava, Basque-Navarre, Chato
Wai Chow: Lung Kong
Wannan Spotted: Lantian Spotted
Welsh: Old Glamorgan
Wessex Saddleback: Belted, Sheeted Wessex
Xinjin: Sitsin
Yorkshire Blue and White: Bilsdale Blue
Yujiang: Yushan Black

BIBLIOGRAPHY

Acharya, R.M., Bhat, P.N.: *Livestock and Poultry Genetic Resources in India* [IVRI, undated]

Adalsteinsson, S. (1981): Origin and conservation of farm animal populations in Iceland *Z..Tierzuchtg.Zuchtgsbiol.* 98.258

A.D.A.S. (1984): *Pig Production and Welfare* [MAFF]

de Alba, Jorge (1971): *Productivity of Native and Exotic Pig Breeds in Latin America* [FAO]

Alderson, Lawrence (1989): *The Chance to Survive* (rev. ed.) [A.H. Jolly, Northamptonshire]

Alderson, Lawrence (ed) (1989): *Genetic Conservation of Domestic Livestock* [CABI]

Baconwa, E.T. (1985): The Philippines: Livestock marketing [*World Animal Review* 55. 34-41]

Bauer, H.-J. (ed) (1990): *Schweine-produktion* [AMK,Berlin]

Baxter's Library of Agricultural andHorticultural Knowledge (3rd ed., 1834)

Bermejo, J.V.D., Serrano E.R., Vallejo, M.E.C., Franganillo, A.R.: *Razas autoctonas andaluzas en peligro de extincion*

Beynon Brown, G. John (1990): *How farmers attain collection influence, with particular reference to 1992* [Report to Nuffield Farming Scholarships Trust]

Bichard, Maurice (1981): Aspects of the Evolution of the British Pig Industry [*Farm Management* Vol.4 No.7, 267-73]

Bichard, Maurice (1982): Current developments in pig breeding [*Outlook on Agriculture* 11.4 pp159-64]

Bökönyi, S. (1974): *History of Domestic Mammals in Central and Eastern Europe* [Akadémiai Kiadó]

Booth, W.D. (1988): Wild Boar farming in the UK [*The State Veterinary Journal* 42.121, pp167-75]

Booth, W.D. (1991): Wild Boar farming in the UK [Paper to 1st European Conference on Wild Livestock Breeding, Grado]

Bowman, J.C., Aindow, C.T. (1973): *Genetic conservation and the less common breeds of British cattle, pigs and sheep* [University of Reading]

Briggs, Hilton M. (1983: *International Pig Breed Encyclopedia* [Elanco, Indianapolis]

Brooks, Philip (1983): Pigs, Pannage, Pestilence and Pipe Rolls [*Newsletter*, Farnham Museum Society]

Brownlow, Mark (1992): Wild Boar farming in Austria [*Sounder*]

Cheng, Pei-lieu (1985): *Livestock Breeds of China* [FAO/China Academic Publishers]

Clutton-Brock, Juliet (1981): *Domesticated Animals from Early Times* [Heinemann/British Museum (Natural History)]

Coburn, F.D. (1909): *Swine in America* [Orange Judd Co., NY]

Craft, W.A. (1953): *Results of Swine Breeding Research* [USDA]

Crawford, R.D. (1984): Assessment and Conservation of Animal Genetic Resource in Canada [*Can. J .Anim. Sci.* 64:235-51]

Culley, George (1807): *Observations on Livestock*

D'Agaro, E., Haley, C.S., Ellis, M. (1990): Breed and genetic effects for PRE and post-weaning performance in Large White and Meishan pigs and their reciprocal crosses [*Proc. 4th World Congr. Genet. Appl. Livest. Prod., Edinburgh* XV]

Dal Pra, Giorgio (1950): *L'allevamento suino e la razza Cinta* [IPA, Siena]

Davidson, H.R. (1953): *The Production and Marketing of Pigs* [Longmans, Green & Co., 2nd ed.]

Devendra, C., Fuller, M.F. (1979): *Pig Production in the Tropics* [Oxford University Press]

Dickson, R.W. (1822): *Improved Live Stock and Cattle Management*
Dmitriev, N.G. (1987): Conservation of Animal Genetic Resources in the USSR [*An. Gen. Res. Inf.* 6, FAO]
Dmitriev, N.G., Ernst, L.K. (1989): *Animal Genetic Resources of the USSR* [FAO/UNEP]
Downer, John (1991): *Lifesense: Our Lives Through Animal Eyes* [BBC Books]
Duniec, Henryk (1971): Some aspects of pig testing applied in RWPG countries [3rd ad hoc consultation on Animal Genetic Resources, Copenhagen, FAO]
Epstein, H. (1969): *Domestic Animals of China* [Commonwealth Agricultural Bureau]
Epstein, H. (1971): *The Origin of the Domestic Animals of Africa* [Africana Publishing Corporation, NY]
Epstein, H., Bichard, M. (1984): Pig. In Mason, Ian L. (ed): *Evolution of Doesticated Animals* [Longman]
Eusebio, J.A. (1980): *Pig Production in the Tropics* [Longman]
Falvey, L. (1981): Research on native pigs in Thailand [*World Animal Review* 38: 16-22]
Feroci, Stefano (1979): Salvare le razze Italiane! [*Suinicoltura* VIII.13-19]
Fream, William (ed) (1893): *Youtt's Complete Grazier and Farmers' and Cattle-Breeders' Assistant*
Fredeen, H.T., Stothart, J.G. (1969): Development of a new breed of pigs: the Lacombe [*Can. J. Anim. Sci.* 49: 237-73]
Fulgenzi, U.N. (1953): *Attualitá zootecniche della regione Umbra* [Grafica Perugia]
Gaál, L., Gunst, P. (1977): *Animal Husbandry in Hungary in the 19th and 20th Centuries* [Akadémiai Kiadó]
Gilbey, Sir Walter (1910): *Farm Stock of Old* [Spur]
Groves, Colin (1981): Ancestors for the pigs: taxonomy and phylogency of the genus *Sus* [Australian National University]
Hall, S.J.G., Clutton-Brock, J. (1989): *Two Hundred Years of British Farm Livestock* [British Museum (Natural History)]
Hankó, B. (1954): *The History of Hungarian Domestic Animals* [Akadémiai Kiadó, Budapest]
Harris, Joseph (1870): *Harris on the Pig. Breeding, Rearing, Management and Improvement* [Orange Judd Co, NY]
Heise, L., Christman, C. (1989): *American Minor Breeds Notebook* [AMBC, Pittsboro, NC]
Henderson, Andrew (1814): *The Practical Grazier*
Hinrich-Sambraus, Heinz (1989): *Atlas van huisdier-rassen* [Terra, Zutfen, Netherlands]
Hodges, John (1984): Conservation of Animal Genetic Resources [*Livest. Prod. Sci.* 11:1-2]
Hodowli, Stan (1991): *Report on Pig Breeding in Poland in 1990* [Instyt Zootechniki, Kraków]
Hogg, James (ed) (1991): *Lord Emsworth's Annotated Whiffle: The Care of the Pig* [Michael Joseph]
Holness, David H. (1991): *Pigs* [Macmillan Education/CTA]
Hulme, Susan (1979): *Book of the Pig* [Saiga, Hindhead]
Kalk, Bruce H. (1991): The extinction of historic breeds of swine [*AMBC News* Vol.8, No.3]
Kiyoshi Namikawa (1989): Animal Genetic Resources in Japan [Proc. of SABRAO Workshop on Anim. Gen. Res. in Asia and Oceania, Tsukuba]
Lauvergne, J.J. (1980): Le porc indigène de Papouaei Nouvelle Guinée: rapport de mission [INRA]
Layley, G.W., Malden, W.J. (1953): *Evolution of the British Pig* [J. Bolt]
Lemmon, Tess (1991): The Whole Hog [*BBC Wildlife* December]
Long, James (1906): *The Book of the Pig* (2nd ed.) [L. Upcott Gill, London/Charles Scribner's Sons, NY]
Loudon, John C. (1831): *An Encyclopaedia of Agriculture*
Low, Professor D. (1842): *The Breeds of the Domestic Animals of the British Isles*
Lush, Jay. L., Anderson, A.L. (1939): A genetic history of Poland China swine [*J. Hered.* 30:149-156, 219-224]
Maijala, K., Cherekaev, A.V., Devillard, J.-M., et al (1984): Conservation of Animal Genetic Resouces in Europe: Final Report of an EAAP Working Party [*Livest. Prod. Sci.*]
Malden, W.J. (1934/5): The Evolution of the British Pig [*Pig Breeders' Annual, Jubilee Issue*, Vol.14]
Malynicz, George L. (1970): Pig keeping by the subsistence agriculturalist of the New Guinea Highlands [*Search* Vol.1 No.5]
Mariante, A. de S., Trovo, J.B. de F. (1989): The Brazilian Resources Conservation Programme [*Rev. Brasil. Genet.* 12.3]
Mason, Ian L. (1988): *World Dictionary of Livestock Breeds* (3rd rev. ed.) [CAB International]
Mason, Ian L. (ed) (1984): *Evolution of Domestcated Animals* [Longman]
Matassino, Donato, et al (1968): Statistiche vitali in scrofe di razza Casertana [*Produzione Animale* 7:173-246]
Mayer, John J., Brisbin, I. Lehr, Jr., Sweeney, James M. (1989): Temporal Dynamics of Color Phenotypes in an Island Population of Feral Swine [*Acta Theriologica* 34,17:217-252]
Mayer, John J., Brisbin, I. Lehr, Jr. (1991): *Wild Pigs of the United States: Their History, Morphology, and Current Status* [University of Georgia Press]
McIntosh, G.H., Pointon, A. (1981): The Kangaroo Island strain of pig in biomedical research [*Australian Veterinary Journal* 57:182-5]
Meat and Livestock Commission: *Pig Yearbook 1991* [MLC]
Mensch, R. (1986): Thailand: Hog Village [*World Animal Review* 38:16-22]
Molenat, M., Tran The Thong (1988): *La génétique porcine dans un pays endéveloppement:Le Viet Nam*
Molenat, M., Tran The Thong (1990): Le production porcine au Viet Nam et son amélioration

[*World Animal Review* 68:26-37]
Moulias, J. (ed) (1991): *Bulletin de l'élevage français* [SOPEXA, Paris]
Mount, L.E. (1968): *The Climatic Physiology of the Pig* [Edward Arnold]
Murray, J.W. (1977): *Growth and Change in Danish Agriculture* [Hutchinson Benham]
National Research Council (1983): *Little-known Asian Animals with a Promising Economic Future* [National Academy Press, Washington DC]
National Research Council (1991): *Microlivestock* [National Academy Press]
Oliver, William L.R. (1984): Introduced and feral pigs. In: *Feral Mammals - Problems and Potential* [IUCN]
Osinska, Z. (1967): Study on the development and classification of pig breeds in Europe [*World Animal Review* 3:15]
Parkinson, Richard (1810): *Breeding and management of Livestock*
Pathiraja, N. (1986): Improvement of pig-meat production in developing countries [*World Animal Review* 60 and 61]
Pitaro, S.: *La razza casertana e il suo miglioramento* [IPA, Caserta]
Pitt, W. (1813): *General View of the Agriculture of the County of Worcestershire*
Plager, Wilbur L. (1975): *History of Yorkshires and the American Yorkshire Club* [American Yorkshire Club Inc., Lafayette]
Runavot, J-P., Devillard, J-M. (1988): *Aspects actuels du dispostif français d'amélioration génétique du porc*
Ryan, P. (ed) (1972): *Encyclopaedia of Papua and New Guinea* [Melbourne University Press]
Sasimowski, Ewald (1987): *Animal Breeding and Production: An Outline* [PWN, Warsaw/Elsevier]
Sidney, Samuel (1871): *The Pig*
Smith, M.W., Smith, M.H., Brisbin, I. Lehr, Jr. (1980): Genetic variability and domestication in Swine [*J. Mamm.* 61(1): 39-45]
Spencer, Saunders (1905): *Pigs: Breeds and Management* (4th ed) [Vinton & Co.]
Spencer, Saunders (1921): *The Pig: Breeding, Rearing and Marketing* [C. Arthur Pearson]
Texier, C., Luquet, M. (1982): *Le porc de pays: Quatres races oubliées* [ITP, Paris]
Texier, C., et al (1984): Inventaire des quatres dernières races locales porcines continentales [*Journées Rech. Porcine en France* 16:495-5-6]
Thear, Katie (1987): Vietnamese pot-bellied pigs [*Home Farm* 71:26-7]
Tonini, Giulio (1949): I suini di Faenza [*Stab. Tip. Ramo Editoriale degli Agricoltori*]
Tonini, Giulio (1950): *La razza suina Mora e i suoi derivati di incrocio* [IPA, Ravenna]
Towne, Charles Wayland, Wentworth, Edward Norris (1950): *Pigs from Cave to Corn Belt* [University of Oklahama Press]
Trow-Smith, Robert C. (1959): *A History of British Livestock Husbandry: To 1700* [Routledge & Kegan Paul]
Trow-Smith, Robert C. (1960): *A History of British Livestock Husbandry: 1700-1900* [Routledge & Kegan Paul]
Trow-Smith, Robert C. (1980): *History of the Royal Smithfield Club* [Royal Smithfield Club]
Vancouver, Charles (1808):*General View of the Agriculture of the County of Devonshire*
Vu-Thien Thai: Quelques aspects de la production animale au Viet-Nam [*World Review of Animal Production* 3(13)]
Webb, A.J., Carden, A.E., Smith, C., Imlah, P. (1982): Porcine stress syndrome in pig breeding [*2nd World Congr. Genet. Appl. Livest. Prod.* Proc. V:588-608]
Wilkins, J.V., Martínez, L. (1983): Bolivia: An investigation of sow production in humid lowland villages [*World Animal Review* 47:15-18]
Wiseman, Julian (1986): *A History of the British Pig* [Duckworth]
Wood, Gene W. (ed) (1977): *Research and Management of Wild Hog Populations* [Clemson University, S. Carolina]
Youatt, W. (1847): *The Pig*
Young, Rev. Arthur (1807): *General View of the Agriculture of the County of Essex*
Young, Rev. Arthur (1813): *General View of the Agriculture of the County of Sussex*
Zeuner, F.E. (1963): *A History of Domesticated Animals* [Hutchinson]
Erhaltung gefährdeter Nutztierrassen [AMK, Berlin, 1984]
Les Races Porcines [ITP, 1982]
Pig Breeders' Annual Vol.14, 1934/5 [National Pig Breeders Association]
Sonderschau Schweine-produktion [AMK, Berlin, 1990]
The Landrace at Home and Abroad (1971) [Bulgaria]
The Spotted Dermantsi (1964) [Bulgaria]
Results of Swine Breeding Research (1953) [USDA]

INDEX